2020

ADVANCES IN
MOLECULAR PATHOLOGY

EDITOR-IN-CHIEF

Gregory J. Tsongalis, PhD, HCLD

SECTION EDITORS

Ahmad N. Abou Tayoun, PhD, FACMG

Helen Fernandes, PhD

Andrea Ferreira-Gonzalez, PhD,
HCLD(ABB), CC(ABB), FACB

Lawrence J. Jennings, MD, PhD, D(ABHI)

Matthew Lebo, PhD, FACMG

Eric Y. Loo, MD

Ann M. Moyer, MD, PhD

ELSEVIER

Publishing Director, Medical Reference: Dolores Meloni
Editor: Lauren Boyle
Developmental Editor: Laura Fisher

Reprints: For copies of 100 or more of articles in this publication, please contact the Commercial Reprints Department, Elsevier Inc., 360 Park Avenue South, New York, NY 10010-1710. Tel: 212-633-3874; Fax: 212-633-3820; E-mail: reprints@elsevier.com.

Printed in the United States of America.

Editorial Office:
Elsevier, Inc.
1600 John F. Kennedy Blvd,
Suite 1800
Philadelphia, PA 19103-2899

International Standard Serial Number: 2589-515X
International Standard Book Number: 13: 978-0-323-72226-1

ADVANCES IN MOLECULAR PATHOLOGY

EDITOR-IN-CHIEF

GREGORY J. TSONGALIS, PhD, HCLD
Professor, Department of Pathology and Laboratory Medicine, The Audrey and Theodore Geisel School of Medicine at Dartmouth, Hanover, NH, USA; Vice Chair for Research and Director, Laboratory for Clinical Genomics and Advanced Technology (CGAT), Department of Pathology and Laboratory Medicine, Dartmouth Hitchcock Medical Center, Lebanon, NH, USA

SECTION EDITORS

AHMAD N. ABOU TAYOUN, PhD, FACMG – Genetics
Al Jalila Genomics Center, Al Jalila Children's Specialty Hospital, Genetics Department, Mohammed Bin Rashid University of Medicine and Health Sciences, Dubai, UAE

HELEN FERNANDES, PhD - Infectious Disease
Associate Professor of Pathology & Cell Biology, Co-Director Genomic Oncology, Columbia University, New York, NY, USA

ANDREA FERREIRA-GONZALEZ, PhD, HCLD(ABB), CC(ABB), FACB – Solid Tumors
Professor and Chair Molecular Diagnostics Division, Department of Pathology, Virginia Commonwealth University, Richmond, VA, USA

LAWRENCE J. JENNINGS, MD, PhD, D(ABHI) – Identity/HLA
Associate Professor of Pathology, Northwestern University Feinberg School of Medicine, Director,

Division of Genomic Pathology, Medical Director, Diagnostic Molecular Biology, Northwestern Memorial Hospital, Chicago, IL, USA

MATTHEW LEBO, PhD, FACMG - Informatics
Director, Laboratory for Molecular Medicine, Director, Bioinformatics, Mass General Brigham Personalized Medicine, Assistant Professor of Pathology, Brigham and Woman's Hospital and Harvard Medical School, Associate Member – Broad Institute, Cambridge, MA, USA

ERIC Y. LOO, MD - Hematopathology
Assistant Professor of Pathology & Laboratory Medicine, Department of Pathology and Laboratory Medicine, Dartmouth-Hitchcock Medical Center, Lebanon, NH, USA

ANN M. MOYER, MD, PhD – Pharmacogenomics
Associate Professor of Laboratory Medicine and Pathology, Department of Laboratory Medicine and Pathology, Mayo Clinic, Rochester, MN, USA

CONTRIBUTORS

AHMAD N. ABOU TAYOUN, PhD, FACMG
College of Medicine, Mohammed Bin Rashid
University of Medicine and Health Sciences,
Genomics Center, Al Jalila Children's Specialty
Hospital, Dubai, United Arab Emirates

MICHELLE AFKHAMI, MD
Chief, Division of Molecular Genomic Pathology,
Medical Director, Clinical Molecular Diagnostic
Laboratory, Department of Pathology, City of Hope
National Medical Center, Duarte, California, USA

HOSNEARA AKTER, MSc
Genetics and Genomic Medicine Centre, NeuroGen
Children's Genomic Clinic, Department of
Biochemistry and Molecular Biology, University of
Dhaka, Dhaka, Bangladesh

FERAS ALLY, MD
Department of Laboratory Medicine and Pathology,
University of Washington, Seattle, Washington, USA

ANTONIA L. ALTOMARE, DO, MPH
Assistant Professor, Department of Medicine,
Dartmouth Geisel School of Medicine, Infectious
Disease and International Health, Dartmouth-
Hitchcock Medical Center, Lebanon, New Hampshire,
USA

DANIELLE M. ANDRADE, MD, MSc
Division of Neurology, Department of Medicine,
University of Toronto, Epilepsy Genetics Program,
Toronto Western Hospital and Krembil Neuroscience
Centre, University of Toronto, Toronto, Ontario,
Canada

CYRUS BOELMAN, MD
Division of Neurology, Department of Pediatrics,
Faculty of Medicine, University of British Columbia

MICHAEL S. CALDERWOOD, MD, MPH
Associate Professor, Department of Medicine,
Dartmouth Geisel School of Medicine, Associate Chief
Quality Officer, Regional Hospital Epidemiologist,
Infectious Disease and International Health,
Dartmouth-Hitchcock Medical Center, Lebanon, New
Hampshire, USA

DAVID B. CHAPEL, MD
Clinical Fellow, Division of Women's and Perinatal
Pathology, Department of Pathology, Brigham and
Women's Hospital, Boston, Massachusetts, USA

SHIMUL CHOWDHURY, PhD
Clinical Laboratory Director, Rady Children's Institute
for Genomic Medicine, San Diego, California, USA

JOANNA L. CONANT, MD
Assistant Professor, Department of Pathology and
Laboratory Medicine, University of Vermont Medical
Center, The Robert Larner, M.D. College of Medicine,
University of Vermont, Burlington, Vermont, USA

CALEB CORNABY, PhD
McLendon Clinical Laboratories, UNC Hospitals,
Chapel Hill, North Carolina, USA

ANN K. DALY, PhD
Translational and Clinical Research Institute, Faculty
of Medical Sciences, Newcastle University, Newcastle
upon Tyne, United Kingdom

KATHERINE A. DEVITT, MD
Assistant Professor, Department of Pathology and
Laboratory Medicine, University of Vermont Medical
Center, The Robert Larner, M.D. College of
Medicine, University of Vermont, Burlington,
Vermont, USA

LIAM DONNELLY, MD
Department of Pathology and Laboratory Medicine, University of Vermont Medical Center, The Robert Larner, M.D. College of Medicine, University of Vermont, Burlington, Vermont, USA

HELEN FERNANDES, PhD
Associate Professor of Pathology & Cell Biology, Co-Director Genomic Oncology, Columbia University, New York, NY, USA

ANDREA FERREIRA-GONZALEZ, PhD, HCLD(ABB), CC(ABB), FACB
Professor and Chair Molecular Diagnostics Division, Department of Pathology, Virginia Commonwealth University, Richmond, VA, USA

JULI-ANNE GARDNER, MD
Associate Professor, Department of Pathology and Laboratory Medicine, University of Vermont Medical Center, The Robert Larner, M.D. College of Medicine, University of Vermont, Burlington, Vermont, USA

HENK-JAN GUCHELAAR, PharmD, PhD
Professor of Clinical Pharmacy and Department Head, Department of Clinical Pharmacy and Toxicology, Leiden University Medical Center, Leiden Network for Personalised Therapeutics, Leiden, The Netherlands

HOUDA HACHAD, PharmD, MRes
Chief Science Officer, Translational Software Inc, Bellevue, Washington, USA

MICHAEL T. HARHEN, MBA, MT(ASCP)
Administrative Director of the Clinical Laboratories, Department of Pathology and Laboratory Medicine, Dartmouth-Hitchcock Medical Center, Lebanon, New Hampshire, USA

JONATHAN T. HUNTINGTON, MD, PhD, MPH
Assistant Professor, Department of Medicine, Dartmouth Geisel School of Medicine, Chief Medical Officer, Hospital Medicine, Dartmouth-Hitchcock Medical Center, Lebanon, New Hampshire, USA

KIELY N. JAMES, PhD
Clinical Genomics Analyst, Genomics, Rady Children's Institute for Genomic Medicine, San Diego, California, USA

REEM KAIS JAN, PhD
College of Medicine, Mohammed Bin Rashid University of Medicine and Health Sciences, Dubai, United Arab Emirates

LAWRENCE J. JENNINGS, MD, PhD, D(ABHI)
Associate Professor of Pathology, Northwestern University Feinberg School of Medicine, Director, Division of Genomic Pathology, Medical Director, Diagnostic Molecular Biology, Northwestern Memorial Hospital, Chicago, IL, USA

SABAH KADRI, PhD
Director of Bioinformatics, Assistant Professor of Pathology, Department of Pathology, Ann and Robert H. Lurie Children's Hospital, Northwestern University Feinberg School of Medicine, Chicago, Illinois, USA

PRITI KAMBLI
Senior Research Fellow, Microbiology Section, P.D. Hinduja Hospital, Mumbai, India

KAREN KAUL, MD, PhD
Chair, Department of Pathology and Laboratory Medicine, Duckworth Family Chair, NorthShore University HealthSystem, Clinical Professor of Pathology, The University of Chicago Pritzker School of Medicine, Evanston, Illinois, USA

JENNIFER KERKHOF, BSc
Molecular Genetics Laboratory, Molecular Diagnostics Division, London Health Sciences Centre, Department of Pathology and Laboratory Medicine, Western University, London, Ontario, Canada

WAHAB A. KHAN, PhD, FACMG
Department of Pathology and Laboratory Medicine, Dartmouth-Hitchcock Medical Center, Lebanon, New Hampshire, USA; Assistant Professor, Dartmouth Geisel School of Medicine, Dartmouth College, Hanover, New Hampshire, USA

JUSTIN LARACY, MD
NewYork-Presbyterian Hospital/Columbia University Irving Medical Center, New York, New York, USA

YAN LIU, MD, PhD

Department of Pathology and Laboratory Medicine, Division of Hematopathology, David Geffen School of Medicine at UCLA, Los Angeles, California, USA

ERIC Y. LOO, MD
Assistant Professor of Pathology & Laboratory Medicine, Department of Pathology and Laboratory Medicine, Dartmouth-Hitchcock Medical Center Lebanon, NH, USA

EKREM MALOKU, MD
Department of Pathology and Laboratory Medicine, Dartmouth-Hitchcock Medical Center, Lebanon, New Hampshire, USA

EDWARD J. MERRENS, MD, MHCDS
Assistant Professor, Department of Medicine, Dartmouth Geisel School of Medicine, Chief Clinical Officer, Hospital Medicine, Dartmouth-Hitchcock Medical Center, Lebanon, New Hampshire, USA

SUJAL PHADKE, PhD
Clinical Genomics Analyst, Genomics, Rady Children's Institute for Genomic Medicine, San Diego, California, USA

SHEEJA PULLARKAT, MD
Clinical Professor, Department of Pathology and Laboratory Medicine, Division of Hematopathology, David Geffen School of Medicine at UCLA, Los Angeles, California, USA

JACK REILLY, BSc
Molecular Genetics Laboratory, Molecular Diagnostics Division, London Health Sciences Centre, Department of Pathology and Laboratory Medicine, Western University, London, Ontario, Canada

LAUREN L. RITTERHOUSE, MD, PhD
Associate Director, Center for Integrated Diagnostics, Massachusetts General Hospital, Assistant Professor, Harvard Medical School, Boston, Massachusetts, USA

CAMILLA RODRIGUES, MD
Consultant Microbiologist, Microbiology Section, P.D. Hinduja Hospital, Department of Laboratory Medicine, P.D. Hinduja National Hospital and Medical Research centre, Mumbai, India

BEKIM SADIKOVIC, PhD
Molecular Genetics Laboratory, Molecular Diagnostics Division, London Health Sciences Centre, Department

of Pathology and Laboratory Medicine, Western University, London, Ontario, Canada

JESSICA SAVIEO, MPGx
Clinical Implementation Specialist, Translational Software Inc, Bellevue, Washington, USA

MARIE C. SMITHGALL, MD
Department of Pathology and Cell Biology, Columbia University Irving Medical Center, New York, New York, USA

JESSE J. SWEN, PharmD, PhD
Associate Professor of Pharmacogenomics and Section Head Laboratory, Department of Clinical Pharmacy and Toxicology, Leiden University Medical Center, Leiden Network for Personalised Therapeutics, Leiden, The Netherlands

DAVID L. THACKER, PharmD
Clinical Pharmacogenomics Content Specialist, Translational Software Inc, Bellevue, Washington, USA

GREGORY J. TSONGALIS, PhD, HCLD
Professor, Department of Pathology and Laboratory Medicine, The Audrey and Theodore Geisel School of Medicine at Dartmouth, Hanover, New Hampshire, USA; Vice Chair for Research and Director, Laboratory for Clinical Genomics and Advanced Technology (CGAT), Department of Pathology and Laboratory Medicine, Dartmouth Hitchcock Medical Center, Lebanon, New Hampshire, USA

MOHAMMED UDDIN, PhD
Assistant Professor, College of Medicine, Mohammed Bin Rashid University of Medicine and Health Sciences, Dubai, United Arab Emirates; The Centre for Applied Genomics, The Hospital for Sick Children, Toronto, Ontario, Canada

CATHELIJNE H. VAN DER WOUDEN, PharmD
PhD Candidate U-PGx Consortium, Department of Clinical Pharmacy and Toxicology, Leiden University Medical Center, Leiden Network for Personalised Therapeutics, Leiden, The Netherlands

GAIL H. VANCE, MD, FCAP, FACMG
Department of Medical and Molecular Genetics, Indiana University School of Medicine, Professor, Pathology and Laboratory Medicine, Indiana

University School of Medicine, Indianapolis, Indiana, USA

ERIC T. WEIMER, PhD
McLendon Clinical Laboratories, UNC Hospitals, Department of Pathology and Laboratory Medicine, University of North Carolina at Chapel Hill School of Medicine, Chapel Hill, North Carolina, USA

SAMUEL E. WEINBERG, MD, PhD
Department of Pathology and Laboratory Medicine, Northwestern University Feinberg School of Medicine, Chicago, Illinois, USA

WENDY A. WELLS, MD, MSc
Professor and Chair, Department of Pathology and Laboratory Medicine, Dartmouth Geisel School of

Medicine, Dartmouth-Hitchcock Medical Center, Lebanon, New Hampshire, USA

SUSAN WHITTIER, PhD
Department of Pathology and Cell Biology, Columbia University Irving Medical Center, New York, New York, USA

TERENCE C. WONG, PhD
Clinical Genomics Analyst, Genomics, Rady Children's Institute for Genomic Medicine, San Diego, California, USA

JASON ZUCKER, MD
Department of Medicine, Division of Infectious Diseases, Columbia University Irving Medical Center, New York, New York, USA

CONTENTS

Hematopathology

Preface

Molecular Pathology: The Laboratory-Developed Test

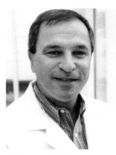

Gregory J. Tsongalis,
PhD, HCLD
Editor-in-Chief

At the time that the majority of this issue was being prepared, our country and the world were facing a severe acute respiratory syndrome coronavirus 2 (SARS-CoV-2) pandemic beyond what many of us have ever experienced before. Although there was a lot of criticism about the laboratory community's slow response, the shining beacon that helped turn the tide on this pandemic was the ability of molecular diagnostic testing laboratories to implement laboratory-developed tests (LDTs). The practice of molecular pathology has been and continues to be dependent upon new and robust molecular diagnostic technologies to interrogate DNA and/or RNA sequences for detection of sequence variants associated with a particular diagnosis, prognosis, or therapeutic response. Many molecular diagnostic tests require nucleic acid extraction, an analytical procedure such as polymerase chain reaction (PCR) or sequencing, and then data analysis and reporting. This 3-step process is combined into the workflow of a single test. Upon completion of the Human Genome Project, the field of molecular diagnostics began to evolve rapidly, and it became clear that the need for more molecular-based tests far outweighed the commercial and financial interests of most vendors to seek Food and Drug Administration (FDA) approval. Many academic and hospital laboratories were left to develop primers/probes targeting genes of clinical interest for their patient population even though test volumes were relatively low compared with other clinical laboratory tests. Southern blot–based testing for linkage analysis and Duchenne muscular dystrophy as well as PCR-based test for cystic fibrosis, parvovirus B19, and cytomegalovirus were only a few examples of tests with clinical utility but no commercial vendor.

Hence, the LDT was born! Initially these tests were called "homebrew" assays, but with regulatory oversight by federal agencies looming, a brand name discouraging a negative perception of the hard work being performed by laboratories to develop and validate these assays as mad scientists huddled around a cauldron of reaction mixture was needed. Laboratory Developed Test or LDT became accepted by those in the field. LDTs represented the "freedom to operate" that laboratories needed to keep up with the pace of new molecular discoveries and to rapidly deliver those to clinical practice. After all, the promises of the Human Genome Project included better diagnostic testing, more accurate

https://doi.org/10.1016/j.yamp.2020.09.001
2589-4080/20/

prognostication, and better therapeutics that would target disease in individuals with specific genetic variants. Under the Clinical Laboratory Improvement Amendment of 1988 and with developing guidelines from various professional organizations, including the College of American Pathologists and the Association for Molecular Pathology, laboratories began validating new tests using a variety of specimen types and technologies that would change the way we assessed patients for genetic diseases, hematologic disorders, infectious diseases, identity, and oncology. As an example, our laboratory performs some 60 different molecular tests of which only 11 are FDA approved or cleared. The majority of these assays are for higher-volume infectious disease tests that were selected by commercial industries based on the number of tests being performed globally in order to help recoup development and regulatory costs.

The LDT played a pivotal role in combating the SARS-CoV-2 pandemic. While some delays were experienced in the United States due to regulatory hurdles, globally many countries were able to mobilize efforts quickly to sequence and identify the virus, establish real-time PCR assays, and implement universal screening strategies. In the United States, the Centers for Disease Control and Prevention and the FDA established a plan for Public Health Laboratories and then hospital-based and private laboratories to begin testing using a variety of different commercially available tests under the Emergency Use Authorization *EUA) ruling. Obtaining EUA status for a particular test was somewhat involved from a validation standpoint due to lack of appropriate positive samples and control materials, but for laboratories using these EUA-marked assays, the "verification" steps involved were very lax compared with traditional LDT validations. In retrospect, there are many lessons to be learned from this experience for the laboratory community. No other scenario could better speak to the importance of LDTs than the crisis we all faced.

In this third issue of *Advances in Molecular Pathology*, we include a special section on COVID-19 experiences and review some of the newest developments in the field of molecular pathology as the need for genetic disease, hematologic disease, infectious disease, pharmacogenomic, solid tumor, and identity testing continues to increase. The articles included in this third issue provide further support for the importance of molecular testing in routine patient care and management, for the continued development of new tests and technologies, and for the appropriate reimbursement and regulation of such testing. As technologies become more robust, faster, and cheaper, we will far exceed the promises of the Human Genome Project.

I am grateful to those friends and colleagues who during the most pressing of times once again agreed to becoming section editors and authors of the fantastic articles presented here.

Happy reading!

Gregory J. Tsongalis, PhD, HCLD
Department of Pathology and
Laboratory Medicine
Dartmouth Hitchcock Medical Center
1 Medical Center Drive
Lebanon, NH 03756, USA

E-mail address: Gregory.j.tsongalis@hitchcock.org

The SARS-CoV-2 Pandemic

Advances in Molecular Pathology 3 (2020) 1–3

ADVANCES IN MOLECULAR PATHOLOGY

The 2020 Wild, Wild West of Diagnostics

Gregory J. Tsongalis, PhD, HCLD[a,b,*], Karen Kaul, MD, PhD[c,d]

[a]Department of Pathology and Laboratory Medicine, The Audrey and Theodore Geisel School of Medicine at Dartmouth, Hanover, NH 03755, USA; [b]Laboratory for Clinical Genomics and Advanced Technology, Department of Pathology and Laboratory Medicine, Dartmouth Hitchcock Medical Center, 1 Medical Center Drive, Lebanon, NH 03756, USA; [c]Department of Pathology and Laboratory Medicine, NorthShore University HealthSystem, Evanston, IL, USA; [d]The University of Chicago Pritzker School of Medicine, Evanston, IL, USA

KEYWORDS
- Pandemic • SARS-CoV-2 • COVID-19 • Laboratory-developed tests • Regulatory oversight
- Emergency use authorization

KEY POINTS
- The COVID-19 pandemic resulted in new insights into regulation of laboratory-developed tests.
- Emergency use authorization status empowered laboratories to provide rapid testing for SARS-CoV-2 albeit with several caveats.
- A much better national response mechanism that is inclusive of state, federal, and academic institutions must be developed.

Regarding regulatory oversight of laboratory-developed tests (LDT) for molecular diagnostics, the Food and Drug Administration (FDA) often refers to the LDT space as the "Wild, Wild West," making it seem like laboratories are all going rogue with respect to Clinical Laboratory Improvement Amendments (CLIA)-defined quality assurance practices. Now, with the challenges of the COVID-19 pandemic in 2020, the FDA finds themselves in a self-created Wild, Wild West regarding molecular and serologic testing for SARS-CoV-2. In December 2019, Chinese officials notified the World Health Organization of a cluster of severe pneumonia cases in Wuhan that had a suspicious origin. On January 7, 2020, the cause was identified, the novel severe acute respiratory coronavirus 2 (SARS-CoV-2), and the first death was reported in China several days later. By the end of January, cases were being reported globally, including the first case in Washington State, and travel bans were issued by some countries. The FDA released a guidance document for designing and validating molecular tests for SARS-CoV-2 and issued the first Emergency Use Authorization (EUA) for a reverse transcriptase, real-time polymerase chain reaction (RT-qPCR) assay to the Centers for Disease Control and Prevention (CDC) on February 4, 2020. The EUA specified that all diagnostic testing for SARS-CoV-2 be reviewed by the FDA, and in effect removed the option to offer testing as an LDT. This changed the landscape of molecular diagnostics for the virus and thrust the nation into a difficult situation because no assays other than the CDC RT-PCR test, available only to public health laboratories (PHLs), were accessible.

---

*Corresponding author, E-mail address: Gregory.j.tsongalis@hitchcock.org

https://doi.org/10.1016/j.yamp.2020.06.001
2589-4080/20/

Soon after distribution of the CDC EUA, assay laboratories noticed failed results, in part because of contaminated reagents. Remanufacturing and redistribution of tests to the PHLs significantly delayed the implementation of wide-scale national testing of symptomatic individuals. Hospital and academic laboratories capable of developing and validating their own assays were forced to do so, and the subsequent tsunami of new molecular SARS-CoV-2 tests submitted for EUA certification overwhelmed the FDA from a regulatory standpoint. One of the advantages of molecular techniques is that they are universal and flexible in their application. This, however, became a disadvantage in the current pandemic as the number of preanalytic variables, including specimen types and different collection tubes, together with the analytical variables associated with different technology platforms, generated an assortment of assays, each requiring review. In addition, the demand to increase testing to include not only well-characterized symptomatic patients but also less well-characterized symptomatic and asymptomatic individuals posed further significant concerns and challenges. To date, no tests are EUA certified for use in asymptomatic patients.

Ideally, a molecular diagnostic procedure for SARS-CoV-2 would call for a specific specimen type or types, a specific extraction method and instrument, and a defined PCR protocol and amplification instrument with published primer/probe sequences and cycling conditions. At first glance, this seems straightforward, but the breadth and depth of methods and instruments available in laboratories across the country makes this very complex; ultimately, these combinations used together in an assay must yield the same result in all laboratories and does, as illustrated by many national proficiency testing programs. The purpose of CLIA is to ensure that all results are correct, regardless of the method or instrument used. This variability was daunting for the FDA (who must remain vendor neutral) to manage through this escalating pandemic. The EUA regulatory process was challenged with increased demand from providers and institutions for more testing using alternative specimens when swabs were in short supply, transport media versus saline versus dry swabs, and multiple methods in the laboratory to ensure supplies for at least 1 EUA assay. Validation/verification data required for EUA were minimal compared with routine validation studies for LDTs or commercial assays. Demonstration of assay performance criteria, especially limit of detection studies, was challenging because of lack of well-characterized control material,

as well as variability in extraction efficiencies and specimen types.

Although the FDA tried to manage the ensuing flood of assays, other federal and state agencies as well as professional societies were calling for new indications for testing of patients. None of these groups willingly recognized the fact that the FDA EUA status granted to all of these tests was for symptomatic patients and that testing beyond that indication would be in direct violation of the EUA. Some noted that there was no information to contradict that the assays should perform the same in asymptomatic versus symptomatic patients forgetting performance characteristics associated with positive and negative predictive values. Others stated that there are no authorized tests for asymptomatic testing, but the health care provider has discretion with ordering tests, and suppliers wishing to seek authorization should contact the FDA and submit a Pre-Emergency Use Authorization request. Nonetheless, the demands from providers and clinical professional societies alike were too great, and many laboratories were forced to perform this testing adding disclaimer after disclaimer to their reports. As with public protests to reopen our country, demands from providers and professional groups to increase testing across all patient populations were due in part to fear of the unknown regarding the virus and to a misunderstanding of good laboratory practices. The system had become a free-for-all.

Some take away lessons from this pandemic for the laboratory are worth mentioning. First, we must have a better, more coordinated national response network in practice, and ready for the next time that we are faced with a pandemic challenge. Second, we need a system that affords certified and licensed clinical laboratories the flexibility to rapidly engage in testing using established protocols in individual laboratories, but continuing to ensure accurate results, ideally with high-quality reference materials available to demonstrate the accuracy of the assay. Third, our supply chain must be more robust across all aspects of our health care system, including laboratory supplies. Fourth, at a time when medical school curricula are being redesigned and reinvented, this pandemic was an amazingly eye-opening experience on how poorly we are training health care providers with regards to diagnostic skills and use of laboratory information. In addition, ongoing national efforts to reduce health care expenditures that include drastic cuts to laboratory reimbursement have hobbled many laboratories. Laboratory results make up only about 2% of health care costs but determine about 80% of subsequent expenditure; modest investment in laboratories provides better information and actually reduces the overall cost of care, as we have seen during the pandemic and in many other situations. Finally, a national mechanism to distribute not only supplies but also help with testing across state borders in support of laboratories in the hot zones is critical to our responsiveness. We have never experienced the impact of a major pandemic such as this, and the hope is that we will be much better prepared for the next one.

DISCLOSURE

The authors have nothing to disclose.

Advances in Molecular Pathology 3 (2020) 5–11

ADVANCES IN MOLECULAR PATHOLOGY

Maintaining Laboratory Services in a Rural Academic Medical Center During the Severe Acute Respiratory Syndrome Coronavirus 2 Pandemic

What Worked and What Did Not (February 29–May 1, 2020)

Wendy A. Wells, MD, MSc[a],*, Michael T. Harhen, MBA, MT(ASCP)[a], Michael S. Calderwood, MD, MPH[b], Antonia L. Altomare, DO, MPH[b], Jonathan T. Huntington, MD, PhD, MPH[c], Edward J. Merrens, MD, MHCDS[c], Gregory J. Tsongalis, PhD, HCLD[a]

[a]Department of Pathology and Laboratory Medicine, Dartmouth-Hitchcock Medical Center, One Medical Center Drive, Lebanon, NH 03756, USA; [b]Infectious Disease and International Health, Dartmouth-Hitchcock Medical Center, One Medical Center Drive, Lebanon, NH 03756, USA; [c]Hospital Medicine, Dartmouth-Hitchcock Medical Center, One Medical Center Drive, Lebanon, NH 03756, USA

KEYWORDS
- Laboratory services • Rural • Academic medical center • SARS-CoV-2

KEY POINTS
- Rural health care systems have their own set of challenges.
- As the only academic medical center in the state of New Hampshire, the recent severe acute respiratory syndrome coronavirus 2 pandemic heightened those challenges.
- Accurate, timely, and clinically relevant statewide testing dictated how patients should be triaged to dedicated treatment areas of the hospital and how health care workers, first responders, employees, and vulnerable members of society should be protected from unnecessary exposures.

In this crisis, leaders are not made, they are revealed
—EDWARD J. MERRENS, MD, CHIEF CLINICAL
OFFICER, DARTMOUTH-HITCHCOCK HEALTH, NH

INTRODUCTION

Rural health care systems have their own set of challenges. As the only academic medical center in the state of New Hampshire, the recent severe acute respiratory syndrome coronavirus 2 (SARS-CoV-2) pandemic heightened those challenges, especially given our close proximity to so many hot-spot states (Massachusetts,

New York, Connecticut) where the prevalence and death rates of SARS-CoV-2 have been very high. Accurate, timely, and clinically relevant statewide testing took center stage early on in this pandemic. It dictated how patients should be triaged to dedicated treatment areas of the hospital and how health care workers, first responders, employees, and vulnerable members of society should be protected from unnecessary exposures. A critical part of our early statewide response to this crisis was the coordinated decision making of laboratory medicine, infectious disease, and epidemiology

---

*Corresponding author, *E-mail address:* Wells.A.Wells@hitchcock.org

https://doi.org/10.1016/j.yamp.2020.07.001
2589-4080/20/

experts at the Dartmouth-Hitchcock Medical Center (DHMC).

PREPARATIONS AND TIMELINES FOR THE DARTMOUTH-HITCHCOCK RESPONSE TO THE SEVERE ACUTE RESPIRATORY SYNDROME CORONAVIRUS 2 PANDEMIC

Dartmouth-Hitchcock Health (DHH), a nonprofit academic health system, provides primary as well as tertiary and quaternary health care to a rural population base of 1.5 million individuals coming from a wide geographic area in New Hampshire and eastern Vermont. Affiliated with Dartmouth College's Geisel School of Medicine and the National Cancer Institute–designated Norris Cotton Comprehensive Cancer Center, DHH employs more than 1500 primary care doctors and specialists and 500 advanced practitioners in almost every area of medicine throughout the health system, with major community practice locations throughout New Hampshire. DHH is the largest employer in New Hampshire aside from the state itself.

In the last decade, the United States has responded to the threats of the H1N1 influenza A pandemic (2009), Middle East respiratory syndrome (2012), H7N9 avian influenza (2013), Ebola virus disease (EVD) in West Africa (2014) and the Democratic Republic of Congo (2018), and Zika virus (2015). DHMC's Readiness and Response to Epidemic Infectious Disease Threats (RARE) subcommittee has monitored each of these emerging infections. We have had an epidemic response plan in place since 2003. A high-threat infection (HTI) team evolved out of Dartmouth-Hitchcock's (DH) response to EVD in 2014. Regularly participating in drills and competency assessments to test DHMC's readiness, the HTI team of doctors, nurses, laboratory technicians, patient-decontamination technicians, and respiratory therapists have all volunteered to be first responders if a patient suspected of having an HTI arrives at DHMC.

The Laboratory for Clinical Genomics and Advanced Technology (CGAT), within the Department of Pathology and Laboratory Medicine at DHMC, is supported by a director, physician-level and doctoral-level assistant directors, and highly trained technologists. CGAT offers a diverse spectrum of high-complexity DNA testing for genetic diseases, infectious diseases, hematologic diseases, oncology, and pharmacogenomics. As a Clinical Laboratory Improvement Amendments (CLIA)–certified, College of American Pathologists (CAP)–accredited clinical laboratory, CGAT maintains a high level of quality assurance through technical, administrative, and structural mechanisms. Institutional investment in this infrastructure over the last 10 years ensured a readiness that was crucial to our rapid response in this pandemic crisis. With this investment and expertise, 5 new diagnostic SARS-CoV-2 molecular assays were developed and validated in-house to meet the needs of high-throughput testing (symptomatic outpatients) and lower-volume rapid testing (symptomatic inpatients and triaging from the emergency department). Choosing the right test, evaluating the best instrument on which to run it, and predicting the availability of reagents and other supplies were all keys to allowing the institution to remain immune to manufacturer and federal promises that could not match demand as the pandemic spread. An appreciation of the technical time and effort needed to offer SARS-CoV-2 testing throughout the state, stretching from covering 1 shift to 3, resulted in a better understanding by many providers of the complexity of the testing.

In mid-February, 2020, as the coronavirus outbreak in Wuhan, Hubei Province, China worsened, laboratory directors in the CGAT laboratory at DHMC started to consider molecular SARS-CoV-2 assay options in terms of the test type, instrument, likely availability of reagents and other supplies, and laboratory workflow [1]. On February 26, 2020, the New Hampshire Department of Health and Human Services (DHHS) released an updated health alert discussing 3 levels of travel advisories, in response to reports that SARS-CoV-2 had spread to 47 other countries, with more than 82,000 cases reported worldwide (95%–96% in mainland China). Even though there were no confirmed SARS-CoV-2 cases in New Hampshire or Vermont at this time, DHMC had begun planning and anticipating potential needs. Supplies were inventoried, including all personal protective equipment (PPE) that health care workers would need to wear while caring for infected patients. Over the next 6 weeks, 3500 employees were trained in all forms of PPE. We started to coordinate a response with our regional system members, as well as with the states of New Hampshire and Vermont. On February 29, 2020, health officials in Washington State confirmed the first US death from SARS-CoV-2, a state that would become an epicenter for the disease early on. The same day, DHMC stood up incident command (DH-IC), which included physician experts in Infectious disease and public health, a planning chief, safety chiefs, operations chiefs, the Chief Medical Officer, the Chief Clinical Officer, an emergency management team, coordinators for ambulatory and inpatient areas as well as the community group practices, a logistics chief, and a public information officer. The timeline of our response from February 29 to May 1 is summarized in Fig. 1.

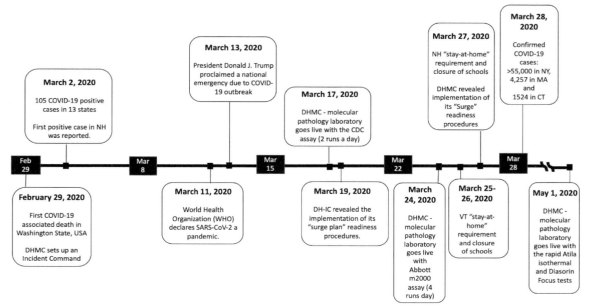

FIG. 1 Timeline for DHH Surge preparations for SARS-CoV-2 patients (February 29–May 1, 2020). CDC, US Centers for Disease Control and Prevention; COVID-19, coronavirus disease 19.

By March 2, 2020, there were about 105 SARS-CoV-2–positive cases in 13 states and the first positive case in New Hampshire was reported. On March 11, 2020 the World Health Organization (WHO) declared SARS-CoV-2 a pandemic. Travel bans from Europe (initially excluding the United Kingdom and Ireland), went into effect on March 13, the same day that President Donald J. Trump proclaimed that the SARS-CoV-2 outbreak in the United States constituted a national emergency. Shortly after, DH made the decision to halt all elective procedures in order to preserve PPE and inpatient capacity. Starting on March 19, DH-IC revealed the implementation of its surge plan readiness procedures. Daily communications to leadership included a DH-IC scorecard detailing numbers of tested and confirmed positive patients with SARS-CoV-2 in New Hampshire and Vermont; numbers of beds and ventilators in use and available statewide; staffing levels; and availability of supplies, PPE, critical medications, and blood products. A dedicated SARS-CoV-2 unit, capable of critical care delivery, was created and the holding capacity of the emergency department (ED) was expanded. Incoming patients and employees were screened at all medical center entrances for coronavirus disease 19 (COVID-19) symptoms and any out-of-state travel. Self-quarantine requirements were instituted for staff with high-risk exposures, requiring coordination with occupational medicine. Staff and faculty reassignment surveys were completed. The emergency management plan was coordinated with other hospitals in both New Hampshire and Vermont, including multistate triage and transfer plan. Preparations were made to augment the number of inpatient beds, including an increase in critical care bed capacity by 250% as well as a morgue expansion.

CGAT went live with the US Centers for Disease Control and Prevention (CDC) assay (2 runs per day, results 12–24 hours after specimen receipt in laboratory) on March 17 and the Abbott m2000 assay (4 runs per day, results in 12–24 hours) on March 24 [1]. In the state of Vermont, a stay-home-stay-safe requirement went into effect on March 25 followed, the next day, by Vermont school closures for the rest of the academic year. On March 27, a New Hampshire stay-at-home requirement and closure of schools went into effect. By March 28, confirmed US deaths from coronavirus doubled from 1000 to 2000 in 2 days, with more than 55,000 confirmed cases in New York, 4257 confirmed cases in Massachusetts, and 1524 in Connecticut. By March 30, 27 states had stay-at-home orders.

As of April 29, 2020, the number of active cases in the United States had risen to 1,012,583 with 58,355 deaths (Table 1). The deaths from SARS-CoV-2 in New Hampshire on that date (n = 60) represented 3% of the total diagnosed cases (n = 2010). Positive cases by county within the state showed many more cases in more densely populated counties of Rockingham, Hillsborough, Strafford, and Merrimack in the south-east of the state bordering with Massachusetts (Fig. 2). Across the 26 hospital sites from which we received specimens for SARS-CoV-2 testing (some from across the Vermont border), the positivity rate increased from 3.37% (the week of 3/17/20–3/23/20) to 6.45% (the week of 4/28/20–5/4/20). On May 1, CGAT went live with a newly validated and readily available rapid Atila isothermal assay (results in 3–4 hours). Limited reagents also became available for the Diasorin Focus assay (results in 3–4 hours).

WHAT WORKED

Clinical laboratories are held accountable by numerous national and federal accrediting bodies (College of American Pathologists [CAP], US Food and Drug Administration, American Association of Blood Banks

[AABB], Foundation for the Accreditation of Cellular Therapy [FACT], Centers for Medicare & Medicaid Services [CMS]). They provide millions of quality test results and interpretations to diagnose, treat, and monitor human disease in a highly efficient environment. They serve the needs of every department by competently operationalizing complex workflows to get specimens delivered to the laboratory for testing. However, they often remain the silent partner. The public (even those in the medical field) do not know what clinical laboratories are and the role they now play in medicine. This pandemic crisis changed that, shining a bright light of public attention and putting testing at the forefront of the national response. The efforts to provide the testing needed to identify, isolate, and treat SARS-CoV-2–positive patients were both facilitated and challenged. The following worked well:

1. DH-IC shaped our laboratory response to the pandemic by recognizing very early on the importance of understanding and leveraging the testing capabilities at DH. The synergistic relationship between experts in infectious disease, epidemiology, and laboratory medicine to facilitate new assay validation and develop evidence-based testing algorithms, ordering menus, and reporting templates was critical in helping the rural health system avoid being overwhelmed. This crucial support to the clinical laboratories was enabled by the following:
   - The appointment of the DH Administrative Director of the Clinical Laboratories as the DH-IC Planning Chief: In this position, this individual's exceptional operational skills and expert advice about all testing ensured optimized laboratory communications with members of the DH-IC, and new and detailed insight by DH-IC into the challenges of selecting, developing, and validating new clinical diagnostic molecular assays.
   - Communication coordination: DH-IC helped to provide regular and consistent decisions regarding testing updates, with evidence-based information, timelines, specific clinical indications, and standardized ordering triages (aligned with state recommendations).
   - New Hampshire state laboratory coordination: DH-IC epidemiologists and laboratorians coordinated policy and procedure updates with colleagues at the state laboratory. This coordination enabled test backlogs throughout the state to be cleared by DHMC to maintain result turnaround times.
   - SARS-CoV-2 test ordering control: early on during the surge planning, DH-IC decided to limit

TABLE 1 Severe acute respiratory syndrome coronavirus 2 cases in New Hampshire and nationally, April 29, 2020	
United States active cases	1,012,583
New Hampshire active cases	2010
Vermont active cases	862
United States deaths	58,355
New Hampshire deaths	60
Vermont deaths	47
In New Hampshire (DHHS data)	
Persons, in total, diagnosed with SARS-CoV-2	2010
Recovered	936 (47%)
Deaths attributed to SARS-CoV-2	60 (3%)
Current cases	1014
Persons, in total, hospitalized for SARS-CoV-2	249 (12%)
Current hospitalizations for SARS-CoV-2	106

Data from NH Division of Public Health Services.

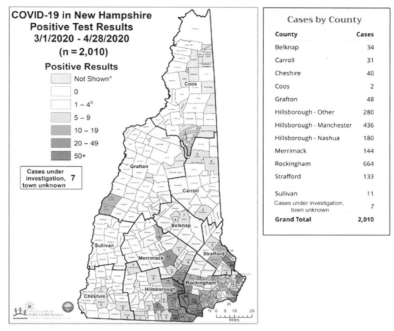

Cases by County	
County	**Cases**
Belknap	34
Carroll	31
Cheshire	40
Coos	2
Grafton	48
Hillsborough - Other	280
Hillsborough - Manchester	436
Hillsborough - Nashua	180
Merrimack	144
Rockingham	664
Strafford	133
Sullivan	11
Cases under investigation, town unknown	7
Grand Total	**2,010**

FIG. 2 Positive test results for SARS-CoV-2 in the state of New Hampshire between March 1, 2020 and April 28, 2020. [a] Positive case counts are suppressed in municipalities with under 100 residents. [b] Exact counts are suppressed for municipalities with 1-4 cases. (*From* NH Division of Public Health Services.)

the providers who were allowed to order a SARS-CoV-2 test. This decision standardized the test requests and provided clean, clinically relevant data. It also helped the institution better understand the need for test assays with shorter and shorter result turnaround time to enable patient triaging from the ED.

• Emergency capital requests: DH-IC immediately approved any capital, test reagents, and supplies purchases to bring up SARS-CoV-2 molecular testing capabilities, serology testing, and convalescent plasma treatment through our departmental Apheresis/Blood Donor Program. By May 1, the products received and invoiced totaled $1,343,275, with additional purchase orders issued for $3,683,849 to sustainably meet the increased need for polymerase chain reaction (PCR)–based and antibody-based SARS-CoV-2 testing (Table 2).

• Supply chain: DH-IC assigned the clinical laboratories a dedicated supply chain representative to facilitate, wherever possible, the rapid acquisition of contracts, capital, reagents, and PPE.

• Access to state relief funds for testing capital and supplies: DH-IC ensured that the clinical

laboratories had immediate access to letters of need from our Chief Legal Officer & General Counsel for State to justify state relief funds.

2. A laboratory COVID task force comprising DHH laboratory managers, section supervisors, a quality manager, the client response team, phlebotomy, and the laboratory specimen receiving staff from every hospital laboratory in the health system helped identify and coordinate responses to staffing shortages, risk assessments, test run times, couriers, and critical supplies such as swabs, universal transport medium, and PPE. Initially meeting by WebEx at the same time daily (March 16–20), the meetings were spread out to 3 times a week, starting March 23. The cooperation between the regional health system laboratories was swift and comprehensive.

3. Research opportunities: research opportunities to collect patient specimens for new assay development and validation, and many epidemiologic studies, highlighted the importance of storing high-quality biospecimens in a CLIA-approved environment to swiftly translate research initiatives into clinical reality. These specimens, collected from consented patients recovering from SARS-CoV-2

TABLE 2
Emergency capital requests for testing capabilities approved by Dartmouth-Hitchcock Health, as of May 1, 2020

Category	Purchase Orders Issued ($)	Product Received and/ or Invoiced ($)
SARS-CoV-2 PCR testing supplies	4,093,050	409,201
Capital	138,728	138,723
Serology testing: clinical chemistry	130,798	130,798
Convalescent plasma: apheresis/ blood donor program	26,951	26,951
Swabs/transport media	637,602	637,602
Total	5,027,124	1,343,275

throughout the state, were used in the development and validation of clinical serology assays as well as evaluating the use of antibody-rich plasma as a COVID-19 treatment. Supported by federal government agencies, including the FDA and the Biomedical Advanced Research and Development Authority, and with the Mayo Clinic serving as the institutional review board, the blood donor program at DHMC collected and processed COVID-19 convalescent plasma to treat patients throughout the state of New Hampshire. The established DHH institutional biorepository, housed in the Department of Pathology and Laboratory Medicine, was capable of accommodating new initiatives such as these.

4. Nimble and responsive laboratory testing and validation: when faced with shortages of swabs, our laboratory worked to validate other potential swabs. With a national shortage of viral transport media, our laboratory developed our own media. In ongoing reductive work, the laboratory developed mechanisms and validations on dry swabs that did not require transport media.

WHAT DID NOT WORK

1. Conflicting recommendations and erroneous information: efforts to combat the SARS-CoV-2 pandemic were hindered by erroneous and conflicting national information as to the availability and validity of the coronavirus diagnostic test. This confused and misled not only our patients but our staff and many providers. Areas of particular confusion included:

- Recognizing the difference between a diagnostic test on symptomatic patients (for which our assays were validated) versus a screening test in an asymptomatic population.
- Trying to explain the nuances of what a robust new assay validation entails so that better comparisons and contrasts can be made with the Emergency Use Authorization products that have flooded the market since March 2020.
- Distinguishing between specimen sampling and testing: specimen sampling took place at sites throughout the state but testing for DH patients was only performed at DHMC.
- Understanding that accurate test results depend on appropriate and competent sampling, and that the result turnaround time depends on the transport time to the laboratory where testing will occur, receipt and preparation of that specimen, the assay and instrumentation used, the technical expertise required to perform these highly complex molecular tests across multiple shifts, and appropriate resulting into the patient's electronic medical record (or other methods of submitting results back to providers if the specimens have come from nonaffiliated collection centers).

2. New Hampshire state politics: while we continued to work collegially and professionally with our New Hampshire state laboratory to clear state-testing backlogs and share reagents and supplies, political decisions about testing sometimes over-ruled sound, evidence-based science. State health alerts and advisories from adjacent New Hampshire and Vermont were often uncoordinated, which resulted in

different testing strategies for hospitals situated on the state borders. Although physically being treated at our institutions in New Hampshire, we were required to abide by the testing requirements of the state of Vermont for residents in that state.

3. Elective surgery planning: carefully considered, evidence-based test triaging by DH-IC, based on CDC published guidelines, was misinterpreted by providers in the name of published statements by their professional associations (American College of Obstetricians and Gynecologists, American College of Surgeons, American Society of Anesthesiologists, Association of Perioperative Registered Nurses, American Heart Association) [2,3]. It took the influence of DH-IC to raise awareness that appropriate PPE was always made available to our providers and that a test performed on an asymptomatic patient coming in for elective surgery was not what the SARS-CoV-2 molecular test was validated for.

4. School and daycare closures: when local school and daycare centers closed, the impact on the ability of both staff and faculty to continue to provide patient services was profound. When elective surgeries were suspended, the reduction in specimen volumes allowed flexibility in coverage in the clinical laboratories. With the return to elective surgeries, and a ramp up in ambulatory testing while schools and daycare centers remained closed, staffing the coverage of key services remained a challenge. Efforts by the College of American Pathologists to get CMS approval for surgical pathologists to sign out patient slides from an office at home, as well as render primary diagnoses from digital images [4], enabled more flexibility for faculty to get back to work.

SUMMARY

Through the early establishment of a DH-IC, planning for a surge in SARS-CoV-2 cases in New Hampshire was highly efficient, building on prior institutional preparations for the monitoring of new, emerging infections. The proactive and visionary work of molecular diagnostic teams in the DH clinical laboratories resulted in us being able to validate an array of new diagnostic test platforms for SARS-CoV-2, to meet the turnaround time and sensitivity needs of the regional population that we serve. We used our existing regional laboratory infrastructure to coordinate testing strategies, reagents, and supplies. A respectful and supportive relationship with the New Hampshire state laboratory maintained a consistently fast SARS-CoV-2 test result turnaround time, statewide. We met the challenges head-on and were not overwhelmed.

DISCLOSURE

The authors have nothing to disclose.

REFERENCES

[1] Lefferts JA, Gutmann EJ, Martin IW, et al. Implementation of an Emergency Use Authorization Test During an Impending National Crisis. J Mol. Diagn 2020;22(7):844–6. https://doi.org/10.1016/j.jmoldx.2020.05.001.

[2] ACOG clinical guidance, practice advisory, novel coronavirus 2019 (COVID-19). 2020. Available at: http://www.acog.org/practice-advisory/articles/2020/03. Accessed April 23, 2020.

[3] Joint Statement: Roadmap for Resuming Elective Surgery after COVID-19 Pandemic: American College of Surgeons, American Society of Anesthesiologists, Association of periOperative Registered Nurses, American Hospital Association. 2020. Available at: https://www.facs.org/covid-19/clinical-guidance/roadmap-elective-surgery. Accessed April 17, 2020.

[4] CAP Secures Remote Work Waiver for Pathologists: College of American Pathologists (CAP) Advocacy Update. 2020. Available at: https://www.cap.org/advocacy/latest-news-and-practice-data/march-26-2020. Accessed March 26, 2020.

Advances in Molecular Pathology 3 (2020) 13–19

ADVANCES IN MOLECULAR PATHOLOGY

Laboratory Testing of Severe Acute Respiratory Virus Coronavirus 2

A New York Institutional Experience

Marie C. Smithgall, MD, Susan Whittier, PhD, Helen Fernandes, PhD*

Department of Pathology & Cell Biology, Columbia University Irving Medical Center, 630 West 168th Street, New York, NY 10032, USA

KEYWORDS
- Laboratory testing • Severe acute respiratory virus coronavirus 2 • COVID-19 • Pandemic

KEY POINTS
- Severe acute respiratory virus coronavirus 2 virus traumatized New York in March and April of 2020 and the coronavirus disease 19 (COVID-19) pandemic left an indelible mark on the majority of individuals particularly, in New York City.
- There are 2 major categories of tests used to detect current or past viral infection: molecular and serologic assays.
- Molecular assays are designed to determine whether a patient is actively infected with a pathogen of interest.
- Serologic assays determine a patient's exposure history.

INTRODUCTION

Throughout March, April, and May 2020, the severe acute respiratory virus coronavirus 2 (SARS-CoV-2) virus traumatized New York and the coronavirus disease 19 (COVID-19) pandemic has affected almost everyone, irrespective of title, status, or ethnicity. It has left an indelible mark on how people regard and conduct everyday life in the midst of the crisis. Clinical molecular laboratory scientists have been frustrated, exhausted, and perplexed at the implementation of diagnostic assays for the detection of SARS-CoV-2 and tests that measure the consequences of infection. Test management has deviated from routine operations under the auspices of regulatory bodies such as the Clinical Laboratory Improvement Amendment (CLIA), US Food and Drug Administration (FDA), College of American Pathologists, and Centers for Medicare & Medicaid Services (CMS). The implication of test validation and

approval has received a new meaning under Emergency Use Authorization (EUA). Perhaps the most noteworthy outcome is that this scenario has made laboratory professionals more visible and respected and induced a deeper sense of ownership of the profession. This brief article provides an overview of the types of testing available for SARS-CoV-2 patient management, as well how testing has affected the situation in New York City.

SARS-CoV-2 first emerged in Wuhan City, Hubei Province, China in December 2019. This novel coronavirus was subsequently isolated and sequenced [1] and has since spread worldwide causing severe disease, termed COVID-19. The World Health Organization (WHO) declared it a pandemic on March 11, 2020 [2]. Since the beginning of the outbreak, clinical laboratories have been developing various assays to aid in detecting SARS-CoV-2 and managing patients with COVID-19, although delays in deploying high-volume

*Corresponding author, *E-mail address:* hf2340@cumc.columbia.edu

diagnostic testing, especially in the United States, have impeded public health containment strategies.

LABORATORY TESTS FOR DETECTION OF SEVERE ACUTE RESPIRATORY VIRUS CORONAVIRUS 2

Clinicians rely on laboratory testing to provide clinically relevant, actionable results that can direct both inpatient and outpatient care. There are 2 main categories of tests used to detect current or past viral infection: molecular and serologic assays. Antigen-detection assays have also been used historically for diagnostic purposes. Molecular assays are designed to determine whether a patient is actively infected with a pathogen of interest, whereas the purpose of serologic testing is to determine prior exposure. The most widely used assays for detection of SARS-CoV-2 use reverse transcriptase polymerase chain reaction (RT-PCR). This technique is already commonly used in microbiology laboratories to detect RNA specific to respiratory viral pathogens, such as influenza and respiratory syncytial virus [3]. The WHO developed the first quantitative RT-PCR test for detecting SARS-CoV-2 and subsequently the US. Centers for Disease Control and Prevention (CDC) began shipping its own RT-PCR test kits after receiving EUA by the FDA on February 4, 2020. However, there were complications that became apparent during the validation process that caused a setback in deploying the assay to the diagnostic community [4]. On February 29, 2020 the Wadsworth Center of the New York State Department of Public Health's RT-PCR assay was the second test to receive EUA. However, this assay was not designed for high-throughput testing, and it analyzed approximately 50 to 60 specimens per day per platform with a turnaround time of 4 to 6 hours from sample to answer. Consequently, testing remained at a minimum until mid-March 2020, when commercially available, fully automated SARS-CoV-2 real-time assays began receiving EUA. These high-throughput automated assays include, but are not limited to, the cobas SARS-CoV-2 Test run on the Roche COBAS 6800/8800 platform and the Abbott RealTime SARS-CoV-2 assay with the m2000 platform. Rapid point-of-care (POC) tests such as Xpert Xpress SARS-CoV-2 (Cepheid) and ID NOW COVID-19 (Abbott), which test single specimens, also became available. These molecular assays detect various viral targets, including SARS-CoV-2–specific targets such as ORF1 a/b, a nonstructural region and N2, a nucleocapsid recombinant protein as well pan-Sarbecovirus targets such as the envelope E-gene.

The ability to batch samples greatly increased testing capabilities in New York City. However, because of significant shortages of testing reagents, positive controls, collection swabs, transport media, and personal protective equipment, only the most critically ill patients presenting to the hospital were being tested. As a result, the biased positive rate of patients tested in New York State was around 50% and New York City was more than 70%. This crucial shortage in testing capacity significantly affected the public health response's ability to contain the virus. The number of SARS-CoV-2–positive cases increased exponentially in New York and adjoining states such as New Jersey, making this region the epicenter of the pandemic (Fig. 1).

With the increase in the number of assays that were verified in several hospitals and laboratories within New York, testing was gradually expanded in April 2020 beyond individuals with a very high pretest probability, to include all symptomatic individuals and people with exposure to known SARS-CoV-2. With this increase in the overall number of tests performed, the overall positive test rate decreased to approximately 20%, a more accurate reflection of the incidence of patients with COVID-19 (Fig. 2). With practicing of social distancing and contact precautions, in addition to expanded testing, the positive rate within the New York community has remained steady since early May 2020, at about 5% to 7%. The overall statistics for New York from early March until May 26th, 2020 can be seen in Fig. 2. Briefly, since the start of the pandemic, more than 2 million tests have been performed with an overall positive rate of approximately 20%. In terms of demographics, not only was incidence higher in men but they also had a much higher fatality rate (58.2%) compared with women (41.8%). Communities of color and lower socioeconomic status also were more seriously affected with higher rates of infection and mortality [5].

Preanalytical Variables of Severe Acute Respiratory Virus Coronavirus 2 Diagnostics

To date there are more than 80 commercial laboratories and/or test kit manufacturers that have received approval for emergency use by the FDA for SARS-CoV-2 testing, with most being molecular assays [6]. Various reports document success with different specimen types ranging from nasopharyngeal (NP), oropharyngeal (OP), anterior nasal, and midturbinate nasal swabs to nasal washes and saliva [7]. In addition, the FDA recently granted EUA for an RT-PCR laboratory-developed test (LDT) for qualitative detection of SARS-CoV-2 in saliva specimens and a test that uses a

CUMULATIVE CASES PER 100,000: ALL STATES

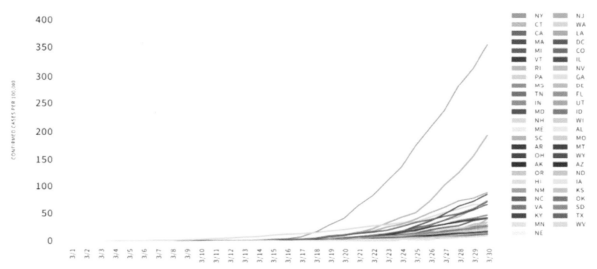

FIG. 1 The number of positive cases statewide in the United States. (*From* March 31 White House briefing presentation. Available at: https://assets.documentcloud.org/documents/6823042/0331-Briefing-BIRX-Final. pdf.)

home collection kit with nasal swabs [6] (for details see https://www.fda.gov/emergency-preparedness-and-response/mcm-legal-regulatory-and-policy-framework/emergency-use-authorization). A recent report showed comparable detection of respiratory viruses by RT-PCR with saliva and NP specimens [8]. Saliva as a specimen type, is appealing for its reduced risk posed at the time of collection; however, larger studies comparing saliva with other validated specimen types are essential for documenting the reliability of this specimen type. In an effort to expand testing capabilities, manufacturers and laboratories have adopted self-collection devices using predominantly anterior nares and midturbinate for sample collection [9]. However, the wide range of specimen types and their varied collection times during the course of COVID-19 infection could contribute to the false-negative rates seen in the RT-PCR assays. A recent study showed that the false-negative rate for SARS-CoV-2 RT-PCR testing can be as high as 67% in individuals tested up to 5 days after exposure and 21% in cases tested 8 days after exposure [10].

Acceptable NP and OP swabs are made with materials such as Dacron and rayon, because they do not inhibit the PCR reaction. Although specimens collected with NP and OP swabs differ in tip size and flexibility, both have been used to successfully collect specimens for identification of SARS-CoV-2 [11]. Other specimens validated by different laboratories include nasal swabs, NP or nasal washes/aspirates, sputum, saliva, and bronchoalveolar lavage [12]. Because each of the specimen types examines different anatomic areas with variable levels of viral inoculum, the possibility of false-negative results should be ruled out for optimal patient management. The NP swab remains the gold-standard specimen source.

Transport media for swabs are reagents that retain virus viability in the specimen and minimize bacterial overgrowth for the time necessary to transport it to the clinical laboratory. Evaluation of different types of transport media, including but not limited to viral transport media and universal transport media, showed that specimens consistently yielded amplifiable RNA with mean cycle threshold differences of less than 3 over the various conditions assayed, thus supporting the use and transport of alternative collection media [13]. For SARS-CoV-2, the FDA has strongly recommended that viral culture not be performed. Thus, alternatives to classic viral transport media have been validated in light of media shortages. These alternatives

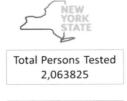

Total Persons Tested
2,063825

Total Tested Positive
370,770

Sex Distribution
Female   48.4%
Male   51.0%
Unknown 0.6%

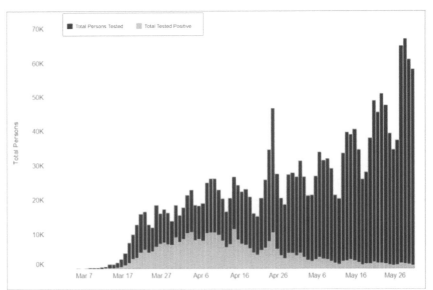

FIG. 2 Number of individuals tested and number of positive cases from March to May 26, 2020. (*Data from* New York State Department of Health. NYSDOH COVID-19 tracker. Available at: https://covid19tracker. health.ny.gov/views/NYS-COVID19-Tracker/NYSDOHCOVID-19Tracker-DailyTracker?%3Aembed=yes&% 3Atoolbar=no&%3Atabs=n.)

include normal saline, Amies transport media, and Hanks balanced salt solution.

A caveat to interpreting molecular results is that it can be difficult to ascertain whether a patient has an active infection or was previously infected. Molecular assays can detect viral RNA both when patients are actively shedding the virus (current infection) and when there is residual viral RNA present. Therefore, these assays are most useful in acute settings to detect patients with SARS-CoV-2, where the results can optimize potential therapy and isolation protocols to ensure that appropriate personal protective equipment protocols are used for containment of the virus.

In addition to RT-PCR, reverse transcription loop-mediated isothermal amplification (RT-LAMP) technologies with increased levels of sensitivity have shown utility in resource-limited settings [14]. Notably, the first test using CRISPR (clustered regularly interspaced short palindromic repeats)-Cas12–based technology for SARS-CoV-2 detection was recently granted EUA (Sherlock Biosciences). The test has a limit of detection of 100 viral copies and involves a 2-step process, where SARS-CoV-2 RNA undergoes RT-LAMP followed by transcription of the amplified DNA, which activates

CRISPR cleavage of reporter genes resulting in a fluorescent readout. The entire process can be completed in an hour [15]. Tests that use high-throughput sequencing of the SARS-CoV-2 genome are also being used in a research setting. These tests give additional information on viral mutations and can trace the global evolution of the pandemic.

RAPID POINT-OF-CARE MOLECULAR ASSAYS

POC testing is beginning to be available for SARS-CoV-2. POC testing refers to a broad category of diagnostic tests that can be performed where patient care occurs. Functionally, these tests have a rapid turnaround time and can potentially be performed by select nonlaboratory clinical personnel. However, at this current time, most clinical laboratories prefer to have all specimens set up by medical technologists in a biosafety cabinet rather than a POC setting. The ID NOW COVID-19 molecular POC test (Abbott) uses isothermal nucleic acid amplification (a technique similar to PCR) to detect SARS-CoV-2 in about 15 minutes. However, because of evidence that samples collected in transport media may be below the assay's limit of detection [16–19], the EUA for this test was modified for testing only from direct swabs. Preliminary data indicates that, despite this modification, the Abbott ID NOW COVID-19 had a significant false-negative rate when using dry nasal swabs [20]. Some additional rapid assays that are commonly used are the Xpert Xpress SARS-CoV2 (Cepheid) and the BIOFIRE COVID-19 test.

SEROLOGIC ASSAYS FOR CORONAVIRUS DISEASE 19

The other major type of diagnostic assay is serologic. These assays determine a patient's exposure history. At this time, it is unknown whether antibody detection equates to immunity. These assays detect the presence of antibodies against SARS-CoV-2 antigens in a patient's serum. There is a delay between the initial viral infection and the production of antibodies by the immune system. During this likely asymptomatic time, termed the window period, a patient who is infected with SARS-CoV-2, but has not yet produced antibodies, would test negative on such an assay. As the immune system mounts a response against the virus, immunoglobulin (Ig) M antibodies are initially produced, which are short lived, followed by a more durable IgG antibody response (Fig. 3). Therefore, serologic tests may be unique to 1 class of immunoglobulins or detect multiple and can typically be completed in 1 to 2 hours.

At present, there are at least 12 EUA serology assays, some of which are automated [6]. Most commercial serologic SARS-CoV-2 assays use a lateral flow assay technique and format, and for many of these there are unsubstantiated, or even false, claims about test performance [21]. The estimated median seroconversion time is 7 to 12 days, with virtually all patients with COVID-19 producing detectable antibodies approximately 15 days after onset of symptoms [22–24]. Therefore, these assays are most helpful in determining an individual's exposure status and perhaps in assessing the individual's immune response to SARS-CoV-2. Going forward, these assays can be particularly helpful in identifying SARS-CoV-2 in individuals who may have had symptoms consistent with SARS-CoV-2 but were never tested with an RT-PCR assay, as well as individuals who may have had asymptomatic infection. Given that ∼80% of SARS-CoV-2 cases are mild to moderate in severity [24,25], and that molecular testing has predominantly been restricted to the most severely ill patients, the true number of SARS-CoV-2 cases is likely to be vastly greater than that available from molecularly confirmed case counts. Thus, serologic testing will help

identify the number of past infections, which can help epidemiologists better understand the true burden of disease to model viral dynamics.

SARS-CoV-2 testing is also important for identifying potential convalescent plasma donors for clinical trials. Studies are currently underway where patients who have recovered from SARS-CoV-2 and have detectable antibodies against SARS-CoV-2 can donate plasma, which can then be transfused to patients who are currently critically ill with COVID-19. Theoretically, the neutralizing antibodies against SARS-CoV-2 present in the plasma will help patients currently infected overcome the illness. Serologic testing to identify anti-SARS-CoV-2 antibodies is now part of the donor work-up to determine eligibility for clinical trials. At some institutions in New York City, potential donors also require RT-PCR testing to determine whether they are still actively shedding virus and, therefore, contagious.

There is now 1 antigen-detection assay available from Quidel that uses a lateral flow CLIA of SARS-CoV and SARS-CoV-2. Information provided by the manufacturer in the package insert indicates an 80% concordance compared with PCR. Historically, antigen-detection kits for viruses have not performed well, so the utility for SARS-CoV-2 remains to be determined. Such tests are used routinely for other viruses: human immunodeficiency virus (HIV) p24 antigen as part of fourth-generation and fifth-generation HIV tests, and also for hepatitis B surface antigen [26].

Considerations for Laboratory Testing During Unprecedented Times of Community Infections

Laboratories regulated by CLIA were able to get EUA for LDTs either directly from the FDA or from the Wadsworth Center of the New York State Department of Health, as in the case of several laboratories in New York. The EUA route permitted the laboratories to implement the LDTs for routine clinical diagnostics. However, in spite of these sanctions, the inability to provide broad diagnostic testing was widely seen as a failing effort to contain the virus. This setback of optimal testing in a crisis was largely caused by the lack of a national laboratory testing strategic plan that brings together the major players in diagnostic testing, including public health, clinical/hospital-based, and commercial laboratories. Clinical hospital-based laboratories play a major role in identification and containment of infectious threats, and a coordinated laboratory network would likely be more effective at damage control earlier in pandemics such as the current one [27].

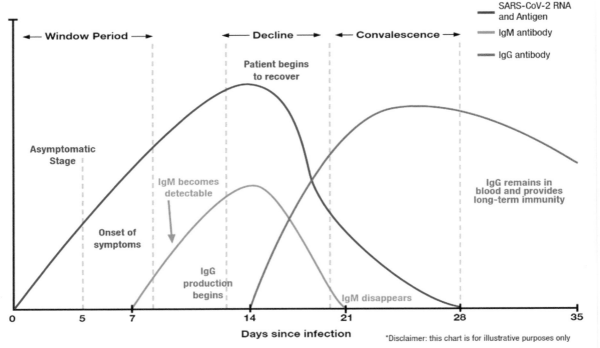

FIG. 3 The antibody response to SARS-CoV-2. (*From* Diazyme Laboratories. Why do we need antibody tests for COVID-19? Available at: https://www.diazyme.com/covid-19-antibody-tests; with permission.)

In summary, testing has been critical to understanding and managing the SARS-CoV-2 pandemic. Although both molecular and serologic tests provide meaningful data for treating patients with SARS-CoV-2, each methodology has a different clinical utility. Moving forward, clinical laboratories will continue to be on the forefront of combating this pandemic by developing new assays and implementing increased testing capabilities to meet the high-volume demands necessitated by this pandemic. A concerted rather than isolated effort may be the best approach to accomplish mass-scale testing.

DISCLOSURE

The authors have nothing to disclose.

REFERENCES

[1] Severe acute respiratory syndrome coronavirus 2 isolate Wuhan-Hu-1, complete genome, in NCBI Reference Sequence: NC_045512.2. 2019. Available at: https://www.ncbi.nlm.nih.gov/nuccore/1798174254.

[2] World Health Organization Coronavirus disease (COVID-19) Pandemic. 2020. Available at: https://www.who.int/emergencies/diseases/novel-coronavirus-2019. Accessed May 26th, 2020.

[3] Mayer LM, Kahlert C, Rassouli F, et al. Impact of viral multiplex real-time PCR on management of respiratory tract infection: a retrospective cohort study. Pneumonia (Nathan) 2017;9:4. https://doi.org/10.1186/s41479-017-0028-z.

[4] Sheridan C. Coronavirus and the race to distribute reliable diagnostics. Nat Biotechnol 2020;38:382–4.

[5] New York State Department of Health COVID-19 Tracker. 2020. Available at: https://covid19tracker.health.ny.gov/. Accessed May 26th, 2020.

[6] U.S. Food and Drug Administration. Emergency Use Authorizations. 2020. Available at: https://www.fda.gov/medical-devices/emergency-situations-medical-devices/emergency-use-authorizations. Accessed May 26th, 2020.

[7] Prevention, C.o.D.C.a., Interim Guidelines for Collecting, Handling, and Testing Clinical Specimens from Persons for Coronavirus Disease 2019 (COVID-19). https://www.cdc.gov/coronavirus/2019-ncov/lab/guidelines-clinical-specimens.html.

[8] Kim Y-g, Yun SG, Kim MY, et al. Comparison between saliva and nasopharyngeal swab specimens for detection of respiratory viruses by multiplex reverse transcription-PCR. J Clin Microbiol 2017;55(1):226–33.

[9] Tu Y-P, Jennings R, Hart B, et al. Patient-collected tongue, nasal, and mid-turbinate swabs for SARS-CoV-2 yield equivalent sensitivity to health care worker collected nasopharyngeal swabs. medRxiv 2020 04.01.20050005.

[10] Kucirka LM, Lauer SA, Laeyendecker O, et al. Variation in false-negative rate of reverse transcriptase polymerase chain reaction–based SARS-CoV-2 tests by time since exposure. Ann Intern Med 2020. https://doi.org/10.7326/M20-1495.

[11] Wölfel R, Corman VM, Guggemos W, et al. Virological assessment of hospitalized patients with COVID-2019. Nature 2020;581(7809):465–9.

[12] Loeffelholz MJ, Tang Y-W. Laboratory diagnosis of emerging human coronavirus infections – the state of the art. Emerg Microbes Infect 2020;9(1):747–56.

[13] Rogers AA, Baumann RE, Borillo GA, et al. Evaluation of Transport Media and Specimen Transport Conditions for the Detection of SARS-CoV-2 Using Real Time Reverse Transcription PCR. J Clin Microbiol 2020. https://doi.org/10.1128/JCM.00708-20.

[14] Park G-S, Ku K, Baek S-H, et al. Development of reverse transcription loop-mediated isothermal amplification assays targeting severe acute respiratory syndrome coronavirus 2. J Mol Diagn 2020;22(6):729–35.

[15] Joung J, Ladha A, Saito M, et al. Point-of-care testing for COVID-19 using SHERLOCK diagnostics. medRxiv 2020. https://doi.org/10.1101/2020.05.04.20091231 05.04.20091231.

[16] Smithgall MC, Scherberkova I, Whittier S, et al. Comparison of cepheid xpert xpress and abbott id now to roche cobas for the rapid detection of SARS-CoV-2. J Clin Virol 2020;128:104428.

[17] Harrington A, Cox B, Snowdon J, et al. Comparison of Abbott ID Now and Abbott m2000 methods for the detection of SARS-CoV-2 from nasopharyngeal and nasal swabs from symptomatic patients. J Clin Microbiol 2020. https://doi.org/10.1128/JCM.00798-20.

[18] Mitchell SL, George KS. Evaluation of the COVID19 ID NOW EUA assay. J Clin Virol 2020;128:104429.

[19] Zhen W, Smith E, Manji R, et al. Clinical evaluation of three sample-to-answer platforms for the detection of SARS-CoV-2. J Clin Microbiol 2020. https://doi.org/10.1128/JCM.00783-20.

[20] Basu A, Zinger T, Inglima K, et al. Performance of the rapid Nucleic Acid Amplification by Abbott ID NOW COVID-19 in nasopharyngeal swabs transported in viral media and dry nasal swabs, in a New York City academic institution. bioRxiv 2020. https://doi.org/10.1128/JCM.01136-20 05.11.089896.

[21] U.S. Food and Drug Administration Beware of Fraudulent Coronavirus Tests, Vaccines and Treatments. 2020. Available at: https://www.fda.gov/consumers/consumer-updates/beware-fraudulent-coronavirus-tests-vaccines-and-treatments. Accessed May 26th, 2020.

[22] Zhao J, Yuan Q, Wang H, et al. Antibody responses to SARS-CoV-2 in patients of novel coronavirus disease 2019. Clin Infect Dis 2020. https://doi.org/10.1093/cid/ciaa344.

[23] To KK, Tsang OT, Leung WS, et al. Temporal profiles of viral load in posterior oropharyngeal saliva samples and serum antibody responses during infection by SARS-CoV-2: an observational cohort study. Lancet Infect Dis 2020;20(5):565–74.

[24] Rokni M, Ghasemi V, Tavakoli Z. Immune responses and pathogenesis of SARS-CoV-2 during an outbreak in Iran: Comparison with SARS and MERS. Rev Med Virol 2020;30(3):e2107.

[25] Chen N, Zhou M, Dong X, et al. Epidemiological and clinical characteristics of 99 cases of 2019 novel coronavirus pneumonia in Wuhan, China: a descriptive study. Lancet 2020;395(10223):507–13.

[26] Gray ER, Bain R, Varsaneux O, et al. p24 revisited: a landscape review of antigen detection for early HIV diagnosis. AIDS 2018;32(15):2089–102.

[27] Kaul KL. Laboratories and pandemic preparedness: A framework for collaboration and oversight. J Mol Diagn 2020;22(7):841–3.

Genetics

Advances in Molecular Pathology 3 (2020) 21–27

ADVANCES IN MOLECULAR PATHOLOGY

Precision Therapies in Neurodevelopmental Disorders

Update on Gene Therapies

Mohammed Uddin, PhD[a,b,*], Ahmad N. Abou Tayoun, PhD[a,c], Reem Kais Jan, PhD[a], Hosneara Akter, MSc[d,e], Danielle M. Andrade, MD, MSc[f,g], Cyrus Boelman, MD[h]

[a]College of Medicine, Mohammed Bin Rashid University of Medicine and Health Sciences, Dubai, UAE; [b]The Centre for Applied Genomics, The Hospital for Sick Children, Toronto, Ontario, Canada; [c]Genomics Center, Al Jalila Children's Specialty Hospital, Dubai, UAE; [d]Genetics and Genomic Medicine Centre, NeuroGen Children's Genomic Clinic, Dhaka, Bangladesh; [e]Department of Biochemistry and Molecular Biology, University of Dhaka, Dhaka, Bangladesh; [f]Division of Neurology, Department of Medicine, University of Toronto, Toronto, Ontario, Canada; [g]Epilepsy Genetics Program, Toronto Western Hospital and Krembil Neuroscience Centre, University of Toronto, Toronto, Ontario, Canada; [h]Division of Neurology, Department of Pediatrics, Faculty of Medicine, University of British Columbia

KEYWORDS

- Precision medicine • Neurodevelopmental disorders • Gene therapy • Antisense oligonucleotide
- Adeno-associated virus

KEY POINTS

- Neurodevelopmental disorders (NDD) refer to a collection of rare disorders that manifest during infancy, characterized by developmental delays across multiple domains, and often manifested with neuropsychiatric and neurologic disorders, including autism spectrum disorder, epilepsy, intellectual disability, movement disorder, and attention-deficit/hyperactivity disorder.
- Genetics play an important role in the cause of NDD, and new genomic technologies have identified more than 100 significant gene associations.
- There are multiple pathways involving neurocognitive functions and other developmental domains that are usually found to be disrupted by pathogenic mutations.
- Although genome-editing technologies (ie, CRISPR/Cas9) are evolving to achieve better accuracy and efficiency, gene therapy is more mature and applicable.
- Gene therapy can stop the impact of a gene mutation at the level of DNA or downstream RNA to preserve the underlying complex functions associated with that gene.

INTRODUCTION

Neurodevelopmental disorders (NDD) refer to a collection of rare disorders that manifest during infancy [1,2], characterized by developmental delays across multiple domains and often manifested with neuropsychiatric and neurologic disorders, including autism spectrum disorder (ASD), epilepsy, intellectual disability (ID), movement disorder, and attention-

Funding: This study is funded by College of Medicine, Mohammed Bin Rashid University of Medicine, Sandooq Al Watan, Al Jalila Foundation, and The Harvard Medical School Center for Global Health Delivery–Dubai.

*Corresponding author. College of Medicine, Mohammed Bin Rashid University of Medicine and Health Sciences, Dubai, UAE. E-mail address: mohammed.uddin@mbru.ac.ae

deficit/hyperactivity disorder (ADHD). The collective prevalence of NDD is high with a global prevalence of between 3% and 5% [3–5].

NDD encompass a spectrum of disorders, and under the *Diagnostic and Statistical Manual of Mental Disorders* (Fifth edition), the diagnostic criteria require assessment of cognitive capacity using the IQ as well as adaptive functioning [6]. The diagnostic complexities of NDD often arise from wide spectrum of comorbidities in NDD; epilepsy is one such comorbidity, with 20% of people with ASD also receiving this diagnosis. Similarly, the prevalence of ASD among Fragile X cases is approximately 50% [7,8]. Apart from IQ, the gold standard for the diagnosis of ASD includes the Autism Diagnostic Observation Schedule, a standardized instrument that uses the observational assessment of social interaction, repetitive behaviors, communication, and play skills [9]. For epilepsy cases, electroencephalography, measuring electrophysiological rhythms of the brain, and high-resolution brain imaging, such as MRI, are typically used to identify brain functional and/or structural abnormalities.

Genetics play an important role in the cause of NDD [1,2,10], and new genomic technologies have identified more than 100 significant gene associations. For numerous NDD comorbidity cohorts (eg, ASD, epilepsy, ID), the genetic contribution to these individual diseases has been independently confirmed through cohort studies [11–13]. Clinical genetic testing is considered a first-tier test for diagnosing rare/de novo genetic variants that may contribute to a patient's NDD [14]. In the last 2 decades, genetic tests have been adopted as highly impactful diagnostic tests in the clinic. A recent report suggests that more than 250 genes reported by multiple independent studies have strong association with NDD [15]. Rare/de novo single nucleotide variants (SNVs) and copy number variations (CNVs) were found to be associated with NDD. Although there is no single high-penetrant mutation found in all NDD cases, a small number of genes (*SCN2A, CHD8, POGZ, STXBP1, mTOR*, and so forth) and loci (16p11.2, 15q13.3, and so forth) have been shown to be enriched for rare/de novo mutations [10,16–18]. In most clinics, exome sequencing is now routinely conducted as a first-tier test. Exome sequencing scans all functional units (exons) in the human genome and identifies SNVs. Similarly, clinical microarray is another genetic test that scans the entire genome to identify large CNVs [2,10]. Large-scale exome or whole-genome sequencing studies suggest that the combined (SNV and CNV) diagnostic yield is greater than 40% for ASD [17,19], epilepsy [20,21], and ID [22,23].

Although the recent progress in genetic diagnosis is significant, there is a lack of therapeutic interventions. The unique phenotypic spectrum of each child and the heterogeneous spectrum of mutations in a large number of genes especially complicate the detection of underlying disease pathways. There is no single common pathway that can explain the clinical manifestation of NDD that can be targeted for drug development. Instead, there are multiple pathways involving neurocognitive functions and other developmental domains that are usually found to be disrupted by pathogenic mutations [2,16,17]. To avoid the complexities of "one-size-fits-all" therapy, the concept of precision medicine has emerged as a major force in accelerating therapeutics in NDD.

Precision medicine is a treatment pathway that uses numerous technologies to guide individually tailored diagnosis and treatment of patients. Precision medicine is a radical shift from the idea of "one-size-fits-all," and gene therapy is one of the most effective technologies that can be used to implement precision medicine. There are currently 2 major precision genetic therapeutic approaches: genome editing (ie, CRISPR/Cas9) and gene therapy. Although genome-editing technologies are evolving to achieve better accuracy and efficiency, gene therapy is more mature and applicable. Gene therapy can stop the impact of a gene mutation at the level of DNA or downstream RNA to preserve the underlying complex functions associated with that gene. Various types of gene replacement and blocking technologies have been tried in past decades to implement precision therapy for NDD.

In this short review, the authors discuss the recent updates and successes of gene therapy technologies in various NDD.

TARGETED GENE THERAPY DRUGS IN NEURODEVELOPMENTAL DISORDERS

Although gene therapy technologies were introduced 4 decades ago, progress has been slow [24,25]. Recently, there have been success stories of the implementation of adeno-associated virus (AAV)-based gene replacement therapy and antisense oligonucleotide therapy (ASO) as potentially targeted treatments. These therapies are discussed later and summarized in Table 1.

Adeno-Associated Virus

In recent years, AAV has been shown to be one of the most effective gene replacement therapies. Despite AAV having a limited cargo capacity (approximately 4.5 kb) for the delivery of genetic material, it has

TABLE 1
List of Gene Therapy Drugs Related to Neurodevelopmental and Neurologic Genetic Disorders

Gene	Coordinate (hg38)	Condition	Drug Type	Drug Name	Targeting Pathway	PMID
SMN1	chr5: 70,925, 030-70,953,012	Spinal muscular atrophy (OMIM 253300)	Adeno-associated virus 9 (AAV9)	Zolgensma	Gene replacement	31371124
			Antisense therapy	Nusinersen	mRNA interference	32180828
MFSD8	chr4: 127,917, 827-127,965,173	Batten disease (OMIM 610951)	Antisense therapy	Malisen	mRNA interference	31597037
DMD	chrX: 31,119,228-33, 211,519 2,092,292	Duchene muscular dystrophy (OMIM 310200)	Antisense therapy	Eteplirsen	mRNA interference	30856119

beneficial advantages (ie, transduction efficiency, long-term DNA persistence) compared with other gene therapy technologies (eg, adenoviral [~36 kb] or lentiviral vectors [~8 kb]). Introducing a wild copy of the faulty gene into the cellular environment in vitro and in vivo through AAV has been shown to be effective to restore gene functions [26,27]. AAV1 serotype was used as a backbone to develop historically the first gene therapy drug "Glybera" for lipoprotein lipase (LPL) deficiency, a multiorgan disorder with triglyceride deposition. The AAV1-based drug successfully delivered a wild-type copy of the LPL gene into human muscle cells [28]. Similarly, AAV9 technology also successfully delivered genetic material crossing the blood-brain barrier targeting neurons and astrocytes [29]. Emerging evidence suggests AAV9 uses laminin receptor for cellular transduction [30]. The AAV9-based drug "Zolgensma" is the first Food and Drug Administration (FDA)-approved AAV-delivered gene therapy used to treat spinal muscular atrophy (SMA), a genetic disorder characterized by loss of motor neurons and progressive muscle wasting owing to mutation in the SMN1 gene. The targeted AAV9 vector replaces the nonfunctioning SMN1 gene with a new, working copy of a human SMN gene. In a clinical trial comprising 12 SMA patients treated with Zolgensma, 11 patients were able to sit independently and 2 patients were able to walk [31].

Antisense Oligonucleotide Therapy

ASOs gene blocking therapy is gaining traction in developing targeted treatments. ASOs are short (21–23 bp), synthetic, single-stranded oligodeoxynucleotides that can impact RNA to reduce, restore, or modify protein expression using several molecular mechanisms. The design of an ASO is the most critical step owing to complexities in genomic context (ie, repeats, mutation) and binding affinity (ie, temperature, ASO structure). This technology allows blocking disease pathogenesis at the source by knocking out the dysfunctional gene as opposed to therapies that target downstream elements of the pathway [32]. The ASO binds with the targeted (complementary) RNA to modulate protein production. The formed DNA-RNA or RNA-RNA duplexes are usually recognized by cellular enzyme RNase H that helps degrade the targeted gene messenger RNAs (mRNAs) [33]. ASO drug development is problematic regarding the in vivo delivery into the biological system owing to rapid ASO degradation by nucleases. To alleviate this problem, scientists are now using chemically modified phosphorothioate and 2′-O-methoxyethyl ASO

backbones that increase the stability against digestion from nucleases [33].

The first FDA-approved ASO drug was introduced in 1998, for the treatment of cytomegalovirus retinitis [34]. Currently, there are 3 ASO therapies that have received FDA approval for the treatment of SMA, Batten disease, and Duchenne muscular dystrophy (DMD). DMD is an X-linked disease of progressive muscle wasting resulting in premature death. Approximately 14% of affected patients carry a stop mutation at exon 51 of the DMD gene. The ASO drug "Exondys 51" or eteplirsen targets this mutation in RNAs and allows for skipping of the mutated exon and production of a shortened protein rather than none. Another ASO therapy "Milasen" was designed for an extremely rare condition, late infantile-onset neuronal ceroid lipofuscinosis, or Batten disease, where a pathogenic mutation in the MFSD8 gene leads to a severe neurodegenerative disorder in the first 5 years of life [35]. This drug was successfully administered to a young girl, and it was designed for an "N of 1" sample, a great example of future precision medicine of NDD. ASO therapy has also recently been approved for SMA; Nusinersen is an ASO-derived drug that redirects the splicing of SMN2 mRNA, the nonfunctional version of SMN1, and promotes inclusion of exon 7 that usually is excluded in patient SMN2 mRNA. The designed ASO binds to the pre-mRNA by Watson-Crick base pairing and through block recognition of splicing factors, thereby controlling the formation of mature mRNA. This mechanism has increased the inclusion of exon 7 to restore production of SMN protein and therefore rescue the phenotype [36]. Animal models and multiphase clinical trials of Nusinersen showed significant increases of SMN protein and the reversal of phenotypes in SMA cases [37].

RISKS AND CHALLENGES OF GENE THERAPY

Gene therapy technologies for the treatment of genetic disorders have been hindered by numerous challenges, including unwanted side effects owing to the immune system invoking innate or adaptive immune responses to the foreign gene product [38]. This issue remains pertinent until today, and technological advancement is necessary to control or avoid immune response against major gene therapy technologies (ie, AAV, ASO) for stable and efficient delivery of gene products. Another major challenge is tissue specificity that hinders transfection rate of gene transport vectors into the cells of different organs. Variability has also been observed within different serotypes of AAV; for example, AAV6 has been shown to have increased transduction rate in skeletal muscle [39], and AAV4 has displayed preference for the central nervous system [40].

There are lingering challenges involving ASO technology also. The most prominent challenge is the short lifespan of ASO in the cellular environment; ASO decays rapidly because of the presence of endogenous nucleases that degrade it, thus reducing its titer within the cellular environment. Despite attempts at improvement of lifespan using modified chemistry, the sensitivity and specificity of ASO are still unknown within most tissue types. Another challenge with ASO technology is the intracellular off target mRNA binding that can lead to specific inhibition of gene expression [41].

Perhaps the main limitation to the utilization of gene therapy in NDD is the large number of chromosomal abnormalities involved in these disorders. For instance, a major risk factor for NDD is CNVs, and each CNV (deletion/duplication) comprises multiple genes, making it impractical to use gene therapy to compensate or mitigate molecular instability causes by multiple gene disruptions. To date, there is no large retrospective study on the long-term effects of using the FDA-approved gene therapy drugs, and there is a lack of gold-standard guidelines for outcome measures. Finally, gene therapy drugs are currently the most expensive drugs globally, and the cost-effectiveness is unlikely to improve because of their limited use in a relatively small number of patients.

FUTURE OF NEURODEVELOPMENTAL DISORDERS GENETIC THERAPIES

Late-stage development of clinical trials is underway for gene therapies for the treatment of several NDD, including Dravet syndrome, Angelman syndrome, and Rett syndrome, targeting *SCN1A*, *UBE3A*, and *MECP2* genes, respectively [42]. Genome editing tools, CRISPR/Cas9 and others, have the potential to design or aid future targeted drugs by manipulation of DNA or RNA. Mutation reversal (alteration) during fetal development may become a possibility when higher accuracy and efficiency are achieved. The combination of gene therapy with CRISPR/Cas9 technology can be a very effective tool for in vivo delivery and precision targeting [43]. These emerging technologies complement each other's strengths and have the potential to accelerate drug development in NDD.

The future therapeutic development should integrate the use of artificial intelligence (AI) to power precision medicine in NDD [4]. AI algorithms have the capacity to handle massive large data sets (ie, genomics,

transcriptomics, proteomics, and clinical records) to decipher information related to a given hypothesis. Machine learning algorithms applying neural networks are becoming a major tool to identify drug molecules for numerous diseases [4,44,45]. Most recently, a new algorithm has been proposed that combines neural networks with a genetic algorithm to conduct massive optimization in search of biological molecules [46]. AI also can be used to best predict repurposed drug candidates for the treatment of NDD.

A combination of CRISPR/Cas9, AI, and gene therapy over the next decade has the potential to significantly accelerate drug development for NDD.

DISCLOSURE

The authors have nothing to disclose.

REFERENCES

[1] Mitchell KJ. The genetics of neurodevelopmental disease. Curr Opin Neurobiol 2011;21(1):197–203.

[2] Uddin M, Pellecchia G, Thiruvahindrapuram B, et al. Indexing effects of copy number variation on genes involved in developmental delay. Sci Rep 2016;6:28663.

[3] Bourke J, de Klerk N, Smith T, et al. Population-based prevalence of intellectual disability and autism spectrum disorders in Western Australia: a comparison with previous estimates. Medicine (Baltimore) 2016;95(21): e3737.

[4] Uddin M, Wang Y, Woodbury-Smith M. Artificial intelligence for precision medicine in neurodevelopmental disorders. NPJ Digit Med 2019;2:112.

[5] Zack MM, Kobau R. National and state estimates of the numbers of adults and children with active epilepsy - United States, 2015. MMWR Morb Mortal Wkly Rep 2017;66(31):821–5.

[6] American Psychiatric Association. Diagnostic and statistical manual of mental disorders (DSM-5®). American Psychiatric Pub; 2013.

[7] Abbeduto L, McDuffie A, Thurman AJ. The fragile X syndrome-autism comorbidity: what do we really know? Front Genet 2014;5:355.

[8] Demark JL, Feldman MA, Holden JJ. Behavioral relationship between autism and fragile X syndrome. Am J Ment Retard 2003;108(5):314–26.

[9] Lord C, Rutter M, Goode S, et al. Autism diagnostic observation schedule: a standardized observation of communicative and social behavior. J Autism Dev Disord 1989;19(2):185–212.

[10] Wassman ER, Ho KS, Bertrand D, et al. Critical exon indexing improves clinical interpretation of copy number variants in neurodevelopmental disorders. Neurol Genet 2019;5(6):e378.

[11] Warrier RP, Azeemuddin S. Aeromonas hydrophilia tenosynovitis in an immunocompromised host. Indian J Pediatr 1984;51(412):609–10.

[12] Tick B, Bolton P, Happe F, et al. Heritability of autism spectrum disorders: a meta-analysis of twin studies. J Child Psychol Psychiatry 2016;57(5):585–95.

[13] Berkovic SF, Howell RA, Hay DA, et al. Epilepsies in twins: genetics of the major epilepsy syndromes. Ann Neurol 1998;43(4):435–45.

[14] Srivastava S, Love-Nichols JA, Dies KA, et al. Meta-analysis and multidisciplinary consensus statement: exome sequencing is a first-tier clinical diagnostic test for individuals with neurodevelopmental disorders. Genet Med 2019;21(11):2413–21.

[15] Coe BP, Stessman HAF, Sulovari A, et al. Neurodevelopmental disease genes implicated by de novo mutation and copy number variation morbidity. Nat Genet 2019;51(1):106–16.

[16] Uddin M, Tammimies K, Pellecchia G, et al. Brain-expressed exons under purifying selection are enriched for de novo mutations in autism spectrum disorder. Nat Genet 2014;46(7):742–7.

[17] Iossifov I, O'Roak BJ, Sanders SJ, et al. The contribution of de novo coding mutations to autism spectrum disorder. Nature 2014;515(7526):216–21.

[18] Uddin M, Sturge M, Peddle L, et al. Genome-wide signatures of 'rearrangement hotspots' within segmental duplications in humans. PLoS One 2011;6(12):e28853.

[19] Jiang YH, Yuen RK, Jin X, et al. Detection of clinically relevant genetic variants in autism spectrum disorder by whole-genome sequencing. Am J Hum Genet 2013; 93(2):249–63.

[20] Helbig KL, Farwell Hagman KD, Shinde DN, et al. Diagnostic exome sequencing provides a molecular diagnosis for a significant proportion of patients with epilepsy. Genet Med 2016;18(9):898–905.

[21] Uddin M, Woodbury-Smith M, Chan A, et al. Germline and somatic mutations in STXBP1 with diverse neurodevelopmental phenotypes. Neurol Genet 2017;3(6): e199.

[22] Chong WW, Lo IF, Lam ST, et al. Performance of chromosomal microarray for patients with intellectual disabilities/developmental delay, autism, and multiple congenital anomalies in a Chinese cohort. Mol Cytogenet 2014;7:34.

[23] Chen X, Li H, Chen C, et al. Genome-wide array analysis reveals novel genomic regions and candidate gene for intellectual disability. Mol Diagn Ther 2018;22(6): 749–57.

[24] Hanna E, Remuzat C, Auquier P, et al. Gene therapies development: slow progress and promising prospect. J Mark Access Health Policy 2017;5(1):1265293.

[25] Rubin GM, Spradling AC. Genetic transformation of Drosophila with transposable element vectors. Science 1982;218(4570):348–53.

[26] Grimm D, Lee JS, Wang L, et al. In vitro and in vivo gene therapy vector evolution via multispecies interbreeding and retargeting of adeno-associated viruses. J Virol 2008;82(12):5887–911.

[27] Bankiewicz KS, Eberling JL, Kohutnicka M, et al. Convection-enhanced delivery of AAV vector in parkinsonian monkeys; in vivo detection of gene expression and restoration of dopaminergic function using pro-drug approach. Exp Neurol 2000;164(1): 2–14.

[28] Ferreira V, Petry H, Salmon F. Immune responses to AAV-vectors, the glybera example from bench to bedside. Front Immunol 2014;5:82.

[29] Foust KD, Nurre E, Montgomery CL, et al. Intravascular AAV9 preferentially targets neonatal neurons and adult astrocytes. Nat Biotechnol 2009;27(1):59–65.

[30] Akache B, Grimm D, Pandey K, et al. The 37/67-kilodalton laminin receptor is a receptor for adeno-associated virus serotypes 8, 2, 3, and 9. J Virol 2006;80(19): 9831–6.

[31] Al-Zaidy SA, Mendell JR. From clinical trials to clinical practice: practical considerations for gene replacement therapy in SMA type 1. Pediatr Neurol 2019; 100:3–11.

[32] Rinaldi C, Wood MJA. Antisense oligonucleotides: the next frontier for treatment of neurological disorders. Nat Rev Neurol 2018;14(1):9–21.

[33] Shen X, Corey DR. Chemistry, mechanism and clinical status of antisense oligonucleotides and duplex RNAs. Nucleic Acids Res 2018;46(4):1584–600.

[34] Marwick C. First "antisense" drug will treat CMV retinitis. JAMA 1998;280(10):871.

[35] Kim J, Hu C, Moufawad El Achkar C, et al. Patient-customized oligonucleotide therapy for a rare genetic disease. N Engl J Med 2019;381(17):1644–52.

[36] Jochmann E, Steinbach R, Jochmann T, et al. Experiences from treating seven adult 5q spinal muscular atrophy patients with Nusinersen. Ther Adv Neurol Disord 2020;13: 1756286420907803.

[37] Claborn MK, Stevens DL, Walker CK, et al. Nusinersen: a treatment for spinal muscular atrophy. Ann Pharmacother 2019;53(1):61–9.

[38] Weeratna RD, Wu T, Efler SM, et al. Designing gene therapy vectors: avoiding immune responses by using tissue-specific promoters. Gene Ther 2001;8(24):1872–8.

[39] Gao GP, Alvira MR, Wang L, et al. Novel adeno-associated viruses from rhesus monkeys as vectors for human gene therapy. Proc Natl Acad Sci U S A 2002; 99(18):11854–9.

[40] Davidson BL, Stein CS, Heth JA, et al. Recombinant adeno-associated virus type 2, 4, and 5 vectors: transduction of variant cell types and regions in the mammalian central nervous system. Proc Natl Acad Sci U S A 2000; 97(7):3428–32.

[41] Corey DR. Synthetic nucleic acids and treatment of neurological diseases. JAMA Neurol 2016;73(10): 1238–42.

[42] Medicine, U. S. N. L. o. Clinical Trials 2020. Available at: https://clinicaltrials.gov/.

[43] Wilbie D, Walther J, Mastrobattista E. Delivery aspects of CRISPR/Cas for in vivo genome editing. Acc Chem Res 2019;52(6):1555–64.

[44] Lima AN, Philot EA, Trossini GH, et al. Use of machine learning approaches for novel drug discovery. Expert Opin Drug Discov 2016;11(3):225–39.

[45] Hessler G, Baringhaus KH. Artificial intelligence in drug design. Molecules 2018;23(10):2520.

[46] Wainberg M, Merico D, Delong A, et al. Deep learning in biomedicine. Nat Biotechnol 2018;36(9): 829–38.

Advances in Molecular Pathology 3 (2020) 29–39

ADVANCES IN MOLECULAR PATHOLOGY

EpiSigns

DNA Methylation Signatures in Mendelian Neurodevelopmental Disorders as a Diagnostic Link Between a Genotype and Phenotype

Jack Reilly, BSc[a,b], Jennifer Kerkhof, BSc[a,b], Bekim Sadikovic, PhD[a,b,*]

[a]Molecular Genetics Laboratory, Molecular Diagnostics Division, London Health Sciences Centre, London, Ontario N6A5W9, Canada; [b]Department of Pathology and Laboratory Medicine, Western University, London, Ontario N6A3K7, Canada

---

KEYWORDS
- DNA methylation • Epigenetics • Episignature • Neurodevelopmental disorders • Molecular diagnosis
- Clinical applications

KEY POINTS
- DNA methylation profiling as episignatures can be used as a biomarker for neurodevelopmental disorders.
- Episignatures are a useful tool for defining patients who lack a diagnosis based on clinical phenotype or previous genetic findings and in assessing variants of uncertain significance.
- DNA methylation microarray data analyzed with the clinical multiclass classification algorithm, EpiSign, permit concurrent assessment of over 40 conditions.

INTRODUCTION

Epigenetics is the study of heritable changes in gene expression that do not involve changes to the underlying DNA sequence, or changes in phenotype without underlying genotype change [1,2]. The most studied and well-understood epigenetic mechanisms include DNA methylation, which refers to addition of a methyl group to cytosine residues, and histone modifications, which refer to chemical modifications of the histone tails [2]. In concert, these modifications affect chromatin, the macromolecular complex of DNA, RNA, and protein machinery. DNA methylation and histone modifications regulate chromatin packaging and compaction, allowing for varying chromatin states, including more open and transcriptionally active and accessible euchromatin, and compacted and transcriptionally inactive heterochromatin. As such, these modifications are able to modulate ability of protein complexes to bind and interact with the underlying DNA structure, rendering epigenetic mechanisms key components of a cell's ability to regulate gene expression.

Although this article primarily focuses on epigenetics of DNA methylation, it is important to briefly discuss key concepts related to histone modification machinery. Histones are protein octamers that are organizational units upon which DNA is wrapped, allowing for compact storage of the human genome's near 3 billion base pairs. This compaction is plastic, with variation occurring as a result of modification of "tail" residues of histone complexes [2]. Histone tail modifications include, but are not limited to, methylation, phosphorylation, acetylation, and ubiquitination, resulting in different chromatin states depending

---

*Corresponding author. Molecular Genetics Laboratory, Molecular Diagnostics Division, London Health Sciences Centre, London, Ontario N6A5W9, Canada. *E-mail address:* bekim.sadikovic@lhsc.on.ca

https://doi.org/10.1016/j.yamp.2020.07.018
2589-4080/20/

on the type and pattern of modification [3]. Genetically identical cells within an organism can thus display diverse patterns of gene expression, resulting in the myriad of cell lines and phenotypes, as well as providing a reversible plastic system of gene regulation, capable of interacting with and responding to environmental stimuli [4]. This epigenetic process provides an organism the ability to diversify spatially, creating unique cell lines, as well as temporally, as variants of histone proteins can be recruited at key developmental stages to allow for preferential gene expression.

Unlike the highly diverse and complex modifications of histone tails, DNA methylation in humans primarily occurs at a DNA cytosine base in Cytosine-Guanine dinucleotides (so-called CpG) by addition of the methyl group (CH3) to the C5 position of the cytosine base [5]. This addition is carried out by DNA methyltransferase enzymes, including DNMT1, DNMT3A, and DNMT3B, whereas the removal process involves Ten-Eleven Translocation (TET) enzymes. The resulting process is plastic (ie, reversible), allowing for epigenetic fine-tuning throughout an organism's life and differentiation between cell lineages. CpG dinucleotides are interspersed throughout the human genome at varying frequencies, including randomly interspersed genomic CpG dinucleotides and gene promoter-associated clusters of increased CpG density, referred to as CpG islands [6]. Although most interspersed CpGs in the human genome are methylated, the CpG island-associated CpGs are predominantly unmethylated and associated with transcriptionally active chromatin configurations in gene promoters [7].

Promoter CpG island hypermethylation is associated with a heterochromatin state, which lessens the ability of proteins to interact with the proximal DNA sequences, thereby reducing and/or silencing the expression of nearby genes [8]. However, epigenomic structure or profiles display regional differences across the human genome. For example, most CpGs in the human genome, with the key exception of CpGs in the CpG islands of gene promoters for housekeeping genes, are methylated during development. Once cells differentiate into separate cell lines, specific genes are differentially methylated in appropriate cells, allowing for expression of the genes that are necessary for differentiation, and subsequently maintenance of their function in these tissues. This plastic system requires several functions for effective regulation of gene expression. Components of this "epigenetic machinery" can be sorted into several classes in relation to the DNA methylation, namely writers, readers, and erasers [9]. Writers, such as the DNMT family, add methyl tags to

cytosine bases. Conversely, erasers, such as the TET family of enzymes, reverse such additions, making the process reversible and therefore more flexible in terms of its functionality. Finally, readers can recognize the presence of methyl groups with specialized methyl binding domains within their structure, allowing the body to accurately modulate methylation at key developmental stages, resulting in spatial and temporal differentiation [10]. Interaction with the microenvironmental and macroenvironmental exposures further adds to the complexity of this system. For example, epigenetic mechanisms have been shown to "respond" to changes in diet, exercise, exposure to chemicals, and a myriad of other environmental stimuli [11]. Epigenomic mechanisms can therefore be described as a conduit between environment and the genotype, and as such, play an active role in cellular and organismal response and adaptation to their environment.

Patterns of methylation modulate key functions within the human body and have been implicated in many aspects of development. For example, when mutations occur in DNMTs and other members of the "epigenetic machinery," the effects are widespread and complex, affecting the entire genome's ability to translate and transcribe its contents [12]. This process is integral to the healthy functioning of an organism, and targeted DNMT gene mutation of embryonic stem cells in mouse models was found to cause an embryonic lethal phenotype when introduced to the germline [13]. When a mutation occurs in the protein machinery related to reading, writing, or erasing methylation marks, histone modifications, or chromatin remodeling complexes, epigenetic and gene expression profiles are consequently disrupted. A recent study involving patients with mutations in *DNMT1*, associated with autosomal dominant cerebellar ataxia, deafness, and narcolepsy (ADCADN; MIM# 604121), demonstrates this principle. Peripheral blood samples of patients with the ADCADN mutations were found to have significant differences in genomic methylation when compared with the controls, primarily increased methylation in areas that normally remain unmethylated [14]. Such hypermethylation in gene promoters can be associated disruption of gene expression and likely plays a part in the observed pathophysiology of this disorder. A large and growing number of human neurodevelopmental disorders are caused by mutations in the epigenetic machinery genes. Major challenges exist in the identification and appropriate diagnosis of the complex neurodevelopmental conditions associated with these genes because of overlapping phenotypes, confounding results from current genomic assays, and a limited ability to detect and interpret non-coding genomic regions. Next-generation sequencing (NGS) assessment practices, including targeted gene analysis and whole-exome sequencing (WES), provide a conclusive genetic diagnosis in approximately 15% to 35% of cases in patients with rare neurodevelopmental disorders [15–19]. Although this is an improvement over the current gold-standard technique of chromosomal microarray (CMA) analysis [20,21], most patients with suspected genetic conditions do not reach a conclusive molecular diagnosis for their condition. As a result, physicians often rely on patients' clinical features to establish a most likely clinical diagnosis, which often has a direct impact on clinical management of these individuals [22]. This process is a difficult one, because many of the disorders in question have overlapping phenotypes. Assessment of dysmorphology or facial abnormalities, for example, can be confounded by many factors, including age, sex, ethnicity, and other genetic and environmental contributing factors. In order to demonstrate the complexity of phenotypic assessment in genetic neurodevelopmental disorders, the authors mapped clinical feature categories to the 49 disorders of epigenetic machinery (Fig. 1, Table 1). These 49 disorders have been previously summarized [9,23].

An additional challenge is that genetic testing commonly results in ambiguous findings, including identification of genetic variants of unknown clinical significance (VUS) [24–26]. Using genomic DNA methylation analysis in conditions that exhibit unique epigenetic signatures associated with specific genetic defects enables resolution of ambiguous genetic findings and uncertain phenotypes in these patients [23]. Where traditional genomic technologies fail to encompass the complexity of phenotypes in relation to the mutation observed in the epigenetic machinery, analysis and comparison of the methylation profile described as an episignature allow for robust classification of the disorder. Rather than assigning the source of pathologic condition to a given mutation or set of mutations, the episignature instead provides a genome-wide view of the downstream epigenetic effects of a defect of a specific gene.

EPISIGNATURES AS DIAGNOSTIC BIOMARKERS IN NEURODEVELOPMENTAL DISORDERS

The investigation of episignatures in the context of inherited disorders has been ongoing over the last 10 years with the earliest reports describing observed patterns of differentially methylated regions (DMRs)

in trisomy 21 (Down syndrome) [27]. Expansion of this work has exploded in more recent years with current literature reporting 34 episignatures for neurodevelopmental disorders resulting from defects in up to 45 genes and chromosomal copy number events (see Table 1). The individual signatures are unique to their associated disorder, which permits use of a multiclass classification algorithm for concurrent analysis of each methylation pattern. These discoveries, in combination with the previous clinically validated imprinting and trinucleotide repeat disorders, has introduced the first clinical genome-wide DNA methylation assay known as EpiSign [12,28–33].

The classic recommended investigative approach for genetic causes of neurodevelopmental disorders, which yields a diagnostic rate of 15% to 20% [34], is CMA with the addition of fragile X testing in males [35] and consideration for single genes, such as *MECP2* and *PTEN* [36]. However, the advancement of NGS, and more recently, the incorporation of copy number detection by NGS data have increased the diagnostic rate to 30% to 43% for the same population through use of targeted gene panels or WES [34]. One of the major challenges of molecular testing, estimated in approximately 25% of diagnostic assessments, is VUS [37,38]. Interpretation of these variants can be aided with population databases and in silico computational prediction methods, but reclassification of genetic VUS in these patients, if possible, is directed by functional in vitro assays, cell and animal model systems, family segregation studies, and expression profiling. Functional studies can be considered strong evidence for determining pathogenicity of a variant, but current methods present limitations of reproducibility because of specimen integrity or true reflection of the biological environment with in vitro systems or animal models. Even with these tools and guidelines, most patients with VUS remain unresolved [39,40]. The benefit of methylation profiling with unique condition episignatures that can be assessed simultaneously on DNA extracted from a patient's peripheral blood, is that it can be applied systematically across large cohorts with data generation similar to current CMA approaches, and that the results are a reflection of the patient's biological environment with a functional assessment of the downstream effects of a VUS. Classification of VUS with the method of episignature matching can stratify variants into the likely benign (not matching the epigenetic signature) or pathogenic (matching the epigenetic signature) categories with the pathogenic classification ultimately increasing the diagnostic yield. Out of 36 patients with a VUS in *KMT2D*, 7 (19%) patients were

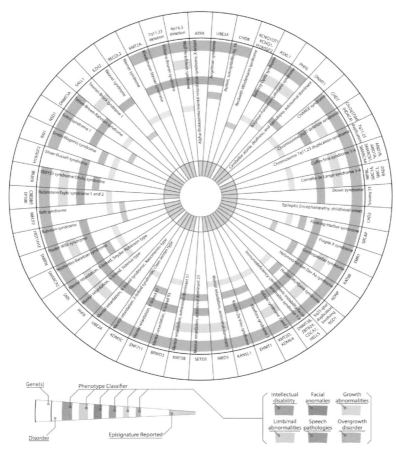

FIG. 1 A comparison of the phenotypic overlap across conditions associated with disruption of epigenetic machinery. Disorders were categorized into 6 classifiers based on descriptions provided in their MIM profile: intellectual disability (n = 42), facial anomalies (n = 36), growth abnormalities (n = 28), limb/nail abnormalities (n = 20), speech pathologies (n = 12), and overgrowth disorders (n = 5). Intellectual disability classifier was applied to disorders whose clinical phenotype contained key words such as intellectual disability, cognitive disability, and mental retardation. Facial anomalies were assigned to disorders described to have malformations of facial features, including descriptions of abnormal nose, eye, eyelid, and mouth features. Growth abnormalities covered a description of deficiencies in development, including short stature, microcephaly, retardation of somatic development, and poor postnatal growth. Overgrowth disorders were assigned to disorders containing descriptors of acromegaly, macroorchidism, and gigantism. Limb/nail abnormalities category contained disorders associated with malformations of the appendicular skeleton, such as brachydactyly, and absence or hypoplasia of various limb features. The speech pathology category was assigned to disorders that were described with speech delay or absence of speech. Other phenotypic key words, including epilepsy, cardiac malformations, immune dysfunction, dental malformation, narcolepsy/dementia and blood disorders, were also observed but were excluded from visualization because of low occurrence (n <4). (Figure produced by Gavin Riddolls, Guildenthaw Design.)

predicted to have a DNA methylation profile matching Kabuki syndrome (MIM# 147920), whereas the remaining 29 samples that matched the control cohort were predicted to carry likely benign variants. In the same study, 8 out of 16 (50%) patients with VUS in NSD1 were predicted as having Sotos syndrome (MIM# 117550) [12]. Assessment of Coffin-Siris (CSS; MIM# 135900, 614607) and Nicolaides-Baraitser (NCBRS; MIM# 601358) syndromes classified 4 of 18 (22%) patients with VUS, in genes encoding subunits

TABLE 1
Episignature Status of Neurodevelopmental Disorders Associated with Epigenetic Machinery or Imprinting Defects and Their Phenotypic Profile

Gene(s)/Locus	Disorder	Phenotype MIM Number	Episignature Reported
ATRX	Alpha-thalassemia/mental retardation syndrome, X-linked	301040	Yes [12,28,29,50]
UBE3A	Angelman syndrome	105830	Yes [33]
CHD8	Autism, susceptibility to, 18	615032	Yes [28,54]
KCNQ1OT1/KCNQ1, H19/IGF2	Beckwith-Wiedemann syndrome	130650	Yes [33]
ASXL1	Bohring-Opitz syndrome	605039	No
PHF6	Borjeson-Forssman-Lehmann syndrome	301900	Yes [28]
DNMT1	Cerebellar ataxia, deafness, and narcolepsy, autosomal dominant	604121	Yes [12,14,28,29]
CHD7	CHARGE syndrome	214800	Yes [12,28,29,45]
Chr2q37del (HDAC4)	Chromosome 2q37 deletion syndrome	600430	No
7q11.23 duplication	Chromosome 7q11.23 duplication syndrome	609757	Yes [28,29,55]
ARID1B, ARID1A, SMARCB1, SMARCA4	Coffin-Siris syndrome 1–4	135900, 614607, 614608, 614609	Yes [25,28,29]
NIPBL, SMC1A, SMC3, RAD2	Cornelia de Lange syndrome 1–4	122470, 300590, 610759, 614701	Yes [28,29]
Trisomy 21	Down syndrome	190685	Yes [28,29,57]
CHD2	Epileptic encephalopathy, childhood-onset	615369	Yes [28]
SRCAP	Floating-Harbor syndrome	136140	Yes [12,28,29,49]
FMR1	Fragile X syndrome	300624	Yes [30]
KAT6B	Genitopatellar syndrome	606170	Yes [12,28,29]
ADNP	Helsmoortel-Van Der Aa syndrome	615873	Yes [28,29]
5q35-qter duplication involving NSD1	Hunter-McAlpine syndrome	601379	Yes [28]
DNMT3B, ZBTB24, CDCA7, HELLS	Immunodeficiency-centromeric instability-facial anomalies syndrome 1–4	242860, 614069, 616910, 616911	Yes [28]
KMT2D, KDM6A	Kabuki syndrome 1 and 2	147920, 300867	Yes [12,28,29,45,51]
EHMT1	Kleefstra syndrome 1	610253	Yes [28]
KANSL1	Koolen-De Vries syndrome	610443	Yes [28]
MBD5	Mental retardation, autosomal dominant 1	156200	No
SETD5	Mental retardation, autosomal dominant 23	615761	No
KMT5B	Mental retardation, autosomal dominant 51	617788	Yes [28]
BRWD3	Mental retardation, X-linked 93	300659	Yes [28]

(continued on next page)

TABLE 1
(continued)

Gene(s)/Locus	Disorder	Phenotype MIM Number	Episignature Reported
ZNF711	Mental retardation, X-linked 97	300803	Yes [28]
KDM5C	Mental retardation, X-linked syndromic, Claes-Jensen type	300534	Yes [12,26,28,29]
UBE2A	Mental retardation, X-linked syndromic, Nascimento-type	300860	Yes [28]
PHF8	Mental retardation, X-linked, Siderius type	300263	No
SMS	Mental retardation, X-linked, Snyder-Robinson type	309583	Yes [28]
SMARCA2	Nicolaides-Baraitser syndrome	601358	Yes [25,28,29,47]
SNRPN	Prader-Willi syndrome	176270	Yes [33]
HIST1H1E	Rahman syndrome	617537	Yes [28,52]
MECP2	Rett syndrome	312750	No
CREBBP, EP300	Rubinstein-Taybi syndrome 1 and 2	180849, 613684	Yes [28]
KAT6B	SBBYSS syndrome/Ohdo syndrome	603736	Yes [12,28]
H19/IGF2	Silver-Russell syndrome	180860	Yes [31–33]
RAI1	Smith-Magenis syndrome	182290	No
NSD1	Sotos syndrome 1	117550	Yes [12,28,29,53]
DNMT3A	Tatton-Brown-Rahman syndrome	615879	Yes [28]
SALL1	Townes-Brock syndrome 1	107480	No
EZH2	Weaver syndrome	277590	No
RECQL2	Werner syndrome	277700	Yes [56]
KMT2A	Wiedemann-Steiner syndrome	605130	Yes [28]
7q11.23 deletion	Williams-Beuren syndrome	194050	Yes [28,29,55]
4p16.3 deletion	Wolf-Hirschhorn syndrome	194190	No

of the SWItch/Sucrose Non-Fermentable (SWI/SNF) chromatin remodeling complex, as good clinical matches [25]. Two additional cohorts of patients with VUS in genes associated with epigenetic machinery were assessed with the EpiSign multiclass classification algorithm and matched a signature with a predicted pathogenic phenotype in 17/44 (39%) [29] and one out of 9 (11%) patients [28].

Episignature analysis is not only enabling reclassification and interpretation of genetic variants but also expanding the knowledge of the types of genetic variants that can cause genetic disorders. Until recently, variant reports for the *ADNP* gene, which is associated with Helsmoortel-van der Aa syndrome (HVDAS; MIM# 615873), have been restricted to truncating loss-of-function variants [41,42]. By matching the episignature defined by patients with truncating loss-of-function mutations, 2 unrelated patients with different missense variants in *ADNP* were shown to be affected by HVDAS (Sadikovic Bekim, 2020), ultimately expanding the variant demographic in this patient population.

Characterizing VUS is one way in which episignature analysis is increasing the molecular diagnostic yield. Another approach is to systematically screen patients with neurodevelopmental conditions that show negative genomic findings. Genomic analyses including Copy Number Variation (CNV) arrays and exome sequencing have limitations, including identification of balanced translocations [20], allele phasing, mapping problems due to Guanine Cytosine (GC) bias, repetitive elements, and homologous sequences, and are normally restricted to assessment of coding regions with minimal coverage of intronic or regulatory elements [43]. Episignature analysis is independent of the specific causative genomic cause because it assesses downstream effects of gene disruption and not the specific cause of the methylation change in the gene itself. As a result, methylation profiling can be used as a biomarker to assess patients with negative genetic findings. Methylation profiling can also help to stratify neurodevelopmental disorders with phenotypic overlap when diagnosis based on clinical features alone is difficult. For example, CHARGE syndrome (MIM# 214800) caused by variants in the *CHD7* gene includes Kabuki syndrome (MIM# 147920, 300867) as one of the differential diagnoses [44,45]. In 1 study, a cohort of 51 patients with a phenotype suggestive of CHARGE syndrome but without molecular confirmation underwent genome-wide DNA methylation analysis. Epigenomic signatures were consistent with CHARGE in 23 patients; 27 patients were ruled out, whereas 1 patient had an episignature consistent with Kabuki syndrome [12]. A larger cohort of 965 subjects with a spectrum of neurodevelopmental delays and congenital anomalies, but negative for routine genetic investigations by CMA, and in some cases, targeted gene panels or WES, underwent genome-wide methylation profiling. Of the 34 episignatures screened, 16 different conditions were matched across 24 unique samples [28,29], further demonstrating the utility of episignature analysis.

EPISIGNATURES AS PHENOTYPIC BIOMARKERS IN NEURODEVELOPMENTAL DISORDERS

Disorders involving either direct or indirect disruption of proteins that regulate the epigenetic machinery display significant phenotypic overlap with one another, which may be associated with the downstream effects of altered gene expression [46]. The DMRs in this group of neurodevelopmental disorders are genome-wide and can range in numbers from hundreds to thousands with both hypermethylation and hypomethylation changes observed. The changes are dispersed both within and outside of gene coding regions. They may involve entire CpG islands or single CpG dinucleotides. The pattern of DMRs within 1 condition is highly reproducible, which permits mapping of their profile for use as potential diagnostic biomarkers [12,14,28,45,47–57]. There are shared DMRs across the epigenetic machinery subclass of neurodevelopmental disorders, but

typically less than 10% are linked to more than 1 condition, and machine learning approaches have been used to accurately classify 1 condition from another, as well as from controls. The process of episignature mapping involves a training cohort consisting of patients with known pathogenic variants to be used for feature selection and model training and has a demonstrated accuracy of up to 99.9% [12,28,29]. Once an episignature is mapped, it is validated with a testing cohort that is also composed of affected individuals. The high accuracy of episignature analysis is demonstrated by validation cohorts shown to have greater than 99% sensitivity for classifying a sample into the correct category (condition or control), whereas assessment of healthy subjects has demonstrated 100% specificity by confidently classifying each as a control [12,28,29]. The importance of an accurate diagnosis in these closely related conditions is necessary for creating an appropriate and direct treatment plan because it has been shown that genetic findings have changed clinical management in up to 55% of individuals with multiple congenital anomalies, developmental delay, intellectual disability, and autism spectrum disorder (ASDs) [58].

Episignatures can distinguish conditions from one another but are also providing insight into the phenotypic variability observed within 1 condition, or perhaps more specifically, the range of phenotypes observed from variants within the same gene. For example, HVDAS is a common cause of ASD and intellectual disability [42,59], but also presents with diverse features of variable expressivity [41]. Variants in the causative *ADNP* gene have been shown to cluster into 2 distinct episignatures dependent on the location of the variant, translating to a spectrum of downstream gene expression effects and ultimately offering a possible explanation to the varied phenotypic range observed in HVDAS [60], although more thorough and detailed phenotyping studies are required to be conclusive. Along the same lines, variants in *SMARCA2* have historically been known to cause NCBRS, but methylation profiling has recently identified a distinct episignature for a subset of *SMARCA2* variants that is predominantly of an opposite pattern to NCBRS and linked to a divergent phenotype.[61]

Although gene-level information is often associated with a defined clinical diagnosis, specific examples of *ADNP* and *SMARCA2* show that nucleotide-level variant features, such as location or variant type, may be required for reaching a correct diagnosis. In addition to defining a distinct phenotype, variant location can be a factor in milder or less expressive variation of the main phenotypes. To revisit *SMARCA2* as a cause of NCBRS, most pathogenic variants map to the ATPase/C-terminal helicase domain [62]. Patients with variants in *SMARCA2* distal to the helicase domain present with milder neurodevelopmental and atypical features compared with typical NCBRS patients. The downstream methylation effects have been shown to represent an intermediate profile that matches neither NCBRS nor controls but overlaps with nearly 50% of control DMRs [47]. The intermediate signature may be a sign of a distinct phenotype or a "signature scale" that could explain variable expressivity observed in some conditions.

Episignatures have started to guide us to more accurately define a patient's diagnosis and provide insight into the explanation behind the idea of 1 gene, multiple phenotypes. Conversely to this idea, DNA methylation profiling is also highlighting the functional relatedness of certain enzyme complexes, evidenced by existence of common episignatures in multiple genes. BAF complex in CSS and NCBRS, cohesin complex in Cornelia de Lange syndrome (MIM# 122470, 300590, 610759, 614701, 300882), and Polycomb repressive complex 2 in Weaver (MIM# 601573) and Cohen-Gibson (MIM# 617561) syndromes are all examples whereby variants in multiple genes map to the common episignature [28].

The recurring theme of phenotypic variability within enzyme complex conditions or within a single gene is further differentiated by conditions with recessive inheritance. Currently, most genes linked to epigenetic machinery are inherited in a dominant fashion [46], and therefore, a single variant can cause changes to the expected methylation profile resulting in the episignature. What is the effect on DNA methylation in the context of recessive inheritance whereby 2 affected alleles underlie the phenotype? One example for this scenario has been reported in Claes-Jensen syndrome (MIM# 300534) caused by variants on the X chromosome gene *KDM5C*, which escapes X-inactivation [63]. Healthy female carriers were shown to exhibit an intermediate pattern between the patient (affected males) and control cohorts [26]. The ability to simultaneously detect carrier and affected populations adds to the power of using episignatures as a diagnostic tool with the potential for use in a prenatal setting as well.

CHALLENGES IN DNA METHYLATION EPISIGNATURE ANALYSIS

Episignature detection works on the model that an inherited pathogenic variant in a gene or within a domain of a gene is associated with a unique methylation profile. The assumption with this model is that the inherited changes are originating early in development, and an episignature observed in peripheral blood is also present in other tissues. The evidence to support this theory is limited, but it has been demonstrated in Sotos syndrome whereby fibroblast samples of affected patients resembled the Sotos episignature derived from blood [53]. Blood is a readily available surrogate tissue that can be used as a biomarker for direct testing when the critical tissues, such as the brain in neurodevelopmental disorders, are unavailable. However, the use of blood for direct testing is challenged by mosaicism when the affected tissues may not include blood as observed in Beckwith-Wiedemann syndrome [64], or if the level of mosaicism produces an episignature that is below the threshold differences of the positive population. This outcome is predicted based on milder profiles observed by carriers of recessive conditions [26] or of carriers with an intermediate pattern when compared with affected individuals [47]. The exact limit of detection of mosaicism for episignature analysis will likely be specific to each signature and is something that has not been systematically investigated to date.

Thus far, episignature discovery work has been focused on genes involved in regulation of the epigenetic machinery. The utility of these episignatures is dependent not only on the robustness of methylation changes but also on the diversity of variants and the number of positive cases in the cohort. Many of the neurodevelopmental disorders are rare, and collection of the appropriate number of cases, or of cases with a diverse variant profile, is not always feasible, which may explain why candidate genes like *MECP2* or *RAI1* have so far evaded episignature detection [28]. The type of variant and the location of it within the gene has shown to impact the episignature profile [28,47,60], and therefore, episignatures based on variants of the same type or within the same protein domain offer challenges in interpreting alternate variant types or regions of the gene. As larger data sets are accumulated, the current episignatures will be further refined, new episignatures will be discovered in both currently described as well as undescribed conditions, and interpretation capabilities will continue to evolve.

Although DNA methylation signatures, or EpiSigns, have clearly evolved beyond scientific concepts to use in diagnosis of patients with a growing number of neurodevelopmental conditions, much more work remains before this technology can reach its full potential. There are more than 25,000 genes and more than 4000 genetic disorders that are, without exception, rare. Collecting cohorts of patients with each of these conditions will take effort and international collaboration for years to come. As technology continues to evolve, it can be expected that targeted approaches, such as methylation microarrays, will be displaced by more comprehensive genomic approaches, such as bisulfite genome sequencing. In that context, reference databases will need to evolve to account for the growing data complexity, which may provide an opportunity to reassess conditions with no existing episignatures based on methylation microarray analysis. Mapping DNA methylation profiles in other tissue types (buccal swabs, fibroblasts, and so forth) will provide further understanding of biology and underpinning mechanisms, but also provide additional opportunities for clinical utilization of this technology. Finally, larger-scale clinical trials of this technology, such as a recently announced Canadian national trial EpiSign-CAN (https://www.genomecanada.ca/en/beyond-genomics-assessing-improvement-diagnosis-rare-diseases-using-clinical-epigenomics-canada), will help develop clinical evidence for more systematic utilization of this testing modality in patients with rare disorders, and form the basis for development of guidelines for technical and clinical adaption of genomic DNA methylation testing in clinical care.

DISCLOSURE

This work was funded in part by the Genome Canada Genomic Application Partnership Program (GAPP) grant awarded to BS, and the London Heath Sciences Molecular Diagnostics Development Fund.

REFERENCES

[1] Berger SL, Kouzarides T, Shiekhattar R, et al. An operational definition of epigenetics. Genes Dev 2009;23(7): 781–3.

[2] Schenkel LC, Rodenhiser DI, Ainsworth PJ, et al. DNA methylation analysis in constitutional disorders: clinical implications of the epigenome. Crit Rev Clin Lab Sci 2016;53(3):147–65.

[3] Kim JH, Lee JH, Lee IS, et al. Histone lysine methylation and neurodevelopmental disorders. Int J Mol Sci 2017; 18(7):1404.

[4] Schenkel LC, Rodenhiser D, Siu V, et al. Constitutional epi/genetic conditions: genetic, epigenetic, and environmental factors. J Pediatr Genet 2017;6(1):30–41.

[5] Tost J. DNA methylation: an introduction to the biology and the disease-associated changes of a promising biomarker. Mol Biotechnol 2010;44(1):71–81.

[6] Hernando-Herraez I, Garcia-Perez R, Sharp AJ, et al. DNA methylation: insights into human evolution. PLoS Genet 2015;11(12):e1005661.

[7] Jung G, Hernandez-Illan E, Moreira L, et al. Epigenetics of colorectal cancer: biomarker and therapeutic potential. Nat Rev Gastroenterol Hepatol 2020;17(2):111–30.

[8] Linner A, Almgren M. Epigenetic programming-the important first 1000 days. Acta Paediatr 2020;109(3): 443–52.

[9] Bjornsson HT. The Mendelian disorders of the epigenetic machinery. Genome Res 2015;25(10):1473–81.

[10] Mullegama SV, Elsea SH. Clinical and molecular aspects of MBD5-associated neurodevelopmental disorder (MAND). Eur J Hum Genet 2016;24(9):1235–43.

[11] Tuscher JJ, Day JJ. Multigenerational epigenetic inheritance: one step forward, two generations back. Neurobiol Dis 2019;132:104591.

[12] Aref-Eshghi E, Rodenhiser DI, Schenkel LC, et al. Genomic DNA methylation signatures enable concurrent diagnosis and clinical genetic variant classification in neurodevelopmental syndromes. Am J Hum Genet 2018;102(1):156–74.

[13] Li E, Bestor TH, Jaenisch R. Targeted mutation of the DNA methyltransferase gene results in embryonic lethality. Cell 1992;69(6):915–26.

[14] Kernohan KD, Cigana Schenkel L, Huang L, et al. Identification of a methylation profile for DNMT1-associated autosomal dominant cerebellar ataxia, deafness, and narcolepsy. Clin Epigenetics 2016;8:91.

[15] Lindy AS, Stosser MB, Butler E, et al. Diagnostic outcomes for genetic testing of 70 genes in 8565 patients with epilepsy and neurodevelopmental disorders. Epilepsia 2018;59(5):1062–71.

[16] Grozeva D, Carss K, Spasic-Boskovic O, et al. Targeted next-generation sequencing analysis of 1,000 individuals with intellectual disability. Hum Mutat 2015;36(12): 1197–204.

[17] Reuter MS, Tawamie H, Buchert R, et al. Diagnostic yield and novel candidate genes by exome sequencing in 152 consanguineous families with neurodevelopmental disorders. JAMA Psychiatry 2017;74(3):293–9.

[18] Evers C, Staufner C, Granzow M, et al. Impact of clinical exomes in neurodevelopmental and neurometabolic disorders. Mol Genet Metab 2017;121(4):297–307.

[19] Redin C, Gerard B, Lauer J, et al. Efficient strategy for the molecular diagnosis of intellectual disability using targeted high-throughput sequencing. J Med Genet 2014; 51(11):724–36.

[20] Miller DT, Adam MP, Aradhya S, et al. Consensus statement: chromosomal microarray is a first-tier clinical diagnostic test for individuals with developmental disabilities or congenital anomalies. Am J Hum Genet 2010;86(5):749–64.

[21] Tammimies K, Marshall CR, Walker S, et al. Molecular diagnostic yield of chromosomal microarray analysis and whole-exome sequencing in children with autism spectrum disorder. JAMA 2015;314(9):895–903.

[22] Moeschler JB, Shevell M, American Academy of Pediatrics Committee on Genetics. Clinical genetic evaluation of the child with mental retardation or developmental delays. Pediatrics 2006;117(6):2304–16.

[23] Sadikovic B, Aref-Eshghi E, Levy MA, et al. DNA methylation signatures in mendelian developmental disorders as a diagnostic bridge between genotype and phenotype. Epigenomics 2019;11(5):563–75.

[24] Nardone S, Sams DS, Reuveni E, et al. DNA methylation analysis of the autistic brain reveals multiple dysregulated biological pathways. Transl Psychiatry 2014;4:e433.

[25] Aref-Eshghi E, Bend EG, Hood RL, et al. BAFopathies' DNA methylation epi-signatures demonstrate diagnostic utility and functional continuum of Coffin-Siris and Nicolaides-Baraitser syndromes. Nat Commun 2018; 9(1):4885.

[26] Schenkel LC, Aref-Eshghi E, Skinner C, et al. Peripheral blood epi-signature of Claes-Jensen syndrome enables sensitive and specific identification of patients and healthy carriers with pathogenic mutations in KDM5C. Clin Epigenetics 2018;10:21.

[27] Kerkel K, Schupf N, Hatta K, et al. Altered DNA methylation in leukocytes with trisomy 21. PLoS Genet 2010; 6(11):e1001212.

[28] Aref-Eshghi E, Kerkhof J, Pedro VP, et al. Evaluation of DNA methylation episignatures for diagnosis and phenotype correlations in 42 Mendelian neurodevelopmental disorders. Am J Hum Genet 2020;106(3):356–70.

[29] Aref-Eshghi E, Bend EG, Colaiacovo S, et al. Diagnostic utility of genome-wide DNA methylation testing in genetically unsolved individuals with suspected hereditary conditions. Am J Hum Genet 2019;104(4):685–700.

[30] Schenkel LC, Schwartz C, Skinner C, et al. Clinical validation of fragile X syndrome screening by DNA methylation array. J Mol Diagn 2016;18(6):834–41.

[31] Prickett AR, Ishida M, Bohm S, et al. Genome-wide methylation analysis in Silver-Russell syndrome patients. Hum Genet 2015;134(3):317–32.

[32] Wu D, Gong C, Su C. Genome-wide analysis of differential DNA methylation in Silver-Russell syndrome. Sci China Life Sci 2017;60(7):692–9.

[33] Aref-Eshghi E, Schenkel LC, Lin H, et al. Clinical validation of a genome-wide DNA methylation assay for molecular diagnosis of imprinting disorders. J Mol Diagn 2017;19(6):848–56.

[34] Srivastava S, Love-Nichols JA, Dies KA, et al. Meta-analysis and multidisciplinary consensus statement: exome sequencing is a first-tier clinical diagnostic test for individuals with neurodevelopmental disorders. Genet Med 2019;21(11):2413–21.

[35] Manning M, Hudgins L, Professional Practice and Guidelines Committee. Array-based technology and recommendations for utilization in medical genetics practice for detection of chromosomal abnormalities. Genet Med 2010;12(11):742–5.

[36] Schaefer GB, Mendelsohn NJ, Professional Practice and Guidelines Committee. Clinical genetics evaluation in identifying the etiology of autism spectrum disorders: 2013 guideline revisions. Genet Med 2013;15(5): 399–407.

[37] Lee H, Deignan JL, Dorrani N, et al. Clinical exome sequencing for genetic identification of rare Mendelian disorders. JAMA 2014;312(18):1880–7.

[38] Trujillano D, Bertoli-Avella AM, Kumar Kandaswamy K, et al. Clinical exome sequencing: results from 2819 samples reflecting 1000 families. Eur J Hum Genet 2017; 25(2):176–82.

[39] Richards S, Aziz N, Bale S, et al. Standards and guidelines for the interpretation of sequence variants: a joint consensus recommendation of the American College of Medical Genetics and Genomics and the Association for Molecular Pathology. Genet Med 2015;17(5): 405–24.

[40] Wang W, Corominas R, Lin GN. De novo Mutations from whole exome sequencing in neurodevelopmental and psychiatric disorders: from discovery to application. Front Genet 2019;10:258.

[41] Helsmoortel C, Vulto-van Silfhout AT, Coe BP, et al. A SWI/SNF-related autism syndrome caused by de novo mutations in ADNP. Nat Genet 2014;46(4): 380–4.

[42] Van Dijck A, Vulto-van Silfhout AT, Cappuyns E, et al. Clinical presentation of a complex neurodevelopmental disorder caused by mutations in ADNP. Biol Psychiatry 2019;85(4):287–97.

[43] Suwinski P, Ong C, Ling MHT, et al. Advancing personalized medicine through the application of whole exome sequencing and big data analytics. Front Genet 2019;10:49.

[44] Hsu P, Ma A, Wilson M, et al. CHARGE syndrome: a review. J Paediatr Child Health 2014;50(7):504–11.

[45] Butcher DT, Cytrynbaum C, Turinsky AL, et al. CHARGE and Kabuki syndromes: gene-specific DNA methylation signatures identify epigenetic mechanisms linking these clinically overlapping conditions. Am J Hum Genet 2017;100(5):773–88.

[46] Fahrner JA, Bjornsson HT. Mendelian disorders of the epigenetic machinery: tipping the balance of chromatin states. Annu Rev Genom Hum Genet 2014; 15:269–93.

[47] Chater-Diehl E, Ejaz R, Cytrynbaum C, et al. New insights into DNA methylation signatures: SMARCA2 variants in Nicolaides-Baraitser syndrome. BMC Med Genomics 2019;12(1):105.

[48] Krzyzewska IM, Maas SM, Henneman P, et al. A genome-wide DNA methylation signature for SETD1B-related syndrome. Clin Epigenetics 2019;11(1):156.

[49] Hood RL, Schenkel LC, Nikkel SM, et al. The defining DNA methylation signature of Floating-Harbor syndrome. Sci Rep 2016;6:38803.

[50] Schenkel LC, Kernohan KD, McBride A, et al. Identification of epigenetic signature associated with alpha thalassemia/mental retardation X-linked syndrome. Epigenetics Chromatin 2017;10:10.

[51] Aref-Eshghi E, Schenkel LC, Lin H, et al. The defining DNA methylation signature of Kabuki syndrome enables functional assessment of genetic variants of unknown clinical significance. Epigenetics 2017;12(11):923–33.

[52] Ciolfi A, Aref-Eshghi E, Pizzi S, et al. Frameshift mutations at the C-terminus of HIST1H1E result in a specific DNA hypomethylation signature. Clin Epigenetics 2020;12(1):7.

[53] Choufani S, Cytrynbaum C, Chung BH, et al. NSD1 mutations generate a genome-wide DNA methylation signature. Nat Commun 2015;6:10207.

[54] Siu MT, Butcher DT, Turinsky AL, et al. Functional DNA methylation signatures for autism spectrum disorder genomic risk loci: 16p11.2 deletions and CHD8 variants. Clin Epigenetics 2019;11(1):103.

[55] Strong E, Butcher DT, Singhania R, et al. Symmetrical dose-dependent DNA-methylation profiles in children with deletion or duplication of 7q11.23. Am J Hum Genet 2015;97(2):216–27.

[56] Guastafierro T, Bacalini MG, Marcoccia A, et al. Genome-wide DNA methylation analysis in blood cells from patients with Werner syndrome. Clin Epigenetics 2017;9:92.

[57] Bacalini MG, Gentilini D, Boattini A, et al. Identification of a DNA methylation signature in blood cells from persons with Down syndrome. Aging 2015;7(2):82–96.

[58] Henderson LB, Applegate CD, Wohler E, et al. The impact of chromosomal microarray on clinical management: a retrospective analysis. Genet Med 2014;16(9):657–64.

[59] Deciphering Developmental Disorders S. Prevalence and architecture of de novo mutations in developmental disorders. Nature 2017;542(7642):433–8.

[60] Bend EG, Aref-Eshghi E, Everman DB, et al. Gene domain-specific DNA methylation episignatures highlight distinct molecular entities of ADNP syndrome. Clin Epigenetics 2019;11(1):64.

[61] Cappuccio G, Sayou C, Tanno PL, et al. De novo SMARCA2 variants clustered outside the helicase domain cause a new recognizable syndrome with intellectual disability and blepharophimosis distinct from Nicolaides-Baraitser syndrome. Genet Med 2020. https://doi.org/10.1038/s41436-020-0898-y.

[62] Van Houdt JK, Nowakowska BA, Sousa SB, et al. Heterozygous missense mutations in SMARCA2 cause Nicolaides-Baraitser syndrome. Nat Genet 2012;44(4):445–9, S441.

[63] Berletch JB, Yang F, Xu J, et al. Genes that escape from X inactivation. Hum Genet 2011;130(2):237–45.

[64] Alders M, Maas SM, Kadouch DJ, et al. Methylation analysis in tongue tissue of BWS patients identifies the (EPI) genetic cause in 3 patients with normal methylation levels in blood. Eur J Med Genet 2014;57(6):293–7.

Hematopathology

Molecular Pathways and Potential for Targeted Therapies in the Treatment of Early T-cell Precursor Acute Lymphoblastic Leukemia

Liam Donnelly, MD[a,b], Juli-Anne Gardner, MD[a,b], Joanna L. Conant, MD[a,b], Katherine A. Devitt, MD[a,b],*

[a]Department of Pathology and Laboratory Medicine, University of Vermont Medical Center, 111 Colchester Avenue, Burlington, VT 05401, USA; [b]Larner College of Medicine at the University of Vermont, Burlington, VT, USA

KEYWORDS

- Early T-cell precursor acute lymphoblastic leukemia • Leukemia • Targeted therapy • Molecular alterations
- Treatment

KEY POINTS

- Early T-cell precursor (ETP) acute lymphoblastic leukemia (ALL) is a higher-risk subtype of T-cell ALL, with pediatric patients requiring intensive therapy regimens with significant toxicity and adult patients having poor treatment responses.
- Several recurrently observed molecular alterations in cell signaling pathways in ETP-ALL have available drug targets that could augment induction/consolidation chemotherapy.
- More preclinical and clinical trials are needed to evaluate the efficacy of targeted therapies in the treatment of ETP-ALL; however, the success of targeted therapies in other hematologic malignancies provides promise for ETP-ALL.

INTRODUCTION

Acute lymphoblastic leukemia (ALL) is a neoplasm of immature lymphoid precursors and includes the categories B-lymphoblastic leukemia/lymphoma and T-lymphoblastic leukemia/lymphoma. T-cell ALL (T-ALL) comprises about 15% of pediatric acute lymphoblastic leukemias and 25% of adult cases [1]. In T-ALL, immature T lymphoblasts infiltrate the blood and bone marrow, with diagnostic cutoffs commonly in the range of 20% to 25% of nucleated cells [2]. Unlike acute myeloid leukemia (AML), there is no defined lower limit for the percentage of blasts required to diagnose ALL. Patients often present with fatigue, mucosal bleeding, and/or recurrent infections caused by disrupted hematopoiesis; however, T-ALL often shows a relative sparing of normal hematopoiesis compared with B-cell ALL (B-ALL). Patients may also have chest pain and respiratory symptoms secondary to an anterior mediastinal mass, which is seen in about 60% of presentations, or neurologic symptoms secondary to central nervous system infiltration by lymphoblasts (10%) [3].

Early T-cell precursor (ETP) ALL is a distinct subtype of T-ALL that gained provisional status from the World Health Organization (WHO) in 2016 [4]. It is defined by its early T-cell immunophenotype (cCD3+, CD1a−, CD5dim, CD8−, CD4−) as well as expression of stem cell and/or myeloid markers (HLA-DR, CD13, CD33, CD34). ETP-ALL has a gene expression profile similar to stem cell/myeloid progenitor cells [1].

---

*Corresponding author. Department of Pathology and Laboratory Medicine, University of Vermont Medical Center, 111 Colchester Avenue, Burlington, VT 05401. *E-mail address:* Katherine.Devitt@uvmhealth.org

https://doi.org/10.1016/j.yamp.2020.07.003
2589-4080/20/

Historically, ETP-ALL has been regarded as a subtype of T-ALL with worse prognosis and higher relapse rates [5].

ETP-ALL has several well-characterized recurrent genetic alterations, including *FLT3*, *IL7R*, *JAK1*, *JAK3*, *STAT5B*, and *RAS*; some of these alterations have existing targeted therapies available. Because of the increased toxicity of high-risk pediatric induction/consolidation regimens and the poor response of adult ETP-ALL, augmentation of traditional chemotherapy regimens with targeted therapies may help reduce chemotherapy-related toxicity and improve outcomes in ETP-ALL.

This article focuses on the molecular pathways altered in ETP-ALL and highlights those that may be more amenable to targeted therapies that already exist for treatment in other diseases.

SIGNIFICANCE
Background

Common lymphocyte progenitor cells destined to become T cells migrate to the thymus where they undergo positive and negative selection and, if they survive, develop into mature T cells. T cells show a characteristic immunophenotype at each stage of their development, and there are several different classification schemes based on marker expression and/or cell location within the thymus. Disruptions of maturation may occur at any stage and can result in T-lymphoblast maturation arrest and uncontrolled proliferation, or T-ALL. Historically, 4 categories of T-ALL were recognized, based on the stages of differentiation: Pro-T, pre-T, cortical T, and medullary T [4]. Another schema based on gene expression profiling studies has been proposed: early immature, which are negative for CD4 and CD8; early cortical, which are positive for CD4, CD8, and CD1a but negative for surface CD3 and typically associated with alterations involving *TLX1*, *TLX3*, *NKX2.1*, and *NKX1.1*; and late cortical, which are positive for CD4, CD8, CD1a, and CD3 and have alterations involving *TAL1* [6,7]. Regardless of classification, there is a subset of early T cells that are negative for both CD4 and CD8 (double negative [DN]). DN T cells can be further broken down into 4 categories: DN1 or ETP (CD44+, CD25−), DN2 (CD44+, CD25+), DN3 (CD44−, CD25+), and DN4 (CD44−, CD25−) [8].

Translocations involving T-cell receptor loci and transcription factors important to thymocyte development are 1 mechanism thought to initiate maturation arrest. These translocations place transcription factors such as *TAL1*, *TLX1*, *TLX3*, *LMO2*, and *NKX2.1* under the control of high-expression T-cell receptor enhancer elements, leading to the arrest of normal thymocyte development. Predictably, the stage of maturation arrest has been associated with specific transcription factors: early immature is associated with *LMO2/LYL1* translocations; early cortical with *TLX1*, *TLX3*, and *NKX2.1* translocations; and late cortical with *TAL1* translocations [6,7]. Once normal maturation is interrupted in this manner, it is hypothesized that additional genetic alterations are acquired, resulting in frank leukemic transformation. These additional genetic alterations have also been found to be associated with specific developmental stages (eg, *PHF6*, *NOTCH-1*, and *CDNK2A* in early cortical).

Despite the ability to classify T-ALL by developmental stage through immunophenotype, transcription factor translocation class, and other recurrent molecular and cytogenetic alterations, none of these categories has been accepted as prognostically relevant, with the exception of ETP-ALL. This lack of agreement is reflected in the current 2016 WHO classification of hematopoietic neoplasms, in which ETP-ALL is highlighted as a provisional subtype of T-ALL [4]. ETP-ALL is a neoplasm of very immature T cells that have limited T-cell markers and also show myeloid and/or stem cell properties. These cells are in the pro-T/pre-T, DN, or early immature categories depending on the classification system used.

T-cell Acute Lymphoblastic Leukemia Outcomes

With newer induction/consolidation therapies (Children's Oncology Group [COG] AALL0434 or United Kingdom ALL [UKALL] 2003), the overall survival (OS) and event-free survival (EFS) for pediatric and young adult patients with T-ALL are approaching 90% and are similar to those seen with B-ALL [5,9]. In adult patients with T-ALL, there is a larger range in OS and EFS depending on the chemotherapy regimen used. In standard regimens used for adults who cannot tolerate more intense pediatric-style regimens, the OS and EFS are lower than in pediatric patients (50%–60% for both) [10]. Newer pediatric-style regimens for adult patients with T-ALL have increased the EFS and OS rates (76% and 82%, respectively). However, these regimens also have increased treatment-related toxicity, especially in patients more than 45 years of age [11,12].

The OS of relapsed T-ALL is significantly lower for all ages, estimated at 25% [13]. Although many clinical, immunophenotypic, and genetic factors have been analyzed for prognostic value in order to risk stratify patients with T-ALL, minimal residual disease (MRD) remains the only widely accepted prognostic factor [1,7]. Compared with B-ALL, patients with T-ALL are more likely to have detectable MRD at the end of induction. Patients with T-ALL with detectable MRD at the end of induction and end of consolidation have both been shown to have lower EFS and OS [1,9]. Patients with MRD that fails to decrease at end of consolidation have been shown to have lower OS, suggesting that end of consolidation MRD may be a better prognostic marker than end of induction MRD in T-ALL [1].

Early T-cell Precursor Acute Lymphoblastic Leukemia

Historically, ETP-ALL was regarded as a subtype of T-ALL with a worse prognosis and higher relapse rates [5]. However, newer treatment protocols in pediatric patients that risk stratify patients into different therapy regimens (Fig. 1) have improved the EFS and OS rates of ETP-ALL (UKALL 2003 and COG AALL0434) to rates that are similar to conventional T-ALL. Despite these comparable OS rates, more patients with ETP-ALL are stratified into high-risk treatment protocols because of factors such as poor morphologic induction response and detectable end of induction MRD (UKALL 2003 and COG AALL0434) (see Fig. 1) [5], which translates into pediatric patients with ETP-ALL undergoing more toxic induction/consolidation regimens with higher rates of adverse events. In adults with ETP-ALL, the clinical outcome data are less well established because of fewer trials with smaller enrollment numbers. However, some trials have found adult ETP-ALL to represent a higher-risk subtype with worse OS [14].

Compared with typical T-ALL, ETP-ALL more often has a lower white blood cell count at presentation and less frequent CDKN2A and NOTCH-1 alterations [5]. Furthermore, patients with ETP-ALL have recurrent genetic alterations similar to those seen in AML, including FLT3 and IL7R activating alterations, and loss-of-function (LoF) mutations involving genes in the PRC2 complex [15]. This finding may be caused by ETP-ALL thymocytes arresting at the early immature stage of development, before the cell is committed to 1 lineage while both myeloid and lymphoid gene expression are still present [16].

Molecular Pathways in Early T-cell Precursor Acute Lymphoblastic Leukemia: Polycomb Repressive Complex 2

Mutations in the PRC2 (polycomb repressive complex 2) core proteins EZH2, SUZ12, and EED are recurrently identified in an estimated 42% of patients with ETP-ALL, and all of these may be amenable to existing targeted therapy [15]. PRC2 is a complex of proteins that regulate chromatin structure and, therefore, gene expression. PRC2 components EZH1/2, SUZ12, EED, and RbAp46/48 function by placing methyl groups on histone 3 at lysine 27 residues (H3K27me3), which are thought to repress gene expression [17]. Interestingly, in a mouse model with EZH2 and p53 LoF alterations that form an ETP-ALL–like phenotype, loss of EZH2 leads to hypermethylation of the promotor regions of genes critical for T-cell development [16]. Loss of H3K27me3 through EZH2 LoF mutations promotes hypermethylation of gene promotors, including BCL11B and RUNX1. BCL11B and RUNX1 are 2 critical transcription factors that induce the D2 to D3 thymocyte transition, and loss of these transcription factors has been shown to lead to ETP-ALL–like thymocytes [18,19]. Thus, EZH2 alterations seem to cause hypermethylation of the promotors of transcription factors critical for T-cell differentiation, leading to a halt in maturation (Fig. 2). Additional acquired mutations, such as FLT3, are then thought to induce leukemic transformation [19].

In an EZH2, FLT3, and RUNX1 LoF mouse model, EZH2 and FLT3 mutations synergize to produce a leukemic ETP-ALL–like malignancy with a highly activated mitogen-activated protein kinase (MAPK)–extracellular signal-regulated kinase (ERK) pathway expression pattern, which was higher than that of FLT3 LoF or wild-type controls [19]. Further, it was observed that EZH2, FLT3, and RUNX1 LoF thymocytes lost H3K27me3 histone marks and gained H3K27ac (acylation) in many gene loci, including the FLT3 receptor, possibly showing that loss of EZH2 also leads to increased histone acylation and gene upregulation, especially in the MAPK-ERK pathway. Bromodomain and extraterminal (BET) proteins recognize histone acylation marks and help modulate gene expression. Use of the BET inhibitor JQ1 in this EZH2, FLT3, RUNX1 thymocyte model as well as human-derived ETP-ALL clones with PRC2 alterations led to growth inhibition and downregulation of many MAP-ERK–related genes, showing that BET inhibitors could benefit patients with ETP-ALL (Fig. 3) [19]. BET inhibitors for ETP-ALL could be particularly effective because mutations in epigenetic regulators and transcription factors are frequently observed in ETP-ALL [7]. This therapy could help modulate the aberrant gene expression signatures that underlie ETP-ALL malignancies.

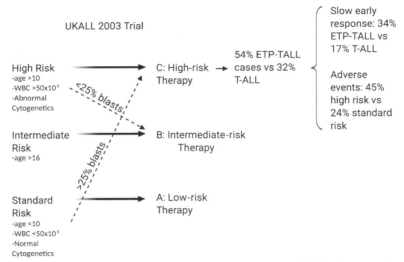

FIG. 1 UKALL 2003 trial risk-based treatment stratification methodology. Initial clinical criteria were used to assign patients to 3 treatment regimens (A, B, and C) with increasing treatment regimen intensity, C being the most intensive. Standard risk: age less than 10 years, noncomplex cytogenetics, white blood cell (WBC) count less than 50×10^9/L. Intermediate risk: age greater than 16 years, high risk/complex cytogenetics, WBC count greater than 50×10^9/L. Further, induction bone marrow response (day 8 or 15) was used to stratify patients: those with blast counts greater than or equal to 25% were moved to high-risk treatment C. High-risk patients with induction response (<25% blasts) were moved to treatment B. Most (54%) of the patients with ETP-ALL in this trial were stratified to high-risk treatment C because of poor induction response and National Cancer Institute risk [5,28]. Further, 34% of patients with ETP-ALL have slow early responses to induction chemotherapy. Significant adverse events were seen in 45% of high-risk group patients (includes ETP-ALL and T-ALL cases).

Molecular Pathways in Early T-cell Precursor Acute Lymphoblastic Leukemia: Janus Kinase–Signal Transducers and Activators of Transcription

Another pathway that is recurrently altered in ETP-ALL is the Janus kinase (JAK)–signal transducers and activators of transcription (STAT) pathway, which also has several drug targets readily available (see Fig. 3). Specifically, activating mutations are recurrently seen in *IL7R*, *JAK1* or *JAK3*, or *STAT5B* [15]. This signaling locus is activated by the cytokine interleukin 7 (IL7) binding to receptor IL7R, causing associated JAK1 and JAK3 kinases to transphosphorylate, allowing the SH2 domain of STAT5 to bind and become an active dimmer, thus acting as a transcription factor. Gene targets in traditional T-ALL include *PIM1*, *OSM*, *IKZF4*, and *BCL2*, which promote cell survival and cell cycle progression [20]. In T-ALL mouse models with induced *IL7R*, *JAK1* or *JAK3*, or *STAT5B* mutations, all were inhibited by selective JAK1/3 inhibitors [20]. Interestingly, in ETP-ALL lines derived from patient samples, ETP-ALL clones show a highly active JAK-STAT pathway relative to normal T-ALL clones. Further, these ETP-ALL clones were all inhibited by ruxolitinib, a JAK inhibitor selective for JAK1 and JAK2, independent of JAK-STAT pathway activating mutations. This finding suggests that epigenetic or other transcription factors or enhancers may be promoting the JAK-STAT pathway in ETP-ALL, and ETP-ALL may be particularly sensitive to JAK inhibitors (see Fig. 3). In addition, the JAK-STAT pathway downstream effectors upregulated by *STAT5* (such as the antiapoptotic factor BCL2) are also potential drug targets, and in mouse models of JAK-STAT activated T-ALL, show synergy with JAK inhibitors [20].

Molecular Pathways in Early T-cell Precursor Acute Lymphoblastic Leukemia: FLT3

As mentioned earlier, *FLT3* mutations are observed frequently in ETP-ALL, with internal tandem duplication (ITD) alterations found more commonly than tyrosine kinase domain (TKD) mutations [21]. FLT3 is a receptor tyrosine kinase that can activate the JAK-

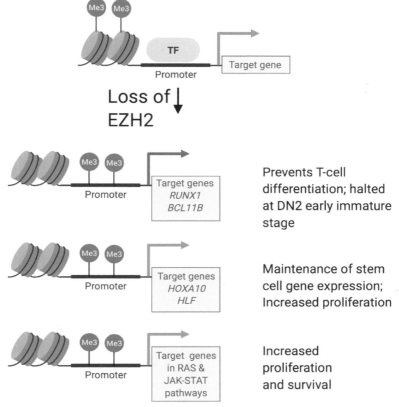

FIG. 2 PRC2 component LoF leads to developmentally vital gene promoter hypermethylation and maturation arrest. PRC2 components *EZH1/2*, *SUZ12*, *EED*, and *RbAp46/48* normally methylate histone 3 lysine residues. Loss of histone methylation is thought to lead to hypermethylation of promotors of genes vital for lymphoblast maturation, including *BCL11B* and *RUNX1*. Additional acquired alterations then promote leukemic transformation. Increased expression of stem cell genes (*HOXA10*, *HLF*) and upregulation in RAS and JAK-STAT pathway components are observed in *EZH2* LoF mouse models; however, the mechanism of upregulation is not known. TF, transcription factor.

STAT, MAPK-ERK, and phosphatidylinositol 3 kinase (PI3K)-protein kinase B (AKT) pathways [22]. In AML, *FLT3*-ITD mutations have been shown to have high basal levels of STAT5 activation [22]. Because AML and ETP-ALL share several recurrent alterations, ETP-ALL with *FLT3*-ITD alterations may also share this STAT5 signaling pathway predilection. Further, in T-ALL, JAK inhibitors may be able to block both active JAK and STAT signaling [20], making *FLT3*-ITD altered ETP-ALL clones sensitive to JAK inhibitors. In addition, there are FLT3 inhibitors available for treatment in patients with AML [23], which may also be effective in ETP-ALL with FLT3 alterations (see Fig. 3) [21].

Molecular Pathways in Early T-cell Precursor Acute Lymphoblastic Leukemia: RAS

Another pathway altered frequently in ETP-ALL is the RAS signaling pathway with activating alterations seen in *NRAS*, *KRAS*, and *PTPN11*. The MAPK-RAS-ERK pathway has several drug targets, including mitogen-activated protein kinase kinase (MEK) inhibitors, which are in phase I/II trials for AML [24]. MEK and other RAS pathway inhibitors, especially in combination with another pathway inhibitor (JAK-STAT or PI3K-AKT) may improve ETP-ALL responses to induction chemotherapy in cases with RAS pathway alterations (see Fig. 3).

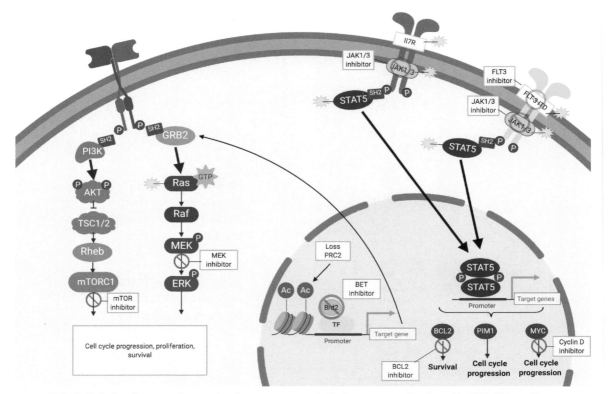

FIG. 3 Cell signaling receptors and pathway components that are recurrently altered in ETP-ALL and have available targeted therapies. Recurrently altered proteins are indicated by the yellow bursts. Pathway-specific targeted therapies are indicated by a red stop circle icon with the drug indicated in a text box. Recurrently altered signaling pathways include the JAK-STAT5 pathway, which can be targeted with JAK1/3 inhibitors and inhibitors of downstream pathway effectors BCL2 and cyclin D. *FLT3* internal tandem duplication (ITD) alterations can be targeted with FLT3 inhibitors. Further, it seems *FLT3*-ITD alterations may preferentially signal through JAK-STAT5, making *FLT3*-ITD altered ETP-ALL susceptible to JAK1/3 inhibition. Loss of PRC2 components leads to widespread histone acylation, and oncogene upregulation (including MAPK-RAS-ERK pathway components), facilitated by BET family transcriptional effectors (BRD2), which recognize histone acylation and promote gene expression. BET inhibitors could block aberrant gene expression in ETP-ALL. Recurrent *RAS* alterations can be targeted with downstream MEK inhibitors. Multiple pathway targets may be required in ETP-ALL because MAPK-ERK, JAK-STAT, and phosphatidylinositol 3 kinase (PI3K)–mammalian target of rapamycin (mTOR) pathways all can coactivate each other through SH2 domain recognition of receptor tyrosine kinase phosphorylation.

Role of Multiagent Targeted Therapy

Single-agent targeted therapy approaches, such as inhibiting solely JAK1/JAK3 with ruxolitinib, may be insufficient in ETP-ALL. Not only can the JAK-STAT pathway activate other pathways, such as MAPK-ERK and PI3K-AKT, but ETP-ALL clones may have codominant activating alterations in multiple pathways, necessitating the use of combined inhibitors (such as JAK and MEK inhibitors) [6,25]. In 1 analysis of a T-ALL cohort, approximately 20% of patients had multiple signaling pathway mutations (such as JAK-STAT and MAPK-RAS-ERK pathway alterations) that likely were within the same immature lymphocyte clone [6]. Further, in AML and many other malignancies, use of single-agent pathway inhibitors generally drives resistance mechanisms, preventing sustained response. In AML, for instance, 1 mechanism of FLT3 inhibitor resistance discovered in patient-derived in vitro models was *RAS* gain-of-function alterations [26]. Therefore, targeting multiple signaling pathways at the start of targeted therapy may help prevent selection of clones with multiple signaling pathway alterations or the development of resistance clones. The validity of this approach has a precedent in solid tumors, such as metastatic colorectal cancer with class 1 *BRAF* alterations, where standard of care is now treatment with combination MEK, BRAF, and epidermal growth factor receptor (EGFR) targeted inhibitors [27].

PRESENT RELEVANCE AND FUTURE AVENUES TO CONSIDER OR TO INVESTIGATE

Given the success of targeted therapies in conjunction with induction/consolidation chemotherapy in other hematologic malignancies such as AML, more preclinical studies treating ETP-ALL xenograft models with targeted combination therapies are needed to assess the validity of this approach in ETP-ALL. Subsequent human clinical trials using targeted therapies in ETP-ALL are vital. Several current active clinical trials are available, including NCT03553238, which is investigating a histone deacetylase inhibitor chidamide in adult ETP-ALL; NCT04000698, where targeted therapy will be trialed in children with chemotherapy-resistant ALL; and NCT03613428, where chemotherapy in conjunction to ruxolitinib will be tested in patients with relapsed/refractory ETP-ALL.

SUMMARY

ETP-ALL is an uncommon subtype of T-ALL that affects both children and adults, and historically has been thought to have a worse prognosis in both groups. Newer data suggest that, with appropriate therapy, prognosis may not be as poor as originally thought, but this appropriate therapy often involves more intensive and toxic regimens. Because of the significant treatment-related toxicity of high-risk induction/consolidation chemotherapy regimens that patients with ETP-ALL frequently require, alternative treatment strategies for ETP-ALL are desirable and necessary. The augmentation of induction/consolidation therapy with therapies targeting tumor-specific molecular alterations holds promise because of the expanding array of drugs with molecular targets. As described in this article, ETP-ALL frequently shows disruption of pathways involving JAK-STAT and MAPK-RAS-ERK, in addition to cell cycle regulators (BCL2, cyclin D), cell receptor FLT3, and PRC2 components. These conditions may be particularly sensitive to therapies that target these recurrent alterations. The success of this approach has already been proved in solid tumors and in other hematologic malignancies, and it is hope that it will allow less toxic chemotherapy regimens while improving the response rates of pediatric and adult patients with ETP-ALL.

DISCLOSURE

The authors have nothing to disclose.

REFERENCES

[1] Hefazi M, Litzow MR. Recent advances in the biology and treatment of T cell acute lymphoblastic leukemia. Curr Hematol Malig Rep 2018;13(4):265–74.

[2] Litzow MR, Ferrando AA. How I treat T-cell acute lymphoblastic leukemia in adults. Blood 2015;126(7): 833–41.

[3] Karrman K, Johansson B. Pediatric T-cell acute lymphoblastic leukemia. Genes Chromosomes Cancer 2017; 56(2):89–116.

[4] Steven H, Swerdlow EC, Lee Harris N, et al. WHO classification of tumors of haematopoietic and lymphoid tissues. 4th edition. Lyon (France): International Agency for Research on Cancer (IARC); 2017.

[5] Patrick K, Wade R, Goulden N, et al. Outcome for children and young people with Early T-cell precursor acute lymphoblastic leukaemia treated on a contemporary protocol, UKALL 2003. Br J Haematol 2014;166(3):421–4.

[6] Liu Y, Easton J, Shao Y, et al. The genomic landscape of pediatric and young adult T-lineage acute lymphoblastic leukemia. Nat Genet 2017;49(8):1211–8.

[7] Van Vlierberghe P, Ferrando A. The molecular basis of T cell acute lymphoblastic leukemia. J Clin Invest 2012; 122(10):3398–406.

[8] Shah DK, Zuniga-Pflucker JC. An overview of the intrathymic intricacies of T cell development. J Immunol 2014;192(9):4017–23.

[9] Wood BL, Winter SS, Dunsmore KP, et al. T-Lymphoblastic leukemia (T-ALL) shows excellent outcome, lack of significance of the early thymic precursor (ETP) immunophenotype, and validation of the prognostic value of end-induction minimal residual disease (MRD) in Children's Oncology Group (COG) Study AALL0434. Blood 2014;124(21):1.

[10] Marks DI, Paietta EM, Moorman AV, et al. T-cell acute lymphoblastic leukemia in adults: clinical features, immunophenotype, cytogenetics, and outcome from the large randomized prospective trial (UKALL XII/ECOG 2993). Blood 2009;114(25):5136–45.

[11] Trinquand A, Tanguy-Schmidt A, Ben Abdelali R, et al. Toward a NOTCH1/FBXW7/RAS/PTEN-based oncogenetic risk classification of adult T-cell acute lymphoblastic leukemia: a Group for Research in Adult Acute

Lymphoblastic Leukemia study. J Clin Oncol 2013; 31(34):4333–42.

[12] Huguet F, Leguay T, Raffoux E, et al. Pediatric-inspired therapy in adults with Philadelphia chromosome-negative acute lymphoblastic leukemia: the GRAALL-2003 study. J Clin Oncol 2009;27(6):911–8.

[13] Raetz EA, Teachey DT. T-cell acute lymphoblastic leukemia. Hematology Am Soc Hematol Educ Program 2016;2016(1):580–8.

[14] Jain N, Lamb AV, O'Brien S, et al. Early T-cell precursor acute lymphoblastic leukemia/lymphoma (ETP-ALL/LBL) in adolescents and adults: a high-risk subtype. Blood 2016;127(15):1863–9.

[15] Tavakoli Shirazi P, Eadie LN, Heatley SL, et al. The effect of co-occurring lesions on leukaemogenesis and drug response in T-ALL and ETP-ALL. Br J Cancer 2019; 122(4):455–64.

[16] Wang C, Oshima M, Sato D, et al. Ezh2 loss propagates hypermethylation at T cell differentiation-regulating genes to promote leukemic transformation. J Clin Invest 2018;128(9):3872–86.

[17] Margueron R, Reinberg D. The Polycomb complex PRC2 and its mark in life. Nature 2011;469(7330):343–9.

[18] Li L, Leid M, Rothenberg EV. An early T cell lineage commitment checkpoint dependent on the transcription factor Bcl11b. Science 2010;329(5987):89–93.

[19] Booth CAG, Barkas N, Neo WH, et al. Ezh2 and Runx1 mutations collaborate to initiate lympho-myeloid leukemia in early thymic progenitors. Cancer Cell 2018;33(2): 274–91.e8.

[20] Govaerts I, Jacobs K, Vandepoel R, et al. JAK/STAT pathway mutations in T-ALL, including the STAT5B N642H Mutation, are Sensitive to JAK1/JAK3 Inhibitors. Hemasphere 2019;3(6):e313.

[21] Neumann M, Coskun E, Fransecky L, et al. FLT3 mutations in early T-cell precursor ALL characterize a stem cell like leukemia and imply the clinical use of tyrosine kinase inhibitors. PLoS One 2013;8(1):e53190.

[22] Choudhary C, Muller-Tidow C, Berdel WE, et al. Signal transduction of oncogenic Flt3. Int J Hematol 2005; 82(2):93–9.

[23] Wu M, Li C, Zhu X. FLT3 inhibitors in acute myeloid leukemia. J Hematol Oncol 2018;11(1):133.

[24] Smith AM, Zhang CRC, Cristino AS, et al. PTEN deletion drives acute myeloid leukemia resistance to MEK inhibitors. Oncotarget 2019;10(56):5755–67.

[25] Cante-Barrett K, Spijkers-Hagelstein JA, Buijs-Gladdines JG, et al. MEK and PI3K-AKT inhibitors synergistically block activated IL7 receptor signaling in T-cell acute lymphoblastic leukemia. Leukemia 2016;30(9): 1832–43.

[26] McMahon CM, Ferng T, Canaani J, et al. Clonal Selection with RAS pathway activation mediates secondary clinical resistance to selective FLT3 inhibition in acute myeloid leukemia. Cancer Discov 2019;9(8):1050–63.

[27] Kopetz S, Grothey A, Yaeger R, et al. Updated results of the BEACON CRC safety lead-in: Encorafenib (ENCO) + binimetinib (BINI) + cetuximab (CETUX) for BRAFV600E-mutant metastatic colorectal cancer (mCRC). J Clin Oncol 2019;37(4_suppl):688.

[28] Vora A, Goulden N, Wade R, et al. Treatment reduction for children and young adults with low-risk acute lymphoblastic leukaemia defined by minimal residual disease (UKALL 2003): a randomised controlled trial. Lancet Oncol 2013;14(3):199–209.

Advances in Molecular Pathology 3 (2020) 49–55

ADVANCES IN MOLECULAR PATHOLOGY

Molecular Genomic Advances in Chronic Myelomonocytic Leukemia

Feras Ally, MD[a], Michelle Afkhami, MD[b],*

[a]Department of Laboratory Medicine and Pathology, University of Washington, 1959 NE Pacific Street, Box 357110, Seattle, WA 98195, USA; [b]Division of Molecular Genomic Pathology, Clinical Molecular Diagnostic Laboratory, Department of Pathology, City of Hope National Medical Center, 1500 North Duarte Road, Room 2287D, Duarte, CA 91010, USA

KEYWORDS

- Chronic myelomonocytic leukemia (CMML) • Monocytosis • Myelodysplastic/myeloproliferative neoplasm
- Next-generation sequencing (NGS)

KEY POINTS

- Chronic myelomonocytic leukemia (CMML) is a heterogeneous disease at the molecular level.
- Next-generation sequencing can help define clonal monocytosis, including CMML.
- Most patients with CMML harbor at least 1 mutation in the *TET2*, *SRSF2*, or *ASXL1* genes.
- Despite some commonality of mutations in CMML, the molecular signature of this entity overlaps with other myeloid neoplasms, and a diagnostically specific molecular profile is yet to be defined.

INTRODUCTION

Chronic myelomonocytic leukemia (CMML) has clinical characteristics that overlap between myelodysplastic syndrome (MDS) and myeloproliferative neoplasm (MPN). CMML is the most common disorder within the MDS/MPN disease category, has an unknown cause, and higher prevalence in men. The criteria required to diagnose this entity include persistent peripheral blood (PB) monocytosis greater than or equal to 1000 monocytes/µL and greater than 10% monocytes in the bone marrow (BM) differential count. Because some MPNs can present with monocytosis, other required criteria for diagnosis are absence of *BCR-ABL1*, *PDGFRA*, *FGFR1*, or *PCM1-JAK2* alterations and certain *PDGFRB* rearrangements. Dysplasia in 1 or more lineage is also expected, but the diagnosis of CMML can still be made if MDS is absent or minimal when an acquired clonal genetic abnormality is present, or if the monocytosis has persisted for at least 3 months and all other causes for monocytosis have been excluded. Initial presentation with more than 20% blasts or blast equivalents excludes the diagnosis of CMML [1–4].

Based on morphology, the disease is subclassified into CMML-0, CMML-1, and CMML-2, replacing the previous subcategorization of CMML into just type I and type II [1]. CMML can also be classified into a myeloproliferative (MP) type with white blood cell count (WBC) greater than or equal to 13,000/µL, or a myelodysplastic (MD) type with WBC less than 13,000/µL. Acquired clonal cytogenetic or molecular genetic abnormalities present in hematopoietic cells can aid in the diagnosis of CMML even when myelodysplasia is absent or minimal [5–8].

Molecular signature of the CMML has been widely studied in the past decade, which revealed more than 90% of CMMLs, tested by focused gene assays with relevant myeloid genes to whole-exome assays, have clinically significant mutations [1–5]. Clonal cytogenetic abnormalities are seen in about 30% of patients with CMML [6,7].

---

*Corresponding author, *E-mail address:* mafkhami@coh.org

https://doi.org/10.1016/j.yamp.2020.07.004
2589-4080/20/   Crown Copyright © 2020 Published by Elsevier Inc. All rights reserved.

Based on clinical laboratory testing, including hematologic indices (such as percentage monocytes), morphology, cytogenetics abnormalities, and mutational signature, multiple prognostic scoring systems have been introduced for prediction of individual patient risk in de novo and even posttransplant CMML. Therefore, it is essential to guide both pathologists and clinicians to incorporate the molecular genomic approach in diagnosis, prognosis, and therapy for CMML.

MORPHOLOGIC FINDINGS IN CHRONIC MYELOMONOCYTIC LEUKEMIA

PB monocytosis is the hallmark of CMML [1]. The monocytic cells range in maturity from mature, normal-appearing monocytes to promonocytes and immature monoblasts. Promonocytes and monoblasts are considered myeloblast equivalents, and quantification of these 2 types of cells is essential in CMML grading. Dysplasia is commonly found in PB and BM and can involve any lineage. Dysgranulopoiesis and dyserythropoiesis can be seen in more than half of the cases. Megakaryocyte dysplasia is seen often. The reported frequency of reticulin fibrosis is variable between studies; some require grade MF-2, whereas other studies allowed MF-1 for inclusion in the f-CMML (CMML with reticulin fibrosis) category [9–12]. In addition to PB and BM involvement, extramedullary sites commonly affected by CMML include the spleen, liver, skin, and lymph nodes.

CMML is further subcategorized as follows:
- CMML-0
  - Blasts (including promonocytes) less than 2% in PB, less than 5% in BM
- CMML-1
  - Blasts (including promonocytes) 2% to 4% in PB or 5% to 9% in BM
- CMML-2
  - Blasts (including promonocytes) 5% to 19% in PB or 10% to 19% in BM
  - Auer rods: upgrade to CMML-2 regardless of blast count

In addition to the recently described MP and MD types [1,13], therapy-related CMML (t-CMML) has been described as representing about 10% of all cases. t-CMML has been associated with poor prognosis and a higher frequency of high-risk cytogenetic abnormalities than de novo CMML, similar to what has been found in therapy-related acute myeloid leukemia (AML) or MDS [14–18].

BM biopsy and careful morphologic evaluation are still required to assign disease grade and exclude the possibility of AML. Progression to AML occurs in approximately 20% of patients with CMML; such cases have a poor prognosis, with median overall survival of 6 months [14]. Risk factors include high-risk karyotype; higher PB and BM blast percentage; absolute monocyte count greater than 10×10^9/L; and presence of *ASXL1*, *RUNX1*, *NRAS*, *SETBP1*, *DNMT3A*, or *NPM1* mutations [3,19,20].

CYTOGENETIC ABNORMALITIES IN CHRONIC MYELOMONOCYTIC LEUKEMIA

Karyotypic abnormalities are found in 30% of patients [7], but none are diagnostically specific for CMML. Such and colleagues [21] showed that patients with an abnormal karyotype (110 patients, 27%) had poor overall survival and higher risk of progression to AML. The most frequent cytogenetic abnormalities in their study were trisomy 8 (n = 30; isolated in 24 patients and with 1 additional abnormality in 6), isolated loss of Y chromosome (n = 18), abnormalities of chromosome 7 [n = 6; isolated in 4 patients and with 1 additional abnormality in 2; monosomy 7 in 5 and del(7q) in 1], and a complex karyotype (n = 12) [21]. That study also found that chromosomal abnormalities were more frequently seen in patients with CMML-2 subtype, 10% or more blasts in BM, presence of blasts in PB, dyserythropoiesis, and dysgranulopoiesis. The median time to 25% probability of AML evolution was 59 months. A higher probability of AML progression was noted if presenting with complex karyotype, and to a lesser extent in patients with trisomy 8. In contrast, patients with normal cytogenetics had lower probability of AML development. Such and colleagues [8,21,22] developed a CMML-specific cytogenetic risk classification where patients were separated into 3 prognostic subgroups related to their cytogenetic pattern: low, intermediate, and high risk.

In 2014, Wassie and colleagues [7] also introduced a step-wise survival analysis resulting in 3 distinct cytogenetic risk categories:
- High (complex and monosomal karyotypes)
- Intermediate (all abnormalities not high or low risk)
- Low [normal, sole -Y, and sole der(3q)]
- Median survivals of 3, 21, and 41 months, respectively

MUTATIONS IN CHRONIC MYELOMONOCYTIC LEUKEMIA

The molecular heterogeneity of CMML has been well established. As ranked by the Cancer Genome Atlas and Catalogue Of Somatic Mutations In Cancer (COS-MIC) databases, the 20 genes most frequently altered in CMML are *TET2, ASXL1, SRSF2, CBL, RUNX1, NRAS, KRAS, U2AF1, EZH2, ZRSR2, JAK2, NF1, SETBP1, IDH2, DNMT3A, NPM1, SF3B1, FLT3, PTPN11,* and *CSF3R.* It is estimated that more than 95% of patients harbor a combination of these mutations [19,20]. Similar to the cytogenetic abnormalities, the spectrum of molecular alterations are not specific for diagnosis in CMML. Nevertheless, the affected genomic pathways overlap between those seen in MDS and MPN, akin to what is observed morphologically.

The DNA methylation pathway contributes to epigenetic regulation of transcription without changing the DNA sequence. This pathway includes *TET2* ($\sim$60%), which is the most common mutated gene in CMML. Other mutated genes from this pathway in CMML are *ASXL1* (40%), *EZH2* (9%), *SETBP1* (6%), *IDH2* (5%), and *DNMT3A* (5%). Some of these genes, such as *TET2,* encode epigenetic modifiers involved in the reversal of the DNA methylation marks, a crucial process for proper gene regulation [5,23–31].

The *ASXL1* gene encodes a chromatin-binding protein required for normal determination of segment identity in the developing embryo. The *ASXL1* gene is frequently altered in myeloid diseases, including 45% of CMML [32–34]. The *EZH2* gene encodes a member of the Polycomb-group (PcG) family. PcG family members form multimeric protein complexes, involved in maintaining the transcriptional repressive state of genes [35,36].

Alterations in the epigenetic modifier genes may be found at low allele frequency in about 5% to 20% of older adults without disease, a situation termed clonal hematopoiesis of indeterminate potential. When a person undergoes molecular work-up for an idiopathic cytopenia of undetermined significance and these genes are determined to be altered in the absence of morphologic dysplasia, this situation is referred to as clonal cytopenia of undetermined significance [37]. Therefore, when the MD-type CMML is in the differential diagnosis, careful interpretation of the molecular findings with criteria such as allele frequency of the mutated genes and precise BM evaluation with clinical correlation is recommended.

In the CMML pathway, *TET2* alterations are most commonly found paired with *SRSF2* mutations. *SRSF2* is the second most commonly mutated gene in CMML. This gene belongs to the spliceosome pathway and is important for splice-site selection, spliceosome assembly, and constitutive and alternative splicing. Clinically significant genes in the spliceosome pathway include *SRSF2* ($\sim$50%), *U2AF1* (9%), *ZRSR2* (9%), and *SF3B1* (4%), and alteration results in dysregulated RNA splicing. This dysregulated splicing causes impairment in the formation of spliceosome, which can result in protein and mitochondrial dysfunction [6,14,35,38–44].

Signaling pathways are also affected, and the most common altered genes include *CBL* (17%), *NRAS* (13%), *KRAS* (9%), *JAK2* (9%), and *CSF3R* (2%). These genes are more commonly altered in patients with MP-CMML [45–47]. The *RAS* gene encodes a family of 3 highly homologous isoforms: *NRAS, HRAS,* and *KRAS.* These membrane-associated proteins regulate signal transduction on binding of ligand to a variety of membrane receptors. *RAS* gene mutations at codons 12, 13, and 61 confer constitutive activation of the *RAS* protein. *NRAS* is commonly altered in hematologic malignancies and is affected in 20% to 30% of patients with CMML. Activating mutations in *NRAS* have been implicated in the differentiation of progenitor cells into leukemic cells. Activating mutations of *KRAS* have been linked with a poorer prognosis and increased resistance to some cancer therapies, and codon 12 is a commonly mutated hotspot [43,44,48].

JAK2 and *MPL* mutations commonly drive MPNs and are infrequently seen in MP-CMML, but their presence rules out reactive conditions. However, in most cases of MDS/MPN, they are comutated with other genes [49,50]. The *JAK2* p.V617F mutation is typically found in the context of polycythemia vera and other MPNs, but rarely in MDS and AML. In the context of CMML, studies have shown that the *JAK2* p.V617F mutation is associated with an aggressive clinical course. This alteration has been described as a driver mutation associated with poor prognosis [51,52]. *MPL* encodes the thrombopoietin receptor and plays an essential role in megakaryocytic differentiation.

In addition, transcription pathway genes, including *RUNX1* (13%), *CUX1, BCOR, BCOR-L1,* and *CEBPA,* are recurrently affected in CMML. The *RUNX1* gene encodes the DNA binding unit of the heterodimeric core binding factor (CBF), a critical regulator of definitive hematopoiesis. In addition to CMML, *RUNX1* mutations are frequently observed in MDS and leukemias of myeloid and lymphoid lineages. *RUNX1, NRAS, SETBP1,* and/or *ASXL1* pathogenic mutations are correlated with poor clinical outcomes [35,44,45,48,53–55].

Gene fusions are uncommon in CMML. Patients with eosinophilia should be screened with chromosome analysis and fluorescence in situ hybridization (FISH) studies to exclude myeloid/lymphoid neoplasms with *PDGFRA/B, FGFR1,* and *PCM1-JAK2* rearrangement. The authors also recommend broader spectrum RNA-sequencing assay evaluation because of reported patients with CMML with eosinophilia [1,56–59].

APPROACH TO DIAGNOSIS AND WORK-UP

To make a definite diagnosis of CMML, the authors recommend the approach shown in Fig. 1. Reactive causes for persistent monocytosis can often be identified through obtaining a detailed history of the duration of absolute monocytosis, medication review, autoimmune disorder or infectious disease history, physical examination, comprehensive blood count, and PB smear review.

When necessary, molecular testing can help determine clonality and identify pathogenic mutations or fusions. The results can be helpful in differentiating between CMML and other hematologic disorders, such as MDS, MPN, and other MDS/MPN. Next-generation sequencing (NGS), PCR, or FISH studies for presence of BCR-ABL1 fusion can exclude the diagnosis of CMML and establish a chronic myeloid leukemia diagnosis. The authors recommend extracting and

storing DNA and RNA from BM or/and PB, to be used if a negative BCR-ABL1 status is established. At this point, an extended NGS assay including fusions, mutations, and expressions can be performed to rule out the myeloid/lymphoid neoplasms with eosinophilia and rearrangement of PDGFRA, PDGFRB, FGFR1, or PCM-JAK2. Morphologic evaluation of the BM and PB with assessment for the previously mentioned fusions needs to be undertaken in all cases of monocytosis before rendering the diagnosis of CMML [56,58,59].

In addition to gene fusions, extended molecular panels can detect mutations in most patients with CMML. Identifying a somatic variant can support disease clonality and exclude a reactive processes. Myeloproliferative neoplasms with monocytosis usually only have alterations in 1 of JAK2, MPL, or CALR genes, whereas affected patients with CMML generally have 2 or more alterations in the genes discussed earlier in relation to mutation.

Even with the presence of these genomic alterations, a morphologic evaluation of the BM is essential because of the significant overlap between myeloid neoplasms at the molecular level, because there is no specific genetic or molecular signature in CMML. Most importantly,

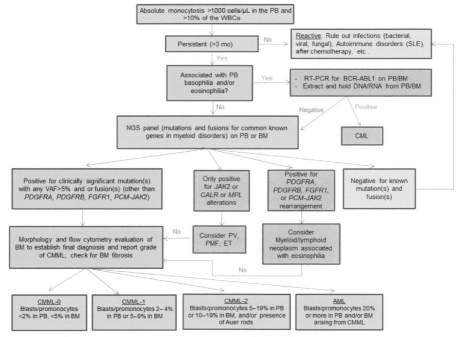

FIG. 1 Algorithm for the approach in the diagnostic workflow of CMML: pivotal role of molecular/cytogenetics testing combined with morphologic examination. CML, chronic myeloid leukemia; ET, Essential Thrombocythemia; NGS, next-generation sequencing; PMF, primary myelofibrosis; PV, polycythemia vera; RT-PCR, reverse transcription polymerase chain reaction; SLE, systemic lupus erythematosus.

the morphologic evaluation for blast proportion is the gold, and sole, standard in defining the grade of the disease, distinguishing CMML from AML.

SUMMARY

Detection of mutations is extremely helpful in the evaluation of unexplained PB monocytosis. Diagnostically, it is helpful in establishing clonality and to rule out a wide variety of reactive monocytosis. Cargo and colleagues [60] recently showed that patients presenting with non-CMML monocytosis carrying 1 or more mutations with high allele frequency have an overall survival comparable with patients with CMML. Survival correlated strongly with the number of mutations; patients without a mutation had a significantly better overall survival, with even the presence of a single mutation resulting in a worse prognosis [60]. A variety of genes also carry prognostic significance, because many variants have been associated with increased risk of progression to AML, such as the *NPM1* mutation. Some other mutations are more commonly associated with the proliferative type of CMML (*NRAS* and *KRAS*), and this subtype has a worse prognosis and unique gene expression profile [45]. Furthermore, many mutations found in CMML are actionable, such as (*TET2*, *FLT3*, and *JAK2*), although whether targeting these mutations in CMML can slow down or affect survival is yet to be investigated. Because of the nonspecific molecular genomic signature in CMML, determination of driver genes and planning targeted therapies have not yet been well established. Allogeneic hematopoietic cell transplant (HCT) is currently the only therapeutic option that can substantively alter CMML's natural history or result in a cure. Symptom-directed therapy with either cytoreductive therapy (eg, hydroxyurea) or hypomethylating agents (eg, azacitidine) is used in patients who are not candidates for allogeneic HCT. Detection of mutations can theoretically also be used in the assessment of response, although the molecular findings are not part of the proposed criteria for measurement of treatment response in adults with CMML [61]. In addition, the frequency of fibrosis in CMML varies between different studies and no clear data about the molecular signature associated with this finding have yet been elucidated. However, it seems that *JAK2* and *TP53* mutations are associated with increased risk of fibrosis in CMML, which can affect survival [9–11].

DISCLOSURE

The authors have nothing to disclose.

REFERENCES

[1] Swerdlow SH, Campo E, Harris NL, et al. WHO classification of tumors of haematopoietic and lymphoid tissues. Lyon (France): IARC; 2017.
[2] Arber DA, Orazi A, Hasserjian R, et al. The 2016 revision to the World Health Organization classification of myeloid neoplasms and acute leukemia. Blood 2016; 127(20):2391–405.
[3] Patnaik MM, Pierola AA, Vallapureddy R, et al. Blast phase chronic myelomonocytic leukemia: Mayo-MDACC collaborative study of 171 cases. Leukemia 2018;32(11):2512–8.
[4] Patnaik MM, Padron E, LaBorde RR, et al. Mayo prognostic model for WHO-defined chronic myelomonocytic leukemia: ASXL1and spliceosome component mutations and outcomes. Leukemia 2013;27(7):1504–10.
[5] Kosmider O, Gelsi-Boyer V, Ciudad M, et al. TET2 gene mutation is a frequent and adverse event in chronic myelomonocytic leukemia. Haematologica 2009;94(12): 1676–81.
[6] Meggendorfer M, Roller A, Haferlach T, et al. SRSF2 mutations in 275 cases with chronic myelomonocytic leukemia (CMML). Blood 2012;120(15):3080–8.
[7] Wassie EA, Itzykson R, Lasho TL, et al. Molecular and prognostic correlates of cytogenetic abnormalities in chronic myelomonocytic leukemia: a Mayo Clinic-French Consortium Study. Am J Hematol 2014;89:1111–5.
[8] Such E, Cervera J, Costa D, et al. Cytogenetic risk stratification in chronic myelomonocytic leukemia. Haematologica 2011;96:375–83.
[9] Petrova-Drus K, Chiu A, Margolskee E, et al. Bone marrow fibrosis in chronic myelomonocytic leukemia is associated with increased megakaryopoiesis, splenomegaly and with a shorter median time to disease progression. Oncotarget 2017;8(61):103274–82.
[10] Khan M, Muzzafar T, Kantarjian H, et al. Association of bone marrow fibrosis with inferior survival outcomes in chronic myelomonocytic leukemia. Ann Hematol 2018;97(7):1183–91.
[11] Gur H, Loghavi S, Garcia-Manero G, et al. Chronic myelomonocytic leukemia with fibrosis is a distinct disease subset with myeloproliferative features and frequent JAK2 p.V617F mutations. Am J Surg Pathol 2018;42(6):799–806.
[12] Arber DA, Orazi A. Update on the pathologic diagnosis of chronic myelomonocytic leukemia. Mod Pathol 2019;32(6):732–40.
[13] Loghavi S, Sui D, Wei P, et al. Validation of the 2017 revision of the WHO chronic myelomonocytic leukemia categories. Blood Adv 2018;2(15):1807–16.
[14] Takahashi K, Pemmaraju N, Strati P, et al. Clinical characteristics and outcomes of therapy-related chronic myelomonocytic leukemia. Blood 2013;122(16): 2807–11.
[15] Johan MF, Goodeve AC, Bowen DT, et al. JAK2 V617F Mutation is uncommon in chronic myelomonocytic leukaemia. Br J Haematol 2005;130:968.

[16] Boiocchi L, Espinal-Witter R, Geyer JT, et al. Development of monocytosis in patients with primary myelofibrosis indicates an accelerated phase of the disease. Mod Pathol 2013;26:204–12.

[17] Wang SA, Galili N, Cerny J, et al. Chronic myelomonocytic leukemia evolving from preexisting myelodysplasia shares many features with de novo disease. Am J Clin Pathol 2006;126:789–97.

[18] Cervera N, Itzykson R, Coppin E, et al. Gene mutations differently impact the prognosis of the myelodysplastic and myeloproliferative classes of chronic myelomonocytic leukemia. Am J Hematol 2014;89:604–9.

[19] Patnaik MM, Wassie EA, Padron E, et al. Chronic myelomonocytic leukemia in younger patients: molecular and cytogenetic predictors of survival and treatment outcome. Blood Cancer J 2015;5:e280.

[20] Vallapureddy R, Lasho TL, Hoversten K, et al. Nucleophosmin 1 (NPM1) mutations in chronic myelomonocytic leukemia and their prognostic relevance. Am J Hematol 2017;92(10):E614–8.

[21] Such E, Germing U, Malcovati L, et al. Development and validation of a prognostic scoring system for patients with chronic myelomonocytic leukemia. Blood 2013;121:3005–15.

[22] Onida F, Kantarjian HM, Smith TL, et al. Prognostic factors and scoring systems in chronic myelomonocytic leukemia: a retrospective analysis of 213 patients. Blood 2002;99(3):840–9.

[23] Ito S, D'alessio AC, Taranova OV, et al. Role of Tet proteins in 5mC to 5hmC conversion, ES-cell self-renewal and inner cell mass specification. Nature 2010;466(7310):1129–33.

[24] Delhommeau F, Dupont S, Della Valle V, et al. Mutation in TET2 in myeloid cancers. N Engl J Med 2009;360(22):2289–301.

[25] Patnaik MM, Zahid MF, Lasho TL, et al. Number and type of TET2 mutations in chronic myelomonocytic leukemia and their clinical relevance. Blood Cancer J 2016;6(9):e472.

[26] Pérez C, Martínez-calle N, Martín-subero JI, et al. TET2 mutations are associated with specific 5-methylcytosine and 5-hydroxymethylcytosine profiles in patients with chronic myelomonocytic leukemia. PLoS ONE 2012;7(2):e3160.

[27] Patnaik MM, Lasho TL, Vijayvargiya P, et al. Prognostic interaction between ASXL1 and TET2 mutations in chronic myelomonocytic leukemia. Blood Cancer J 2016;6:e385.

[28] Cui Y, Tong H, Du X, et al. TET2 mutations were predictive of inferior prognosis in the presence of ASXL1 mutations in patients with chronic myelomonocytic leukemia. Stem Cell Investig 2016;3:50.

[29] Mulligan CG. TET2 mutations in myelodysplasia and myeloid malignancies. Nat Genet 2009;41(7):766–7.

[30] Chiba S. Significance of TET2 mutations in myeloid and lymphoid neoplasms. Rinsho Ketsueki 2016;57(6):715–22.

[31] Abdel-Wahab O, Pardanani A, Patel J, et al. Concomitant analysis of EZH2 and ASXL1 mutations in myelofibrosis, chronic myelomonocytic leukemia and blast-phase myeloproliferative neoplasms. Leukemia 2011;25(7):1200–2.

[32] Gelsi-Boyer V, Brecqueville M, Devillier R, et al. Mutations in ASXL1 are associated with poor prognosis across the spectrum of malignant myeloid diseases. J Hematol Oncol 2012;5:12.

[33] Gelsi-boyer V, Trouplin V, Roquain J, et al. ASXL1 mutation is associated with poor prognosis and acute transformation in chronic myelomonocytic leukaemia. Br J Haematol 2010;151(4):365–75.

[34] Gelsi-boyer V, Trouplin V, Adélaïde J, et al. Mutations of polycomb-associated gene ASXL1 in myelodysplastic syndromes and chronic myelomonocytic leukaemia. Br J Haematol 2009;145(6):788–800.

[35] Patnaik MM, Tefferi A. Cytogenetic and molecular abnormalities in chronic myelomonocytic leukemia. Blood Cancer J 2016;6:e393.

[36] Patnaik MM, Vallapureddy R, Lasho TL, et al. EZH2 mutations in chronic myelomonocytic leukemia cluster with ASXL1 mutations and their co-occurrence is prognostically detrimental. Blood Cancer J 2018;8(1):12.

[37] Steensma DP, Bejar R, Jaiswal S, et al. Clonal hematopoiesis of indeterminate potential and its distinction from myelodysplastic syndromes. Blood 2015;126(1):9–16.

[38] Liang Y, Tebaldi T, Rejeski K, et al. SRSF2 mutations drive oncogenesis by activating a global program of aberrant alternative splicing in hematopoietic cells. Leukemia 2018;32(12):2659–71.

[39] Patnaik MM, Lasho TL, Finke CM, et al. Spliceosome mutations involving SRSF2, SF3B1, and U2AF35 in chronic myelomonocytic leukemia: prevalence, clinical correlates, and prognostic relevance. Am J Hematol 2013;88(3):201–6.

[40] Arbab jafari P, Ayatollahi H, Sadeghi R, et al. Prognostic significance of SRSF2 mutations in myelodysplastic syndromes and chronic myelomonocytic leukemia: a meta-analysis. Hematology 2018;23(10):778–84.

[41] Federmann B, Abele M, Rosero cuesta DS, et al. The detection of SRSF2 mutations in routinely processed bone marrow biopsies is useful in the diagnosis of chronic myelomonocytic leukemia. Hum Pathol 2014;45(12):2471–9.

[42] Saez B, Walter MJ, Graubert TA. Splicing factor gene mutations in hematologic malignancies. Blood 2017;129(10):1260–9.

[43] Gunby RH, Cazzaniga G, Tassi E, et al. Sensitivity to imatinib but low frequency of the TEL/PDGFRbeta fusion protein in chronic myelomonocytic leukemia. Haematologica 2003;88(4):408–15.

[44] Gelsi-boyer V, Trouplin V, Adélaïde J, et al. Genome profiling of chronic myelomonocytic leukemia: frequent alterations of RAS and RUNX1 genes. BMC Cancer 2008;8:299.

[45] Ricci C, Fermo E, Corti S, et al. RAS mutations contribute to evolution of chronic myelomonocytic leukemia to the proliferative variant. Clin Cancer Res 2010;16:2246–56.

[46] Schuler E, Schroeder M, Neukirchen J, et al. Refined medullary blast and white blood cell count based classification of chronic myelomonocytic leukemias. Leuk Res 2014;38:1413–9.

[47] Williamson PJ, Kruger AR, Reynolds PJ, et al. Establishing the incidence of myelodysplastic syndrome. Br J Haematol 1994;87:743–5.

[48] Prior IA, Lewis PD, Mattos C. A comprehensive survey of Ras mutations in cancer. Cancer Res 2012;72(10):2457–67.

[49] Kiladjian JJ. The spectrum of JAK2-positive myeloproliferative neoplasms. Hematology Am Soc Hematol Educ Program 2012;2012:561–6.

[50] Malcovati L, Rumi E, Cazzola M. Somatic mutations of calreticulin in myeloproliferative neoplasms and myelodysplastic/myeloproliferative neoplasms. Haematologica 2014;99(11):1650–2.

[51] Steensma DP, Mcclure RF, Karp JE, et al. JAK2 V617F is a rare finding in de novo acute myeloid leukemia, but STAT3 activation is common and remains unexplained. Leukemia 2006;20(6):971–8.

[52] Steensma DP, Dewald GW, Lasho TL, et al. The JAK2 V617F activating tyrosine kinase mutation is an infrequent event in both "atypical" myeloproliferative disorders and myelodysplastic syndromes. Blood 2005; 106(4):1207–9.

[53] Itzykson R, Kosmider O, Renneville A, et al. Prognostic score including gene mutations in chronic myelomonocytic leukemia. J Clin Oncol 2013;31(19):2428–36.

[54] Kohlmann A, Grossmann V, Klein HU, et al. Next-generation sequencing technology reveals a characteristic pattern of molecular mutations in 72.8% of chronic myelomonocytic leukemia by detecting frequent alterations in TET2, CBL, RAS, and RUNX1. J Clin Oncol 2010;28(24):3858–65.

[55] Geissler K, Jäger E, Barna A, et al. Chronic myelomonocytic leukemia patients with RAS pathway mutations show high in vitro myeloid colony formation in the absence of exogenous growth factors. Leukemia 2016; 30(11):2280–1.

[56] Savage N, George TI, Gotlib J. Myeloid neoplasms associated with eosinophilia and rearrangement of PDGFRA, PDGFRB, and FGFR1: a review. Int J Lab Hematol 2013; 35(5):491–500.

[57] Bain BJ, Fletcher SH. Chronic eosinophilic leukemias and the myeloproliferative variant of the hypereosinophilic syndrome. Immunol Allergy Clin North Am 2007;27: 377–88.

[58] Parikh SA, Tefferi A. Chronic myelomonocytic leukemia: 2012 update on diagnosis, risk stratification, and management. Am J Hematol 2012;87(6):610–9.

[59] Cheah CY, Burbury K, Apperley JF, et al. Patients with myeloid malignancies bearing PDGFRB fusion genes achieve durable long-term remissions with imatinib. Blood 2014;123(23):3574–7.

[60] Cargo C, Cullen M, Taylor J, et al. The use of targeted sequencing and flow cytometry to identify patients with a clinically significant monocytosis. Blood 2019; 133(12):1325–34.

[61] Savona MR, Malcovati L, Komrokji R, et al. An international consortium proposal of uniform response criteria for myelodysplastic/myeloproliferative neoplasms (MDS/MPN) in adults. Blood 2015;125:1857.

Advances in Molecular Pathology 3 (2020) 57–64

ADVANCES IN MOLECULAR PATHOLOGY

Erdheim-Chester Disease

A Review of Molecular Genetic and Clinical Features

Ekrem Maloku, MD, Eric Y. Loo, MD*

Department of Pathology and Laboratory Medicine, Dartmouth-Hitchcock Medical Center, One Medical Center Drive, Lebanon, NH 03756, USA

KEYWORDS
• Erdheim-Chester disease • Histiocytosis • BRAF V600E mutation • MAP kinase pathway

KEY POINTS
• Erdheim-Chester disease is a neoplastic histiocytosis driven by abnormal activation of the MAPK and PI3K/AKT signaling pathways.
• About 55-70% of all ECD cases are associated with a driving *BRAF* p.V600E alteration.
• Molecular evaluation of Erdheim-Chester disease has broad value for diagnosis confirmation, guidance of therapy, and clarification of the disorder's ontology.

INTRODUCTION

Cells of the mononuclear phagocyte system (MPS) have traditionally been grouped into monocytes, macrophages, and dendritic cells. Recent distinctions in the phenotype, ontogeny, and function of these cells have led to an ongoing reformation of the nomenclature and classification framework for the MPS [1,2]. Notwithstanding these changes, "histiocyte" (a general morphologic term referring to tissue-based macrophages) remains in medical vernacular as a generic "catch-all" for cells within this lineage. The so-called neoplastic histiocytoses are among the rarest of the World Health Organization recognized myeloid lineage malignancies, and they represent less than 1% of soft tissue and lymph node malignancies [3].

Erdheim-Chester disease (ECD) is one of these malignant histiocytoses, associated with chronic but extremely variable clinical manifestations, depending on sites of involvement. About 1500 ECD cases have been reported since its initial description in 1930 by William Chester, with recent increases in the last 2 decades that are likely related to improved diagnostic guidelines with better recognition of this rare entity [4–7]. Until recently, ECD was generally considered to have a very poor prognosis with less than half of patients surviving beyond 3 years; most casualties resulted from complications related to extraskeletal involvement [8]. Poor disease recognition and delayed diagnosis still remain a substantial challenge, resulting in failure to provide appropriate and timely intervention. Delayed diagnosis is of particular consequence because recent insights into the genetic drivers of disease can facilitate the use of targeted therapies in most cases.

SUMMARY OF CLINICAL-PATHOLOGIC FEATURES

ECD affects mostly adults, with a male predominance of 3:1. Virtually any organ or tissue can be involved, and infiltration of multiple organ systems is typical.

Funding: No funding was received for this article.

*Corresponding author, *E-mail address:* Eric.Y.Loo@Hitchcock.org

Microscopically the process is characterized by a fibrosing histiocytic infiltrate with a xanthomatous component that often includes Touton giant cells. The neoplastic histiocytes typically have a protein expression profile that is positive for CD68, CD163, and factor XIIIa; is negative for CD1a and Langerin; and may have mixed expression of S100 and *BRAF* p.V600E by mutation-specific antibody immunohistochemistry.

The symptoms of ECD are contingent on the mixture of involved sites when the patient presents for medical evaluation and the degree to which they are affected. Bone involvement with lower-extremity bone pain is a common presenting symptom, and osteosclerosis of the metadiaphyseal bones around the knee is seen in nearly all cases and is essentially pathognomonic for ECD [5,9]. Lymph nodes are typically not involved, whereas numerous other sites throughout the body may be affected, including (but not limited to) the skin, mediastinum, pleura, heart, pericardium, periaortic tissue, visceral and renal arteries, retroperitoneum, liver, spleen, testes, and orbital/periorbital tissues [3,5,9–13]. The central nervous system (CNS) is involved in 30% to 40% of cases, often within the posterior fossa compartment, but dural and pituitary stalk involvement is also described, and CNS involvement has been reported to be an independent predictor of death [5,14,15].

The diversity of involved sites gives rise to the variety of presenting organ system manifestations, negatively impacting disease recognition through mimicry of a multitude of other conditions. For example, cases with pituitary involvement may present with increased urinary frequency associated with diabetes insipidus (20%–30% of cases) or other endocrine abnormalities, such as growth hormone and corticotrophin deficiencies [5,16]. In essentially all cases, suspicion for an ECD requires an astute synthesis of clinic and imaging features, and the diagnosis should be properly established by the expected histologic findings in a procured tissue biopsy.

THE GENOMIC LANDSCAPE IN ERDHEIM-CHESTER DISEASE

Although there was some debate as to its ontology, until fairly recently, ECD and similar processes, such as Langerhans cell histiocytosis (LCH), were considered to be nonneoplastic inflammatory disorders. In 1999, Chetritt and colleagues [17] evaluated the X-chromosome inactivation pattern in the human androgen receptor gene from microdissected formalin-fixed paraffin-embedded tissues in ECD cases and provided initial evidence supporting the clonal nature of this disease process. The first reported documentation of a clonal cytogenetic finding in ECD was reported at Mayo Clinic in 2007 [18]. However, the balanced chromosomal translocation that was found was not generalizable to other cases of ECD, but did provide additional support to the idea that at least some cases of ECD were clonal proliferations.

A significant advance in understanding for the related entity LCH came in 2010, when *BRAF* p.V600E was initially described in LCH by Badalian-Very and colleagues [19]. *BRAF* p.V600E is a well-characterized missense variant that is known to drive tumorigenesis in a variety of human neoplasms, primarily through deregulated activation of downstream of mitogen-activated protein kinase kinase (MEK)/extracellular signal-regulated kinase (ERK) effectors. About half of all LCH cases were found to carry this driving *BRAF* variant, and subsequent work found downstream *MAP2K1* mutations in approximately 25% of the *BRAF*-wild-type cases [20–22]. In this way, the mitogen-activated protein (MAP) kinase (MAPK) signaling pathway became a target for investigation in ECD and other neoplastic histiocytoses. Two years after the discovery of driver *BRAF* mutations in LCH, Haroche and colleagues [23] demonstrated that recurrent *BRAF* p.V600E could also be found in a significant subset of ECD cases, more conclusively proving its clonal origins.

It is now recognized that about 55% to 70% of all ECD cases are associated with a driving *BRAF* p.V600E variant [7]. In BRAF-wild-type cases, ensuing case reports and series found recurrent *PIK3CA* and *NRAS* mutations in ~ 10.9% and 3.7% of cases, respectively [24–26]. The central role of MAPK pathway in ECD was also revealed, with aberrant signaling now known to drive greater than 80% of cases. Finally, protein kinase B/mammalian target of rapamycin (PI3K/AKT/MTOR) pathway activation has also been implicated as a potential contributor to disease pathogenesis. In addition to *BRAF* assessment, inherent value in more extensive multigene mutation profiling is becoming increasingly evident.

Relatively recent whole-exome sequencing and RNA-based fusion analysis studies undertaken in a 2016 multicenter investigation further expanded the understanding of the genomic landscape underscoring ECD [27]. Bolstering the MAPK and PI3K/AKT/MTOR pathways' role in ECD pathogenesis, Diamond and colleagues [27] described recurrent activating variants in *MAP2K1* (32%), *NRAS* (16%), *KRAS* (11%), *PIK3CA* (8%), and *ARAF* (3%) in *BRAF*-wild-type cases. Other sequence variants that have been described in these pathway-related genes include GNAS, MAP2K2, NF1, and atypical BRAF mutations [28]. Indeed, with appropriate breadth of testing, most *BRAF*-wild-type non-Langerhans cell histiocytoses will carry at least 1 MAPK or PI3K/AKT/MTOR pathway mutation [27,28]. A summary of selected genetic variants in ECD are aggregated in Table 1.

Pathologic signaling through these pathways is not limited to driver gene sequence variation. Amplification of the *RAF1* and *ERBB2* genes has been described [28]. A subset of *BRAF* p.V600E negative cases are now also known to carry kinase fusions involving the *BRAF*, *ALK*, and *NTRK1* genes [27,28]. In vitro work in cytokine-dependent murine pro-B cells revealed that introduction of the *BRAF* fusions led to activation of ERK and MEK phosphorylation and cytokine-independent growth. Introduction of the *ALK* fusion showed clear ALK, MAP kinase, STAT3, and PI3K-AKT pathway activation as well as cytokine-independent growth. Finally, the identified *NTRK1*-fusion had

---

TABLE 1

Select Mitogen-Activated Protein Kinase/Extracellular Signal-Regulated Kinase and Protein Kinase B/ mammalian Target of Rapamycin Pathway Genes Affected in Erdheim-Chester Disease

Gene	Encoded Protein	Reported Somatic Mutations Have Included	Estimated Incidence, %
MAPK/ERK Pathway			
KRAS	K-Ras	*Missense* in codons G12, Q61, R149 *Nonsense*	4–8
NRAS	N-Ras	*Missense* in codon G12, G13, Q61 *Frameshift/truncating*	4–8
ARAF	A-Raf	*Missense* in codons S214, P216, A225, D228, P539	4
BRAF	B-Raf	*Missense* in codon V600 *Frameshift/truncating* *Deletions*	55–70
RAF1	C-Raf	*Missense* in codon K106	1
MAP2K1 (MEK1)	MAPK kinase 1 (ERK)	*Missense* in codons F53, Q56, K57, F68, C121, S123, P124, E144 *Deletions* of codons E51-Q58, Q58-E62, E102-I103, P105-I107 *Frameshift/truncating*	14–18
MAP2K2	MAPK kinase 2	–	1
MAP3K1	MAPK kinase 3	–	<1
PI3K/AKT/MTOR pathway			
PIK3CA	p110α protein	*Missense* in codons E542, E545, A1046, H1047	11
Gene Fusions			
BRAF fusions	–	Reported partners have included *RNF11* and *CLIP2*	2
ALK fusions	–	Reported partners have included *KIF5B*	3
NTRK1	–	Reported partners have included *LMNA*	1
ETV3-NCOA2	–	–	–

This list of genes is not exhaustive, and other genes in these signaling pathways may potentially be affected by pathologically significant sequence variants or fusions.

Gathered from Refs [9,24,26–28,38,48,53–57].

previously been reported in Spitzoid neoplasms, and these prior studies did demonstrate fusion-associated aberrant NTRK1 expression with consequent MAPK and PI3K-AKT pathway activation [27,29].

THE MITOGEN-ACTIVATED PROTEIN KINASE/EXTRACELLULAR SIGNAL-REGULATED KINASE PATHWAY

The mitogen-activated protein kinase (MAPK) pathway is a critical regulator of cell physiology. These conserved kinase systems link extracellular signals to cellular machinery that regulates major physiologic processes, including cell growth, differentiation, migration, and apoptosis [30]. Stimuli, such as mitogens, growth factors, stress-related cytokines, and other factors, use the MAPK pathways to induce their effects, and normally signal transmission is tightly controlled. The MAPK pathway and other transduction cascades typically also contain numerous points of interaction with other signaling pathways cascades, and this continual crosstalk adds another layer of regulation (Fig. 1).

The RAS family of GTPases is the first cytosolic intermediary to activate the MAPK phosphorylation cascade and includes HRAS, KRAS, NRAS, and others.

Downstream and activated by RAS are the RAF proteins (ARAF, BRAF, CRAF, and so forth), a family of serine/threonine kinases. RAF proteins initiate the successive activation of MEK (MAPK or ERK kinase) and ERK1/2. Three MAPK families have been characterized: "classic" ERK, Jun kinase (JNK/SAPK), and p38 MAPK. ERK1/2, activates a variety of transcription factors, including CREB, c-Myc, and NF-κB. Dysregulation of these signaling cascades is estimated to occur in about one-third of all human malignancies and renders them attractive and important foci for targeted therapy [31,32].

MITOGEN-ACTIVATED PROTEIN KINASE, PROTEIN KINASE B/MAMMALIAN TARGET OF RAPAMYCIN, AND OTHER PATHWAY INTERACTIONS

The PI3K/AKT/MTOR pathway has similar signaling architecture to the MAPK pathway, in that that they both transduce an extracellular stimulus through a cascade that terminates with nuclear translocation of factors that modulate gene expression. In addition, PI3K/AKT/MTOR signaling is known to interact with the MAPK cascade. Emphasizing its important role in

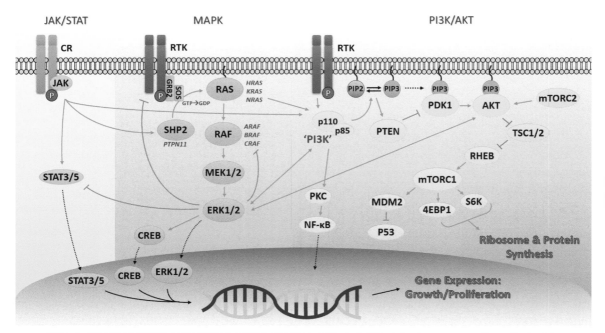

FIG. 1 Simplified MAPK and selected related signaling pathways. Green line/arrow, promoting effect; pink terminal line, inhibitory effect; blue line/double arrow, bidirectional; CR, cytokine receptor; RTK, receptor tyrosine kinase; PIP, phosphatidylinositol; PIP2, PIP biphosphate; PIP3, PIP triphosphate.

human malignancy, RAS activates both the MAPK and PI3K/AKT/MTOR pathways.

The dynamic interaction between RAS/ERK and RAS/PI3K is bidirectional, with both positive and negative feedback loops [31]. These feedback networks can negatively affect the effectiveness of single-agent targeted therapy. For example, a study in EGFR- and HER2-driven cancers discovered a therapy-pertinent mechanism after MEK inhibition led to activation of PI3K/AKT signaling by relieving a negative feedback response to ERBB receptors [33]. Because the MAPK and PI3K cascades are also known to have complex interactions with additional pathways, such as JAK/STAT and Notch-1, it becomes readily apparent why acquired resistance to single-agent pathway inhibitor therapy is of significant concern [34,35].

MOLECULAR DIAGNOSTICS IN THE EVALUATION OF ERDHEIM-CHESTER DISEASE

Given that ECD is rare and that microscopic identification of malignant histiocytoses is often challenging, clonal molecular markers substantially corroborate a diagnosis. Discriminating one or more pathologic intracellular pathway aberrancies is also germane to selection of targeted therapy. As such, assessment for underlying genetic drivers of disease is standard and essential for the initial evaluation of ECD [3,5,6,36]. Standard techniques that can be used to identify gene sequence aberrancies include immunohistochemical (IHC) analysis, polymerase chain reaction (PCR), or next-generation sequencing (NGS). Fusion analysis is also recommended and fluorescence in situ hybridization or RNA-based molecular techniques may be used.

In many instances, the tissue procured for laboratory evaluation will arrive in fixative (precluding traditional chromosome analysis) and will be of insufficient quantity for extensive workup. Because most cases are driven by BRAF p.V600E, IHC staining with a mutation-specific antibody is available as a fast and cost-effective diagnostic tool. IHC has a high degree of concordance compared with DNA-based molecular methods [37] and may greatly assist in helping to confirm ECD or other neoplastic histiocytosis. However, the high concordance between IHC and molecular testing is limited only to the V600E mutation. Other BRAF variants and mutation in other genes will not be detected. Thus, negative or equivocal IHC results must be confirmed by at least 1 other molecular method.

In BRAF-wild-type ECD cases, abnormal MAPK and PI3K/AKT/MTOR pathway activation can be caused by a variety of sequence variants and mutation types across numerous genes. Essentially all recent expert consensus statements recommend molecular profiling several of the more common genes involved in these pathways [3,5,36]. Thus, initial evaluation by NGS using a gene panel that sufficiently covers MAPK and PI3K/AKT/MTOR pathway genes is a more practical, expedient, and economical approach, especially when compared with expending time, resources, and tissue to several different stand-alone molecular assays. RNA-based gene-fusion NGS testing is also increasing in availability, which further augments the attractiveness of this testing method.

Although not a recommended tissue source for primary molecular evaluation, the use of plasma-derived cell-free DNA has been described, both as viable means to detect BRAF p.V600E and other mutations and also for monitoring response to therapy in ECD and other systemic histiocytic neoplasms [28,38]. However, regardless of the method used, a standard workup for suspected ECD should include MAPK and PI3K/AKT/MTOR pathway mutation analysis, as well as evaluation for relevant kinase fusions and gene amplification. This molecular workup is in addition to the other laboratory and radiographic assessment required to render a confident ECD diagnosis.

ERDHEIM-CHESTER DISEASE MOLECULAR PATHOLOGY AS A GUIDE FOR TARGETED THERAPY

Interferon-alpha has been the recent initial therapy of choice in ECD, but its efficacy is variable by patient and site of disease involvement [14,39]. However, before interferon therapy, there were no interventions that improved survival in this disease. On November 6, 2017, the Food and Drug Administration granted regular approval for the use of vemurafenib in the treatment of adult patients with ECD with BRAF p.V600 mutation [40,41].

Vemurafenib is a small-molecule BRAF inhibitor, and positive clinical responses have been demonstrated in greater than 90% of treated adult and pediatric patients with BRAF p.V600E-positive histiocytoses [38,42–44]. Of particular note, the efficacy of BRAF inhibitor therapy is reported to be particularly robust in severe forms of non-LCH [7]. In other common MAPK-pathway–driven malignancies, targeted inhibitor therapy is frequently limited because of acquired resistance, typically caused by activation of compensatory feed-back loops in tumor cells and tumor microenvironment components [35]. Quite remarkably, their use in ECD has demonstrated prolonged durability of response with no reports of acquired resistance to date [7].

Some groups recommend application of vemurafinib only for disease with severe manifestations or in interferon-refractory cases, whereas others advocate for its use as first-line therapy. Dabrafenib (a BRAF p.V600E inhibitor) and trametinib (an inhibitor of MEK downstream of BRAF) are both undergoing evaluation for efficacy in ECD, but some preliminary studies have already reported cases with progressive and sustained responses to these agents [45,46]. Other treatment options being evaluated include immunomodulatory and immunosuppressive agents, such as sirolimus or anakinra, antimetabolites like cladribine, and various targeted therapies, including various MEK inhibitors [7,47,48]. Regardless, therapy is recommended at diagnosis for all patients, along with referral to an academic center for enrollment in clinical trial.

MOLECULAR PATHOLOGY AND ERDHEIM-CHESTER DISEASE/LANGERHANS CELL HISTIOCYTOSIS DISEASE ONTOGENY

Before the general acceptance of ECD as a neoplastic disorder via the discovery of BRAF p.V600E, Chetritt and colleagues [17] showed remarkable insight when postulating that, "…Chester-Erdheim [sic] disease may be considered as the 'macrophage' counterpart of Langerhan's cell histiocytosis in the histiocytosis spectrum." Indeed, the clinical manifestation of these abnormal histiocytic proliferations exists on a spectrum. For example, it is recognized that a subset of mixed infiltrates will have features that overlap between ECD and either LCH or Rosai-Dorfman disease (RDD) [5,36,49].

A study by Hervier and colleagues [50] found that overlapping forms of ECD and LCH appear to occur in approximately 10% to 15% of patients with ECD. The cases with mixed/concomitant ECD and LCH had a phenotype that was generally closer to that of isolated ECD and higher frequency of BRAF p.V600E mutations in the LCH (69%) and ECD (82%) lesions compared with the incidence for either entity alone (50%–60%). The chronology of ECD diagnosis was also noted to follow or have simultaneous identification with LCH, but was never noted to come first. A separate study found RDD cooccurrence to be a less frequent finding at only 2% to 4% of ECD cases, seen mostly in men, almost always extranodal, with frequent involvement of the testes, and commonly driven by MAP2K1 mutation [51].

In a later study, Milne and colleagues [52] would use BRAF p.V600E allele-specific PCR to map the presence of a neoplastic clone within flow-sorted cells derived only from the mononuclear fraction of blood leukocytes. The tracked circulating leukocyte fractions included marrow progenitor, classical monocyte, nonclassical monocyte, and CD1c + myeloid dendritic cells. The mutant allele in blood was associated with multisystem disease in LCH and was found as expected in cases of ECD, which typically presents systemically. Notably, the pattern of involvement in the various cell fractions was indistinguishable between diseases, with mutant BRAF alleles traceable to marrow progenitors, monocytes, and myeloid dendritic cells. The nonspecific mutant allele distribution notwithstanding, they further demonstrated that the circulating BRAF + precursors had distinct LCH-like and macrophage differentiation capacities depending on exogenous signals. Both the CD1c + dendritic cells and the CD14$^+$ classical monocytes could acquire an LCH-like profile with high Langerin and CD1a. In contrast, classical and nonclassical monocytes, but not CD1c + dendritic cells, made foamy macrophages (an ECD feature) easily in vitro with macrophage colony-stimulating factor and human serum.

The 2016 whole-exome and transcriptome study in histiocytic neoplasms by Diamond and colleagues [27] should also be considered, showing that these histiocytic neoplasms had no clear differences in the pattern of mutational frequencies for specific genes or affected signaling pathways between LCH and non-LCH cases. Although no significant differences could be discerned upstream in transcription, total RNA profiling of ECD and LCH reveals dissimilar gene expression signatures. LCH shows enrichment of gene sets highly expressed in classic dendritic cells, whereas in contrast ECD shows upregulation of hematopoietic stem cell and core macrophage-associated genes.

Taken together, the comparable genetic profiles, indistinguishable pattern of involvement in affected peripheral myeloid cell fractions, and relatively high incidence of overlap cases, reinforces the concept that ECD and LCH are closely related malignancies. Hypothetically, the distinctive pathologic features of ECD and LCH may be explained in part by the divergence in phenotypic differentiation fostered by the individual cellular microenvironment. A multitude of other factors could influence phenotypic variation between LCH and ECD, including germline variation, presence of other age-related myeloid hematopoietic aberrancies such as clonal hematopoiesis of indeterminate potential (CHIP), or extrinsic inflammatory signals unique to the local tissue environment whereby dysregulated MAPK or PI3K/AKT signaling may offer a selective advantage.

SUMMARY

Molecular diagnostics have unequivocally improved early diagnosis and prognosis for this rare disorder. Although ECD remains a challenging disease to recognize and diagnose, the last 2 decades have seen meaningful advancement in the understanding of its underlying pathogenesis. The practical value of these insights can be seen unambiguously by recent alterations in therapeutic approach, but may also herald shifts in disease classification and nomenclature.

DISCLOSURE

The authors have nothing to disclose.

REFERENCES

[1] Guilliams M, Ginhoux F, Jakubzick C, et al. Dendritic cells, monocytes and macrophages: a unified nomenclature based on ontogeny. Nat Rev Immunol 2014;14(8):571–8.

[2] Ziegler-Heitbrock L, Ancuta P, Crowe S, et al. Nomenclature of monocytes and dendritic cells in blood. Blood 2010;116(16):e74–80.

[3] Swerdlow SH, Campo E, Harris NL, et al, editors. WHO classification of tumours of haematopoietic and lymphoid tissues. Revised 4th edition. Lyon (France): IARC; 2017.

[4] Chester W. Über Lipoidgranulomatose. Virchows Archiv für pathologische Anatomie und Physiologie und für klinische Medizin 1930;279:561–602.

[5] Goyal G, Young JR, Koster MJ, et al. The Mayo Clinic Histiocytosis Working Group consensus statement for the diagnosis and evaluation of adult patients with histiocytic neoplasms: Erdheim-Chester disease, Langerhans cell histiocytosis, and Rosai-Dorfman disease. Mayo Clin Proc 2019;94(10):2054–71.

[6] Diamond EL, Dagna L, Hyman DM, et al. Consensus guidelines for the diagnosis and clinical management of Erdheim-Chester disease. Blood 2014;124(4):483–92.

[7] Haroche J, Cohen Aubart F, Amoura Z. Erdheim-Chester disease. Blood 2020;135(16):1311–8.

[8] Haroche J, Arnaud L, Cohen-Aubart F, et al. Erdheim-Chester disease. Rheum Dis Clin North Am 2013;39(2):299–311.

[9] Estrada-Veras JI, O'Brien KJ, Boyd LC, et al. The clinical spectrum of Erdheim-Chester disease: an observational cohort study. Blood Adv 2017;1(6):357–66.

[10] Chasset F, Barete S, Charlotte F, et al. Cutaneous manifestations of Erdheim-Chester disease (ECD): clinical, pathological, and molecular features in a monocentric series of 40 patients. J Am Acad Dermatol 2016;74(3):513–20.

[11] Brun AL, Touitou-Gottenberg D, Haroche J, et al. Erdheim-Chester disease: CT findings of thoracic involvement. Eur Radiol 2010;20(11):2579–87.

[12] Gianfreda D, Palumbo AA, Rossi E, et al. Cardiac involvement in Erdheim-Chester disease: an MRI study. Blood 2016;128(20):2468–71.

[13] Mazor RD, Manevich-Mazor M, Shoenfeld Y. Erdheim-Chester disease: a comprehensive review of the literature. Orphanet J Rare Dis 2013;8:137.

[14] Arnaud L, Hervier B, Néel A, et al. CNS involvement and treatment with interferon-α are independent prognostic factors in Erdheim-Chester disease: a multicenter survival analysis of 53 patients. Blood 2011;117(10):2778–82.

[15] Parks NE, Goyal G, Go RS, et al. Neuroradiologic manifestations of Erdheim-Chester disease. Neurol Clin Pract 2018;8(1):15–20.

[16] Courtillot C, Laugier Robiolle S, Cohen Aubart F, et al. Endocrine manifestations in a monocentric cohort of 64 patients with Erdheim-Chester disease. J Clin Endocrinol Metab 2016;101(1):305–13.

[17] Chetritt J, Paradis V, Dargere D, et al. Chester-Erdheim disease: a neoplastic disorder. Hum Pathol 1999;30(9):1093–6.

[18] Vencio EF, Jenkins RB, Schiller JL, et al. Clonal cytogenetic abnormalities in Erdheim-Chester disease. Am J Surg Pathol 2007;31(2):319–21.

[19] Badalian-Very G, Vergilio JA, Degar BA, et al. Recurrent BRAF mutations in Langerhans cell histiocytosis. Blood 2010;116(11):1919–23.

[20] Chakraborty R, Hampton OA, Shen X, et al. Mutually exclusive recurrent somatic mutations in MAP2K1 and BRAF support a central role for ERK activation in LCH pathogenesis. Blood 2014;124:3007–15.

[21] Brown NA, Furtado LV, Betz BL, et al. High prevalence of somatic MAP2K1 mutations in BRAF V600E-negative Langerhans cell histiocytosis. Blood 2014;124:1655–8.

[22] Nelson DS, van Halteren A, Quispel WT, et al. MAP2K1 and MAP3K1 mutations in Langerhans cell histiocytosis. Genes Chromosomes Cancer 2015;54:361–8.

[23] Haroche J, Charlotte F, Arnaud L, et al. High prevalence of *BRAF V600E* mutations in Erdheim-Chester disease but not in other non-Langerhans cell histiocytoses. Blood 2012;120(13):2700–3.

[24] Diamond EL, Abdel-Wahab O, Pentsova E, et al. Detection of an NRAS mutation in Erdheim-Chester disease. Blood 2013;122(6):1089–91.

[25] Aitken SJ, Presneau N, Tirabosco R, et al. An NRAS mutation in a case of Erdheim-Chester disease. Histopathology 2015;66(2):316–9.

[26] Emile JF, Diamond EL, Hélias-Rodzewicz Z, et al. Recurrent RAS and PIK3CA mutations in Erdheim-Chester disease. Blood 2014;124(19):3016–9.

[27] Diamond EL, Durham BH, Haroche J, et al. Diverse and targetable kinase alterations drive histiocytic neoplasms. Cancer Discov 2016;6(2):154–65.

[28] Janku F, Diamond EL, Goodman AM, et al. Molecular profiling of tumor tissue and plasma cell-free DNA from patients with non-Langerhans cell histiocytosis. Mol Cancer Ther 2019;18(6):1149–57.

[29] Wiesner T, He J, Yelensky R, et al. Kinase fusions are frequent in Spitz tumours and spitzoid melanomas. Nat Commun 2014;5:3116.

[30] Junttila MR, Li SP, Westermarck J. Phosphatase-mediated crosstalk between MAPK signaling pathways in the regulation of cell survival. FASEB J 2008;22(4):954–65.

[31] Burotto M, Chiou VL, Lee JM, et al. The MAPK pathway across different malignancies: a new perspective. Cancer 2014;120(22):3446–56.

[32] Dhillon AS, Hagan S, Rath O, et al. MAP kinase signalling pathways in cancer. Oncogene 2007;26(22):3279–90.

[33] Turke AB, Song Y, Costa C, et al. MEK inhibition leads to PI3K/AKT activation by relieving a negative feedback on ERBB receptors. Cancer Res 2012;72(13):3228–37.

[34] El-Habr EA, Levidou G, Trigka EA, et al. Complex interactions between the components of the PI3K/AKT/mTOR pathway, and with components of MAPK, JAK/STAT and Notch-1 pathways, indicate their involvement in meningioma development. Virchows Arch 2014;465(4):473–85.

[35] Braicu C, Buse M2, Busuioc C, et al. A comprehensive review on MAPK: a promising therapeutic target in cancer. Cancers (Basel) 2019;11(10) [pii:E1618].

[36] Emile JF, Abla O, Fraitag S, et al. Revised classification of histiocytoses and neoplasms of the macrophage-dendritic cell lineages. Blood 2016;127(22):2672–81.

[37] Loo E, Khalili P, Beuhler K, et al. BRAF V600E mutation across multiple tumor types: correlation between DNA-based sequencing and mutation-specific immunohistochemistry. Appl Immunohistochem Mol Morphol 2018;26(10):709–13.

[38] Hyman DM, Diamond EL, Vibat CR, et al. Prospective blinded study of BRAFV600E mutation detection in cell-free DNA of patients with systemic histiocytic disorders. Cancer Discov 2015;5(1):64–71.

[39] Haroche J, Amoura Z, Trad SG, et al. Variability in the efficacy of interferon-alpha in Erdheim-Chester disease by patient and site of involvement: results in eight patients. Arthritis Rheum 2006;54(10):3330–6.

[40] Diamond EL, Subbiah V, Lockhart AC, et al. Vemurafenib for BRAF V600-mutant Erdheim-Chester disease and Langerhans cell histiocytosis: analysis of data from the histology-independent, phase 2, open-label VE-BASKET Study. JAMA Oncol 2018;4(3):384–8.

[41] Oneal PA, Kwitkowski V, Luo L, et al. FDA approval summary: vemurafenib for the treatment of patients with Erdheim-Chester disease with the BRAFV600 mutation. Oncologist 2018;23(12):1520–4.

[42] Haroche J, Cohen-Aubart F, Emile JF, et al. Dramatic efficacy of vemurafenib in both multisystemic and refractory Erdheim–Chester disease and Langerhans cell histiocytosis harboring the BRAF V600E mutation. Blood 2013;121(9):1495–500.

[43] Haroche J, Cohen-Aubart F, Emile JF, et al. Reproducible and sustained efficacy of targeted therapy with vemurafenib in patients with BRAF(V600E)-mutated Erdheim-Chester disease. J Clin Oncol 2015;33(5):411–8.

[44] Héritier S, Jehanne M, Leverger G, et al. Vemurafenib use in an infant for high-risk Langerhans cell histiocytosis. JAMA Oncol 2015;1(6):836–8.

[45] Bhatia A, Ulaner G, Rampal R, et al. Single-agent dabrafenib for BRAFV600E-mutated histiocytosis. Haematologica 2018;103(4):e177–80.

[46] Al Bayati A, Plate T, Al Bayati M, et al. Dabrafenib and trametinib treatment for Erdheim-Chester disease with brain stem involvement. Mayo Clin Proc Innov Qual Outcomes 2018;2(3):303–8.

[47] Goyal G, Shah MV, Call TG, et al. Efficacy of biological agents in the treatment of Erdheim-Chester disease. Br J Haematol 2018;183(3):520–4.

[48] Diamond EL, Durham BH, Ulaner GA, et al. Efficacy of MEK inhibition in patients with histiocytic neoplasms. Nature 2019;567(7749):521–4.

[49] Liersch J, Carlson JA, Schaller J. Histopathological and clinical findings in cutaneous manifestation of Erdheim-Chester disease and Langerhans cell histiocytosis overlap syndrome associated with the BRAFV600E mutation. Am J Dermatopathol 2017;39(7):493–503.

[50] Hervier B, Haroche J, Arnaud L, et al. Association of both Langerhans cell histiocytosis and Erdheim-Chester disease linked to the BRAFV600E mutation. Blood 2014;124(7):1119–26.

[51] Razanamahery J, Diamond EL, Cohen-Aubart F, et al. Erdheim-Chester disease with concomitant Rosai-Dorfman like lesions: a distinct entity mainly driven by MAP2K1. Haematologica 2020;105(1):e5–8.

[52] Milne P, Bigley V, Bacon CM, et al. Hematopoietic origin of Langerhans cell histiocytosis and Erdheim-Chester disease in adults. Blood 2017;130(2):167–75.

[53] Picarsic J, Pysher T, Zhou H, et al. BRAF V600E mutation in juvenile xanthogranuloma family neoplasms of the central nervous system (CNS-JXG): a revised diagnostic algorithm to include pediatric Erdheim-Chester disease. Acta Neuropathol Commun 2019;7(1):168.

[54] Emile JF, Charlotte F, Amoura Z, et al. BRAF mutations in Erdheim-Chester disease. J Clin Oncol 2013;31(3):398.

[55] Nordmann TM, Juengling FD, Recher M. Trametinib after disease reactivation under dabrafenib in Erdheim-Chester disease with both BRAF and KRAS mutations. Blood 2017;129(7):879–82.

[56] Diamond EL, Abdel-Wahab O, Durham BH, et al. Anakinra as efficacious therapy for 2 cases of intracranial Erdheim-Chester disease. Blood 2016;128(14):1896–8.

[57] Goyal G, Lau D, Nagle AM, et al. Tumor mutational burden and other predictive immunotherapy markers in histiocytic neoplasms. Blood 2019;133(14):1607–10.

Advances in Molecular Pathology 3 (2020) 65–75

ADVANCES IN MOLECULAR PATHOLOGY

Utility of Fluorescence *In Situ* Hybridization in Clinical and Research Applications

Gail H. Vance, MD[a,b], Wahab A. Khan, PhD[c,d,*]

[a]Department of Medical and Molecular Genetics, Indiana University School of Medicine, 975 West Walnut Street IB 354, Indianapolis, IN 46202, USA; [b]Department of Pathology and Laboratory Medicine, Indiana University School of Medicine, 350 West 11th Street, Indianapolis, IN 46202-5120, USA; [c]Department of Pathology and Laboratory Medicine, Dartmouth-Hitchcock Medical Center, Williamson Translational Research Building–4th Floor, 1 Medical Center Drive, Lebanon, NH 03766, USA; [d]Geisel School of Medicine at Dartmouth College, Hanover, NH, USA

KEYWORDS
- Fluorescence *in situ* hybridization (FISH)   • Cytogenomics   • Microscopy   • Chromosome biology
- Medical genetics   • Chromosomal microarray   • Copy number alterations   • FISH research applications

KEY POINTS
- Fluorescence *in situ* hybridization (FISH) permits nucleic acid sequences to be detected directly on metaphase chromosome or interphase nuclei.
- The FISH assay is a powerful tool in visualizing simple and complex chromosomal rearrangements at single-cell resolution.
- The FISH assay provides cell-based diagnosis and monitoring of abnormal clones in hematological malignancies.
- FISH provides rapid diagnosis in subset of constitutional disorders and complements microarray findings.
- Emerging research applications for FISH are providing novel insights into chromosome biology.

INTRODUCTION

Fluorescence *in situ* hybridization (FISH) has proven to be a key tool in diagnostic molecular cytogenetics along with research applications in chromosome and cell biology. FISH allows the ability to contextually define and localize nucleic acid sequences directly on human metaphase chromosomes and interphase nuclei. From its earliest inception in the late 1960s [1] to the first use of nonradioisotopic techniques [2], the impact of FISH has been vast. In particular, in cytogenetics, FISH has provided diagnostic and prognostic information for prenatal and constitutional disorders as well as hematological malignancies, and solid tumors. FISH has also complemented genomic studies, such as chromosomal microarray (CMA) [3]. Research applications in FISH technology have evolved to include the use of superresolution microscopy systems for visualizing intranuclear chromosomal organization, and various methods have been used for improving probe labeling efficiency.

SIGNIFICANCE

As either a stand-alone diagnostic method or a molecular method coupled with standard karyotyping, FISH

---

*Corresponding author. Department of Pathology, Dartmouth-Hitchcock Medical Center, Williamson Translational Research Building–4th Floor, 1 Medical Center Drive, Lebanon, NH 03766. *E-mail address:* wahab.a.khan@hitchcock.org

https://doi.org/10.1016/j.yamp.2020.07.006
2589-4080/20/   © 2020 Elsevier Inc. All rights reserved.

has significantly improved the resolution and therefore detection of numerical and structural chromosomal abnormalities beyond the light microscope. A distinct advantage of FISH is the application of fluorescent probes to nondividing cells obtained from cell suspension or paraffin-embedded tissues. FISH can detect tumor heterogeneity for both major and minor clonal abnormalities. The use of multicolor probes enables the localization and detection of multiple targets simultaneously.

FISH performed with probes comprising a lymphoma test panel (*BCL2, BCL6, MYC*) can identify "double-hit" lymphoma in cases with a pathologic diagnosis of diffuse large B-cell lymphoma [4]. FISH is also used to confirm chromosomal rearrangements identified by standard karyotyping or other molecular methods, including CMA. Parental confirmation of copy number gain or loss identified in a proband may be performed with labeled bacterial artificial chromosome DNA probe constructs that capture the copy number abnormality and detect its presence or absence in parental DNA. FISH remains a critical tool for detection and monitoring of genomic abnormalities across the spectrum of prenatal, constitutional, and neoplastic disease.

CLINICAL USE OF FLUORESCENCE *IN SITU* HYBRIDIZATION AND ITS MAJOR AREAS OF ADVANCEMENT

In a clinical context, FISH is typically performed using endpoint analysis because the hybridization kinetics are not observed in real time. However, in order to ensure that hybridization kinetics go to completion, various FISH protocols are validated with respect to probe type (eg, centromeric [repetitive] sequences, single copy unique loci, whole-chromosome paints) and specimen (eg, cell suspension vs tissue blocks). The principles of FISH are analogous to that of Southern blotting whereby single-stranded DNA anneals to its complementary target DNA. The target in FISH is that of DNA (or RNA) within interphase cells or on metaphase chromosomes that are fixed onto a microscope slide. FISH primarily uses DNA fragments that are generated by incorporating fluorophore-coupled nucleotides as probes to examine the absence or presence of complementary sequences with the use of an epifluorescent microscope [5]. This technique may also be performed on fixed and cultured tissue as well as on bone marrow, blood, and cytology smears. Clinical FISH tests that routinely use panels of gene-specific DNA probes targeting pathognomonic deletions, duplications, whole-chromosome gains/losses,

and translocations have been widely used in both somatic and constitutional testing.

The major areas of advancement in FISH have seen improvements in probe labeling chemistries and use of high-resolution imaging modalities [6,7]. The former has relied on a range of approaches included but not limited to digoxigenin/biotin labeling of the probe [8], degenerate oligonucleotide primed PCR [9], *cis*-platinum complex-mediated labeling [10], quantum dots, and click chemistry [11,12]. These advances in probe labeling have led to a natural progression in multiplexing and automating the FISH assay.

DIGITIZING AND AUTOMATING FLUORESCENCE *IN SITU* HYBRIDIZATION IMAGING

One of the first automated FISH systems was able to achieve correct segmentation on at least 89% of interphase nuclei; however, it was not designed to count split FISH signals in a given image [13]. Clinical FISH laboratories use various cocktails of DNA probes that are typically prelabeled in different fluorescence spectrums and can be generalized into 2 major categories (Table 1). Cytogenetic laboratories are also familiar with nuances in preparing specimen slides using fixed cell suspension or other analysis considerations in which cells may be overlapped or fluorescence signals are present in different focal planes. To accommodate this, technological advancements in FISH imaging modalities and microscopy instrumentation have further enabled automated epifluorescence imaging for more end-user functionality. These advancements allow the user to set thresholds before automated capturing of a FISH microscope slide [14]. Automated capturing parameters can be implemented using neural networks and domain-based algorithms to fine-tune fluorescence signal classification in different focal planes [15,16]. Segmentation of clustered overlapped nuclei can be further refined, and morphologic features resulting from image noise can be removed in order to improve on true signal classification [17].

Presently, several companies have commercialized automated FISH capturing. These companies include MetaSystems, CytoVision, Applied Spectral Imaging, and BioView, among others. All platforms permit automated FISH spot counting with built-in classifiers to generate a gallery of cell images. These images may be triaged and further ranked based on chromosome spreading, nuclei quality, probe signal intensity, and background. The metaphase or interphase cells are

TABLE 1
Categories of Labeled Probes for Fluorescence In Situ Hybridization

Direct-Labeled Nucleotides	Indirect-Labeled Nucleotides
FITC-12-dUTP	Biotin 11-dUTP
AMCA-6-dUTP	Digoxigenin-11-dUTP
Rhodamine-6-dUTP	Dinitrophenyl-11-dUTP
Cy3-dCTP	
Texas red-12-dUTP	

scanned from the microscope slide in both Brightfield and fluorescent modes with auto-recorded cell coordinates. These automated platforms are being incorporated into the clinical setting, for example, to provide digital analysis of *HER2* in breast cancer or *ALK* rearrangements in non–small cell lung cancer [18]. As a result, optimizing a given platform's classifiers for proper segmentation of chromosomes and nuclei along with reducing false positive calls is an important consideration for integrating this automation in the laboratory [14,15,17,19]. Despite these advances, however, manual counting and analysis by well-trained technologists remain the predominant procedures in many laboratories; this is in part due to the technologist's ability to quickly determine the quality of an interphase or metaphase cell for further analysis and also to follow unique scanning patterns for specific specimens and probes [20].

CONSIDERATIONS FOR FLUORESCENCE *IN SITU* HYBRIDIZATION DNA PROBE VALIDATION

As molecular cytogenomics continues to expand because of biomarker discovery, new FISH probes and disease panels are continually developed and commercialized. Therefore, it is important to reiterate the process of validation of FISH probes to be used clinically for quality assurance as put forth by the College of American Pathologists and to ensure excellence in patient care.

The process of establishing the analytical validity of FISH testing is typically divided into 4 major categories. These categories involve, but are not limited to, assessing the accuracy, reproducibility, sensitivity, and specificity of the assay. The series of consensus opinions and expert guidelines have evolved over the years as a resource toward validation of DNA probe-based *in situ* hybridization assays. Mainly, these comprise the American College of Medical Genetics technical document, the Clinical Laboratory Standards Institute guidelines, and the College of American Pathologists checklist items pertaining to FISH [21–23]. It is also important to note that FISH probe validation requirements vary depending on whether the probe has been approved/cleared by the Food and Drug Administration (FDA) or whether it is non-FDA approved, such as an analyte-specific reagent.

Of note, probe sensitivity or frequency of hybridization to an intended genomic target and probe specificity, a measure of a given target detected by the probe, will vary in different sample types. These samples can range from suspension cultures, formalin-fixed paraffin-embedded (FFPE) tissue, or fresh tissue preparations, and therefore, the validation process needs to be established for each. Signal truncation during slide sectioning for FFPE specimens should be carefully considered for probes intended to detect a chromosomal deletion when establishing sensitivity, specificity, and reference ranges [24,25].

Other factors to consider during the probe validation process are cross-hybridization and reproducibility of the assay [25]. Fluorescent signal cross-hybridizations are evaluated on metaphase chromosomes, which also speaks to the specificity of the probe. Instances whereby the FISH probe demonstrates significant cross-hybridizations (eg, recurrent signals at unintended chromosomal bands) may be indicative of probe contamination, which may require further repurification protocols and/or a different lot of FISH probe before clinical use [25]. Alternatively, the probe manufacturer may need to create/design a new version of the probe of interest. Precision or reproducibility of different FISH probes during interphase analysis can be measured in several ways. Blinded interassay (ie, microscope slides hybridized on different days) or intraassay (ie, hybridizations performed on the same day) analysis of FISH probe patterns by multiple microscopists can provide a measurement of reproducibility [26]. Finally, a given FISH probe's performance and overall hybridization efficiency should be periodically monitored as part of an ongoing probe validation and quality control plan. To this end, hybridization performance against a set of internal or external controls can be recorded for each *in situ* hybridization analysis, and periodic reevaluation of normal reference range cutoffs is recommended [21].

ROLE OF *IN SITU* HYBRIDIZATION ASSAYS IN HEMATOLOGICAL MALIGNANCIES WITH A CHROMOSOMAL BASIS

Cytogenetics has contributed significant data to the analysis, prognostication, and risk stratification of hematological malignancies. The Word Health Organization recommends cytogenetic studies at diagnosis and at defined intervals thereafter along with incorporation of morphologic and immunophenotyping data for stratifying leukemias and lymphomas [4,27]. The cytogenetic and/or molecular genetics aberrancies in hematological malignancies are defined by banded karyotype analysis of bone marrow or neoplastic blood metaphase cells as well as FISH and reverse transcriptase polymerase chain reaction studies. The molecular studies, with advancements in absolute chimeric transcript quantification, become especially important in monitoring for minimal residual disease after initial diagnosis [28]. Although not a comprehensive discussion, the following text focuses on FISH diagnosis of some of the recurrent hematological malignancies with a chromosomal basis unique to a particular myeloid or lymphoid lineage.

FLUORESCENCE *IN SITU* HYBRIDIZATION PROBE DESIGN STRATEGIES TO ASSESS CHROMOSOMAL CORRELATES IN ACUTE MYELOID LEUKEMIA

In the more common adult form of acute myeloid leukemia (AML), with prevalence of immature forms of myeloid cells, the genes involved in key rearrangements can be detected by FISH. The principal advantage of an *in situ*–based approach is that probe signals are localized at single-cell resolution to interphase nuclei without the need to culture cells. Detection of probe signals in these nondividing nuclei uses primarily 2 strategies in DNA probe design. One involves the use of break-apart FISH whereby probes are differentially labeled with fluorophores flanking genomic sequences at known chromosomal breakpoints. The close spatial proximity of the DNA probes that are differentially labeled, typically in the spectrums of green and red fluorescence, appears to the eye as a mixed yellow signal (Fig. 1A). As a chromosomal translocation occurs, 1 signal is separated (ie, "split signal") into its independent spectrum components: green or red. The remaining yellow (combined red and green fluorophores) signal indicates the nonrearranged chromosome (Fig. 1B).

In a separate fusion strategy of probes labeled with distinct fluorophores, typically dual-color, dual-fusion,

FISH probes target specific chromosomal regions that are known to either form chimeric fusion products or close juxtaposition of translocated segments and genes. If a rearrangement occurs, defined by a reciprocal translocation or intrachromosomal event (ie, inversion or deletion), the dual-color probes that otherwise in a wild-type state show distinct copies of a red fluorophore and a green fluorophore for each locus, emitting an RRGG signal pattern (Fig. 2A), are brought into close proximity. On exchange of the involved chromosomal segments, yellow (combined red and green) signals are visualized (Fig. 2B). Either 1 or 2 yellow fusion signals, depending on the probe placement with respect to the breakpoint, will indicate the fusion product on the derivative chromosome. Analogous to a break-apart strategy, the probe signal that is not rearranged, in a fusion strategy, remains as distinct green and red fluorescent signals.

Another FISH probe strategy, similar to the fusion strategy, involves an extra signal probe. This probe set also incorporates the use of a dual-color differentially labeled probe and is often used in detecting a karyotypically cryptic translocation, such as t(12;21)(*ETV6/RUNX1*), common to childhood leukemia (Fig. 3A; normal scenario). With this strategy, the fusion produces a yellow signal (combination of red and green) on the derivative (abnormal) chromosome. In the same abnormal cell, there are also green and red signals present on chromosomes not involved in the translocation. In addition, there is an "extra" "small" red signal representing a residual portion of one of the involved loci in the translocation on the other derivative chromosome (Fig. 3B). This probe strategy has many applications in diagnosis and monitoring of childhood leukemia. FISH provides analysis of a large number of cells because the abnormality is not detectable by trypsin-Giemsa or G-banded metaphases [29]. Multiple FISH strategies designed for the detection of recurrent genetic abnormalities, such as t(8;21)(q22;q22)(*RUNX1/RUNX1T1*), inv(16)(p13.1q22) in AML, or t(15;17)(q24;q21)(*PML/RARA*) in acute promyelocytic leukemia (APL) among others (Table 2), allow for rapid analysis and reporting. The FISH strategy to detect the t(15;17) in APL is a STAT test (ie, meaning immediately) in many laboratories with reporting of the result within 24 hours. These cytogenetic markers also serve as prognostic indicators of disease. In addition, the rearrangement of *KTM2A* at 11q23.3, with multiple translocation partners, often is associated with an adverse outcome. FISH analysis has supplemented molecular and traditional cytogenetic testing to define a subset of secondary or therapy-related AML [30]. In these cases, deletion or loss of

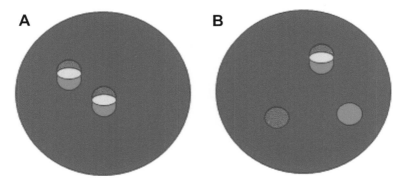

FIG. 1 Expected interphase FISH probe patterns in (**A**) normal and (**B**) rearranged nuclei using a dual-color, break-apart DNA probe strategy. Spectrum yellow is due to juxtaposition of spectrum red and green probe fluorescence.

chromosomes 5/5q or 7/7q and rearrangements of *KMT2A, RUNX1* as well as *PML/RARA* may be detected by FISH enumeration or break-apart probe strategies.

FLUORESCENCE *IN SITU* HYBRIDIZATION PROBE STRATEGIES FOR DETECTING MYELOPROLIFERATIVE NEOPLASMS

Among the myeloproliferative disorders, chronic myeloid leukemia (CML) is well known. CML is most commonly a disease of adults with symptomatic findings, including fatigue, malaise, headache, weight loss, and splenomegaly, developing over time. CML was the first malignancy to be associated with a specific chromosome defect, in which patients were found to have the Philadelphia chromosome translocation, t(9;22)(q34;q11.2) by G-banded analysis [31,32]. The Philadelphia chromosome (derivative chromosome 22) is characterized by a balanced translocation between the long arms of chromosomes 9 and 22. Among CML cases, the well-recognized BCR-ABL1 translocation is pathognomonic and required for the diagnosis. At the molecular level, the gene for *ABL1*, an oncogene on chromosome 9, joins a gene on chromosome 22 named *BCR*. The result of the fusion of these 2 genes is a new fusion protein of about 210 kDa with increased tyrosine kinase signaling that overrides normal cell regulatory mechanism. Cryptic deletions of either distal portion of *BCR* and/or proximal region of *ABL1*, as well as rare cryptic insertions between chromosome 9 and 22,

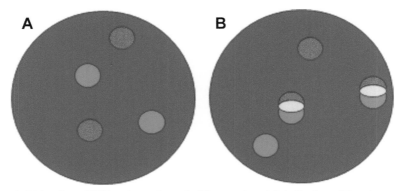

FIG. 2 Expected interphase FISH probe patterns in (**A**) normal nuclei, indicative of the absence of a rearrangement event (translocation/inversion). (**B**) In contrast, a dual-color, dual-fusion DNA probe strategy shows evidence of a reciprocal translocation with fusion signals (*yellow*) on each derivative chromosome. The yellow fluorescence is due to juxtaposition of red and green probe fluorescence.

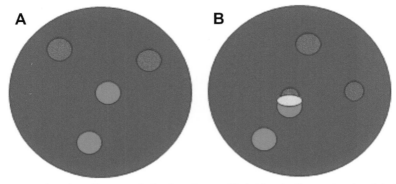

FIG. 3 (**A**) In a normal nucleus, the expected pattern for a cell hybridized with an extra signal dual-color, dual-fusion probe is 2 red and 2 green signals. (**B**) In an abnormal cell containing a fusion event (often seen with *ETV6/RUNX1* using this probe set), the expected signal pattern is 1 green, 1 red (ie, targets not involved in translocation), 1 smaller red signal (ie, residual probe target partially not involved in translocation), and 1 fused yellow signal (translocated product). This strategy increases the sensitivity of the FISH assay in detecting cryptic chromosomal rearrangements.

may occur in cases lacking a Philadelphia chromosome and are detected by FISH often using a 3-color, dual-fusion probe strategy [33,34]. Detection of the translocation is especially relevant in an era of tyrosine kinase inhibitors that target the chimeric protein encoded by the *BCR/ABL1* fusion gene.

Another myeloid disorder for which FISH has played a key role at diagnosis is eosinophilia with rearrangements involving *PDGFRA*, *PDGFRB*, and *FGFR1*. FISH break-apart strategies have proved to be useful in detecting *FGFR1* rearrangements with its many translocation partners. With respect to *PDGFRA*, a deletion of *CHIC2* leads to a cryptic fusion of *FIP1L1/PDGFRA* on chromosome 4q12. This abnormality is sensitive to imatinib mesylate and therefore relevant for rapid identification [35]. Similarly,

TABLE 2
Abbreviated List of Recurring Cytogenetic Abnormalities and Risk Stratifications in Well-Known Hematological Malignancies

Cytogenetics	Classification	Genes Involved	Outcome
t(8;21)(q22;q22)	AML	*RUNX1/RUNX1T1*	Favorable
inv(16)(p13.1q22) or t(16;16)(p13.1;q22)	AML	*CBFB/MYH11*	Favorable
t(15;17)(q24;q21)	APL	*PML/RARA*	Favorable
t(9;11)(p22;q23)	AML	*MLLT3/KMT2A*	Poor to intermediate
t(6;9)(p23;q34)	AML	*DEK/NUP214*	Poor
−7 or del 7q	MDS	—	Poor
−5 and del 5q	MDS	—	Poor
Isolated del 5q or del 20q	MDS	—	Good
Negative	De novo AML	—	Intermediate

All translocations listed are detectable by interphase and/or metaphase FISH.

rearrangements of *PDGFRB* at 5q32, such as the translocation t(5;12)(q32;p13.2), may be detected by FISH and is sensitive to tyrosine kinase inhibitors.

FLUORESCENCE *IN SITU* HYBRIDIZATION PROBE STRATEGIES DETECTING CHROMOSOMAL CORRELATES IN MATURE B-CELL NEOPLASMS

For most hematological aberrations in chronic lymphocytic leukemia (CLL) or plasma cell myeloma (PCM, formerly multiple myeloma), FISH is performed in concert with metaphase analysis. Multiple research groups, including the International Myeloma Working Group and the International Workshop on Chronic Lymphocytic Leukemia, recommend the use of FISH as a priority test for diagnostic workup for patients with CLL and PCM [36].

Various probe strategies (eg, break apart, dual color/dual fusion; enumeration) as discussed above may be applied in the context of CLL and/or PCM. These strategies include enumeration probes, especially in PCM, where hyperdiploidy accounts for approximately 45% of cases, and deletions of *TP53* portend an adverse outcome. Translocations involving the immunoglobulin heavy chain (*IGH*) are frequent in PCM and include partner genes *CCND1* (11q13.3), *MAF* (16q23.2), *FGFR3/NSD2* (*FGFR3/MMSET*)(4q16.3), *CCND2* (12p13.32) and *CCND3* (6p21.1), *MAFA* (8q24.3) and *MAFB* (20q12) [4]. It is understood that several of the PCM translocations are cryptic by standard karyotyping and that FISH is a critical component of the PCM diagnostic workup [37–39].

CLL is a disease of older adults with an incidence of ~20 cases/100,000 individuals aged 70 years or older [40]. Often asymptomatic, clinical signs may include lymphadenopathy, splenomegaly, anemia, and thrombocytopenia. Clonal abnormalities are detected in 80% of CLL cases [41,42]. The frequency of these chromosomal abnormalities depends on immunoglobulin heavy chain variable region (IGHV) mutation status. For example, trisomy 12, found in ~20% of cases, overall has an incidence of 15% in mutated IGHV and 19% in unmutated IGHV. Deletions of 11q are seen in 4% of cases with mutated IGHV and ~27% of cases with unmutated IGHV [40]. Recurring chromosomal translocations are less frequent in CLL. The t(14;18)(q32.33;q21.33) *IGH/BCL2* rearrangement, typically associated with follicular and diffuse large B-cell lymphoma, has been identified in ~2% of CLL cases as the sole aberration [40,41].

ROLE OF SINGLE NUCLEOTIDE POLYMORPHISM CHROMOSOMAL MICROARRAYS IN HEMATOLOGICAL MALIGNANCIES

In the constitutional setting, CMA analysis has achieved great success in delineating new genomic disorders and identifying genes with importance in dosage sensitivity. Application of this methodology to neoplasia has further refined assessment of copy number changes on a genomic scale using single nucleotide polymorphism (SNP) arrays. Having the SNP and copy number content on CMA platforms provides additional genotyping information that may not be achieved with FISH or karyotyping, such as the detection of copy-neutral loss of heterozygosity (cn-LOH), along with copy number changes, amplifications, and imbalances involving whole chromosomes (Fig. 4). CMA has also uncovered masked hypodiploidy related to poor outcomes. For example, SNP-microarray has proved useful in cases of hypodiploid B-cell acute lymphoblastic leukemia (ALL), whereby detection of the duplication of a hypodiploid clone (see Fig. 4) may be limited by traditional cytogenetic methods. In addition, certain focal intragenic deletions can be detected by SNP-microarray and are important for assessing genomic risk in lymphoid malignancies [43]. The detection of intragenic deletions by CMA, such as *IKFZ1*, has also led to changes in treatment protocols in B-cell ALL, especially among the pediatric patient cohort sensitive to relapse [44].

Focal gene amplifications, often associated with features of solid tumors, have also been observed in hematological malignancies by karyotype, FISH, and CMA. For example, the amplification of *RUNX1* (ie, iAMP21), when observed by CMA, revealed in a small number of cases that the amplification was not confined to *RUNX1* but rather spanned a contiguous region encompassing up to ~32 Mb. In these cases, there was also a concomitant deletion of the distal long arm of chromosome 21, including genes *DSCAM*, *AIRE*, and *TSPEAR* [45]. In myeloid malignancies, whole-gene amplifications of *KMT2A*, *MYC* as well as partial tandem duplications of *KMT2A*, sometimes covert by FISH, may be detected by SNP-based CMA [43].

A distinct advantage of SNP-based CMA over karyotyping and FISH is its ability to detect cn-LOH. The presence of cn-LOH can affect prognostication in hematological disease. In myelodysplastic syndrome (MDS), for example, cn-LOH of chromosome 7 has been linked to poor prognostication, similar to deletion of chromosome 7q detected by FISH or karyotype

Log2 Ratio

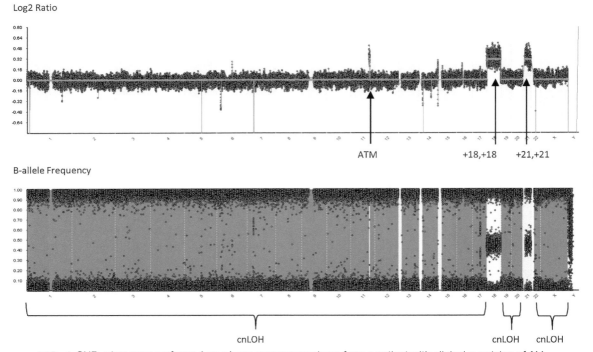

B-allele Frequency

FIG. 4 SNP-microarray performed on a bone marrow specimen from a patient with clinical suspicion of ALL. The top panel indicates the log2 ratio on the y-axis and chromosome number along the x-axis. Gain of *ATM* with 2 additional copies (11q22.3) along with whole-chromosome gains of 18 and 21 are noted. In the bottom panel, the B-allele frequency across the genome suggests cn-LOH for chromosomes 1 to 19, 22, and X. (*From* Berry NK, Scott RJ, Rowlings, et al. Clinical use of SNP-microarrays for the detection of genome-wide changes in haematological malignancies. Crit Rev Oncol Hematol. 2019;142:62; with permission.)

[43,46]. Of particular interest, cn-LOH may lead to loss of tumor suppression transcripts, such as *TP53*, or oncogenes, such as *JAK2* and *FLT3*. The cn-LOH may manifest as a "rescue event" whereby there is loss of the chromosome carrying the wild-type allele with either duplication of the chromosome with the mutated gene or intrachromosomal deletion of the wild-type allele [43]. Currently, detection of balanced chromosomal rearrangements in MDS and other hematological malignancies most frequently requires a metaphase karyotype and/or FISH analysis. However, next-generation sequencing (NGS) -based approaches for translocations with fusion transcript detection are being implemented [47].

EXPANDING TRADITIONAL APPLICATIONS OF FLUORESCENCE *IN SITU* HYBRIDIZATION

FISH in a research context has been applied across broad applications in molecular cytogenetics and

genomics. Coupling immunofluorescence with FISH has led to detection of chromosomal abnormalities in cells by their phenotype [48]. Coupling FISH with DNA halo preparations of linearized DNA has aided in visualization of sequences as little as 10 kb apart along with their chromatin interactions [49]. Applying the use of DNA FISH probes in a 3-dimensional (3D) context has contributed to the field of chromosome nanoscience. To this end, superresolution microscopy approaches, such as 3D structured illumination microscopy or single molecule stochastic optical reconstruction microscopy, that are beyond the diffraction limit of light have been applied to the study of short nonrepetitive genomic targets [6,50,51] as well as large chromosomal targets and proteins [52,53]. Ultimately, these studies shed light on 3D-chromatin organization.

Novel applications of FISH performed in suspension rather than in *in situ* cultures have allowed simultaneous measurements of RNA in conjunction with cell surface protein markers. This "FISH-flow" approach has enabled localization of antigens, messenger RNA (mRNA) expression, and nucleic acid targets in an integrated assay [54]. For example, "FISH-flow" has enabled counting of mRNA molecules per cell and allows differentiating this population of cells from those that do not have any mRNA molecules. "FISH-flow" has also been useful in examining single-cell gene expression in rare circulating cancer cells [54]. In more recent efforts, a technique known as Live-FISH exploited the CRISPR-Cas9 editing system to explore movement of DNA-double-strand breaks as well as concomitant viewing of DNA and RNA transcripts in live cells [55]. The use of chromosome orientation or CO-FISH and parent of origin or POD-FISH on homologous targets of mitotic metaphase chromosomes has further extended the use of the standard FISH assay. Through the use of these techniques, recombination events localized to regions traditionally difficult to interrogate, such as centromeric sites involved in rearrangements in cancer [56], sister chromatid exchange patterns [57], as well as discrimination of homologous chromosomes based on copy number changes [58], can be directly visualized. Taken together, research applications of FISH continue to push the limits of the understanding of chromosome biology.

FUTURE CONSIDERATIONS

The future of FISH will be predicated on its ability to provide on demand rapid single-cell resolution of nucleic acids in the genome for a range of targets and tissue types. Improvements in microscale methods of performing FISH will be important to the success of this approach. Microscale methods will aid in a reduction of FISH probe consumption and time to completion of hybridization reactions for a typical FISH assay [59]. Moreover, diagnostic and prognostic genetic targets in cancer and constitutional disorders will continue to increase with the use of FISH-, CMA-, and NGS-based discovery. Therefore, flexibility in the design of FISH probes as an orthogonal or rapid means of confirmation would be needed in some cases for different targets in the genome. To this end, computational efforts aimed at identifying optimal nucleic acid probe sequences, on demand, instead of relying on collection of preexisting commercial FISH probes will streamline research and clinical applications [60].

SUMMARY

FISH has proven to be a powerful technology with applications in both the clinical and research context. A multitude of FISH probes can be applied in different scenarios ranging from locus-specific targets to whole-chromosome paints. In neoplasia, the utility of FISH has been demonstrated in diagnostics, prognostics, and follow-up studies to monitor abnormal clones. Because the assay is single-cell based, it also provides the ability to rapidly detect low-level clones from uncultured cells. In constitutional studies, FISH serves as a confirmatory assay for microarray-based analysis of copy number variation. Because of its ability to delineate loci directly on chromosome structure, FISH may provide contextual information on gains and losses from metaphase chromosome analysis. Moreover, as a stand-alone test, FISH has enabled the detection of a spectrum of submicroscopic chromosomal abnormalities. As novel genomic targets are discovered, microscopy techniques improve, and genomic science evolves, it is anticipated that molecular cytogenomics will continue to play a key role in cancer and germline diagnostics.

DISCLOSURE

The authors have nothing to disclose.

REFERENCES

[1] Pardue ML, Gall JG. Molecular hybridization of radioactive DNA to the DNA of cytological preparations. Proc Natl Acad Sci U S A 1969;64(2):600–4.

[2] Manning JE, Hershey ND, Broker TR, et al. A new method of in situ hybridization. Chromosoma 1975; 53(2):107–17.

[3] Bi W, Borgan C, Pursley AN, et al. Comparison of chromosome analysis and chromosomal microarray analysis: what is the value of chromosome analysis in today's genomic array era? Genet Med 2013;15(6):450–7.

[4] Swerdlow S, Campo E, Harris N, et al. 4th edition. WHO classification of tumours of haematopoietic and lymphoid tissues, vol. 2. Lyon (France): WHO Press; 2017.

[5] Gozzetti A, Le Beau MM. Fluorescence in situ hybridization: uses and limitations. Semin Hematol 2000;37(4): 320–33.

[6] Khan WA, Rogan PK, Knoll JH. Localized, non-random differences in chromatin accessibility between homologous metaphase chromosomes. Mol Cytogenet 2014; 7(1):70.

[7] Yusuf M, Kaneyoshi K, Fukui K, et al. Use of 3D imaging for providing insights into high-order structure of mitotic chromosomes. Chromosoma 2019;128(1):7–13. https://doi.org/10.1007/s00412-018-0678-5.

[8] Chen TR. Fluorescence in situ hybridization (FISH): detection of biotin- and digoxigenin-labeled signals

on chromosomes. J Tissue Cult Methods 1994;16(1): 39–47.

[9] Telenius H, Pelmear AH, Tunnacliffe A, et al. Cytogenetic analysis by chromosome painting using DOP-PCR amplified flow-sorted chromosomes. Genes Chromosomes Cancer 1992;4(3):257–63.

[10] Wiegant JC, van Gijlswijk RP, Heetebrij RJ, et al. ULS: a versatile method of labeling nucleic acids for FISH based on a monofunctional reaction of cisplatin derivatives with guanine moieties. Cytogenet Cell Genet 1999; 87(1–2):47–52.

[11] Knoll JHM. Human metaphase chromosome FISH using quantum dot conjugates. Methods Mol Biol 2007;374: 55–66.

[12] Müller S, Cremer M, Neusser M, et al. A technical note on quantum dots for multi-color fluorescence in situ hybridization. Cytogenet Genome Res 2009;124(3–4): 351–9.

[13] Netten H, Young IT, van Vliet LJ, et al. FISH and chips: automation of fluorescent dot counting in interphase cell nuclei. Cytometry 1997;28(1):1–10.

[14] Vrolijk H, Sloos WC, van de Rijke FM, et al. Automation of spot counting in interphase cytogenetics using brightfield microscopy. Cytometry 1996;24(2):158–66.

[15] Lerner B, Clocksin WF, Dhanjal S, et al. Automatic signal classification in fluorescence in situ hybridization images. Cytometry 2001;43(2):87–93.

[16] Malpica N, de Solórzano CO, Vaquero JJ, et al. Applying watershed algorithms to the segmentation of clustered nuclei. Cytometry 1997;28(4):289–97.

[17] Kozubek M, Kozubek S, Lukásová E, et al. High-resolution cytometry of FISH dots in interphase cell nuclei. Cytometry 1999;36(4):279–93.

[18] van der Logt EMJ, Kuperus DAJ, van Setten JW, et al. Fully automated fluorescent in situ hybridization (FISH) staining and digital analysis of HER2 in breast cancer: a validation study. PLoS One 2015;10(4): e0123201.

[19] Kajtár B, Méhes G, Lörch T, et al. Automated fluorescent in situ hybridization (FISH) analysis of t(9;22)(q34; q11) in interphase nuclei. Cytometry A 2006;69(6): 506–14.

[20] Abbott Molecular Inc. UroVysion: Bladder Cancer Kit. Available at: https://www.molecular.abbott/us/en/products/oncology/urovysion-bladder-cancer-kit. Accessed March 14, 2020.

[21] Mascarello JT, Hirsch B, Kearney HM, et al. Section E9 of the American College of Medical Genetics technical standards and guidelines: fluorescence in situ hybridization. Genet Med 2011;13(7):667–75.

[22] Mascarello JT, Hirsch B, Kearney HM, et al. ADDENDUM: section E9 of the American College of Medical Genetics Technical Standards and Guidelines: fluorescence in situ hybridization. Genet Med 2019; 21(10):2405.

[23] MM07A2: FISH Methods for Clinical Laboratories - CLSI. Clinical & Laboratory Standards institute. Available at: https://clsi.org/standards/products/molecular-diagnostics/documents/mm07/. Accessed January 6, 2020.

[24] Yoshimoto M, Ludkovski O, Good J, et al. Use of multicolor fluorescence in situ hybridization to detect deletions in clinical tissue sections. Lab Invest 2018;98(4): 403–13.

[25] Gu J, Smith JL, Dowling PK. Fluorescence in situ hybridization probe validation for clinical use. Methods Mol Biol 2017;1541:101–18.

[26] Saxe DF, Persons DL, Wolff DJ, et al. Cytogenetics Resource Committee of the College of American Pathologists. Validation of fluorescence in situ hybridization using an analyte-specific reagent for detection of abnormalities involving the mixed lineage leukemia gene. Arch Pathol Lab Med 2012;136(1):47–52.

[27] Sabattini E, Bacci F, Sagramoso C, et al. WHO classification of tumours of haematopoietic and lymphoid tissues in 2008: an overview. Pathologica 2010;102(3): 83–7.

[28] Maier J, Lange T, Cross M, et al. Optimized digital droplet PCR for BCR-ABL. J Mol Diagn 2019;21(1): 27–37.

[29] Wolff DJ, Bagg A, Cooley LD, et al. Guidance for fluorescence in situ hybridization testing in hematologic disorders. J Mol Diagn 2007;9(2):134–43.

[30] Bueso-Ramos CE, Kanagal-Shamanna R, Routbort MJ, et al. Therapy-related myeloid neoplasms. Am J Clin Pathol 2015;144(2):207–18.

[31] Nowell PC. The minute chromosome (Phl) in chronic granulocytic leukemia. Blut 1962;8:65–6.

[32] Rowley JD. Letter: a new consistent chromosomal abnormality in chronic myelogenous leukaemia identified by quinacrine fluorescence and Giemsa staining. Nature 1973;243(5405):290–3.

[33] Castagnetti F, Testoni N, Luatti S, et al. Deletions of the derivative chromosome 9 do not influence the response and the outcome of chronic myeloid leukemia in early chronic phase treated with imatinib mesylate: GIMEMA CML Working Party analysis. J Clin Oncol 2010; 28(16):2748–54.

[34] Luatti S, Baldazzi C, Marzocchi G, et al. Cryptic BCR-ABL fusion gene as variant rearrangement in chronic myeloid leukemia: molecular cytogenetic characterization and influence on TKIs therapy. Oncotarget 2017;8(18): 29906–13.

[35] Hilal T, Fauble V, Ketterling RP, et al. Myeloid neoplasm with eosinophilia associated with isolated extramedullary FIP1L1/PDGFRA rearrangement. Cancer Genet 2018;220:13–8.

[36] Revised International Staging System for Multiple Myeloma: a report from International Myeloma Working Group. - PubMed - NCBI. Available at: https://www.ncbi.nlm.nih.gov/pubmed/?term=26240224. Accessed February 4, 2020.

[37] Hu Y, Chen W, Wang J. Progress in the identification of gene mutations involved in multiple myeloma. Oncotargets Ther 2019;12:4075–80.

[38] Tan D, Lee JH, Chen W, et al. Recent advances in the management of multiple myeloma: clinical impact based on resource-stratification. Consensus statement of the Asian Myeloma Network at the 16th International Myeloma Workshop. Leuk Lymphoma 2018;59(10): 2305–17.

[39] Avet-Loiseau H, Brigaudeau C, Morineau N, et al. High incidence of cryptic translocations involving the Ig heavy chain gene in multiple myeloma, as shown by fluorescence in situ hybridization. Genes Chromosomes Cancer 1999;24(1):9–15.

[40] Swerdlow SH, Campo E, Pileri SA, et al. The 2016 revision of the World Health Organization classification of lymphoid neoplasms. Blood 2016;127(20):2375–90.

[41] Roos-Weil D, Nguyen-Khac F, Chevret S, et al. Mutational and cytogenetic analyses of 188 CLL patients with trisomy 12: a retrospective study from the French Innovative Leukemia Organization (FILO) working group. Genes Chromosomes Cancer 2018;57(11): 533–40.

[42] Chastain EC, Duncavage EJ. Clinical prognostic biomarkers in chronic lymphocytic leukemia and diffuse large B-cell lymphoma. Arch Pathol Lab Med 2015; 139(5):602–7.

[43] Berry NK, Scott RJ, Rowlings P, et al. Clinical use of SNP-microarrays for the detection of genome-wide changes in haematological malignancies. Crit Rev Oncol Hematol 2019;142:58–67.

[44] Sutton R, Venn NC, Law T, et al. A risk score including microdeletions improves relapse prediction for standard and medium risk precursor B-cell acute lymphoblastic leukaemia in children. Br J Haematol 2018;180(4): 550–62.

[45] Baughn LB, Biegel JA, South ST, et al. Integration of cyto-genomic data for furthering the characterization of pediatric B-cell acute lymphoblastic leukemia: a multi-institution, multi-platform microarray study. Cancer Genet 2015;208(1–2):1–18.

[46] da Silva FB, Machado-Neto JA, Bertini VHLL, et al. Single-nucleotide polymorphism array (SNP-A) improves the identification of chromosomal abnormalities by metaphase cytogenetics in myelodysplastic syndrome. J Clin Pathol 2017;70(5):435–42.

[47] Zhong Y, Beimnet K, Alli Z, et al. Multiplexed digital detection of B-cell acute lymphoblastic leukemia fusion transcripts using the nanoString nCounter System. J Mol Diagn 2020;22(1):72–80.

[48] Fuller KA, Bennett S, Hui H, et al. Development of a robust immuno-S-FISH protocol using imaging flow cytometry. Cytometry A 2016;89(8):720–30.

[49] Elcock LS, Bridger JM. Fluorescence in situ hybridization on DNA halo preparations and extended chromatin fibres. Methods Mol Biol 2010;659:21–31.

[50] Knoll JHM, Rogan PK. Sequence-based, in situ detection of chromosomal abnormalities at high resolution. Am J Med Genet A 2003;121A(3):245–57.

[51] Ni Y, Cao B, Ma T, et al. Super-resolution imaging of a 2.5 kb non-repetitive DNA in situ in the nuclear genome using molecular beacon probes. eLife 2017;6:e21660.

[52] Khan WA, Chisholm R, Tadayyon S, et al. Relating centromeric topography in fixed human chromosomes to α-satellite DNA and CENP-B distribution. Cytogenet Genome Res 2013;139(4):234–42.

[53] Kyriacou E, Heun P. High-resolution mapping of centromeric protein association using APEX-chromatin fibers. Epigenetics Chromatin 2018;11(1):68.

[54] Arrigucci R, Bushkin Y, Radford F, et al. FISH-Flow, a protocol for the concurrent detection of mRNA and protein in single cells using fluorescence in situ hybridization and flow cytometry. Nat Protoc 2017;12(6):1245–60.

[55] Wang H, Nakamura M, Abbott TR, et al. CRISPR-mediated live imaging of genome editing and transcription. Science 2019;365(6459):1301–5.

[56] Giunta S. Centromere chromosome orientation fluorescent in situ hybridization (Cen-CO-FISH) detects sister chromatid exchange at the centromere in human cells. Bio Protoc 2018;8(7):e2792.

[57] Williams ES, Cornforth MN, Goodwin EH, et al. CO-FISH, COD-FISH, ReD-FISH, SKY-FISH. Methods Mol Biol 2011;735:113–24.

[58] Weise A, Gross M, Hinreiner S, et al. POD-FISH: a new technique for parental origin determination based on copy number variation polymorphism. Methods Mol Biol 2010;659:291–8.

[59] Huber D, Kaigala GV. Rapid micro fluorescence in situ hybridization in tissue sections. Biomicrofluidics 2018; 12(4):042212.

[60] Beliveau BJ, Kishi JY, Nir G, et al. OligoMiner provides a rapid, flexible environment for the design of genome-scale oligonucleotide in situ hybridization probes. Proc Natl Acad Sci U S A 2018;115(10):E2183–92.

Advances in Molecular Pathology 3 (2020) 77–85

ADVANCES IN MOLECULAR PATHOLOGY

Germline Mutations with Predisposition to Myeloid Neoplasms

Yan Liu, MD, PhD[a], Sheeja Pullarkat, MD[b],*

[a]Department of Pathology and Laboratory Medicine, Division of Hematopathology, David Geffen School of Medicine at UCLA, AL-111c CHS Building, 10833 Le Conte Avenue, Los Angeles, CA 90095, USA; [b]Department of Pathology and Laboratory Medicine, Division of Hematopathology, David Geffen School of Medicine at UCLA, AL-134 CHS Building, 10833 Le Conte Avenue, Los Angeles, CA 90095, USA

KEYWORDS

- *ETV6* • *RUNX1* • *ANKRD6* • *CEBPA* • *DDX41* • *GATA2*, myeloid neoplasm • Germline mutation

KEY POINTS

- Inherited predisposition to myelodysplastic syndrome/acute myeloid leukemia is more common than previously described.
- Early recognition of germline predisposition in a patient with cytopenias and/or myeloid neoplasms is crucial for optimal care of the patient.
- Myeloid neoplasms MDS or AML are associated with germline mutations of *CEBPA* or *DDX41* and present without a preexisting disorder or organ dysfunction.
- Germline mutations of *RUNX1*, *ANKRD26*, or *ETV6* and other pertinent genes causing platelet dysfunction should be in the differential diagnosis of thrombocytopenia.
- Germline mutations associated with myeloid neoplasms offer a unique opportunity for research to understand the stepwise pathogenesis of these neoplasms.

INTRODUCTION

Myelodysplastic syndrome (MDS) and acute myeloid leukemias (AML) are generally known to have a sporadic onset with typical presentation in older individuals. However, these entities may also arise in the setting of inherited mutations and present with unique clinical findings. These inherited syndromes, often referred to as familial MDS/AML, typically have an earlier age of onset, and include the bone marrow failure syndromes, such as Fanconi anemia, Shwachman-Diamond syndrome, and dyskeratosis congenita. With the advent of newer molecular techniques and easy accessibility for gene sequencing, there is greater awareness of germline mutations with genetic predisposition to AML and MDS. The 2016 edition of the World Health Organization

Classification of Tumors of Haematopoietic and Lymphoid Tissues includes three categories of myeloid neoplasms with germline predisposition: (1) myeloid neoplasms with germline predisposition without a preexisting disorder or organ dysfunction, (2) myeloid neoplasms with germline predisposition and preexisting platelet disorders, and (3) myeloid neoplasms with germline predisposition and other organ dysfunction [1]. The recognition and diagnosis of myeloid malignancies that arise from a germline mutation is critical because some of these patients may present with additional clinical problems that warrant personalized clinical management. For instance, those with germline *ETV6*, RUNX family transcription factor 1 (*RUNX1*), and Ankyrin repeat domain 26 (*ANKRD6*) mutations are susceptible to bleeding

*Corresponding author, *E-mail address:* spullarkat@mednet.ucla.edu

https://doi.org/10.1016/j.yamp.2020.07.007
2589-4080/20/ Published by Elsevier Inc.

because of platelet defects and may need anticipatory transfusion of normal platelets before surgery and childbirth. Knowledge of familial predisposition syndromes is of utmost importance in patients with these conditions who are candidates for allogeneic stem cell transplant because of an underlying hematologic malignancy. Careful donor selection is critical in these patients to avoid family members with deleterious mutations. Herein, we discuss the major myeloid neoplasms with germline predispositions (Table 1). Detailed review on the congenital bone marrow failure syndromes is outside the scope of the current article (Table 2).

MYELOID NEOPLASMS WITH GERMLINE PREDISPOSITION AND PREEXISTING PLATELET DISORDERS

This category is collectively termed familial platelet defect disorders and encompasses three main disorders with germline mutations in *RUNX1*, *ANKRD26*, and *ETV6*.

Myeloid Neoplasms with Germline RUNX1 Mutation

RUNX1 is a gene located in 21q22.12, which contains 13 exons and encodes the DNA-binding α subunit of the core binding factor that is essential for hematopoiesis, including hematopoietic stem cell (HSC) formation and cell differentiation of lymphoid, myeloid, and megakaryocytic lineages [2]. Germline mutations in *RUNX1* include deletions, duplications, frameshift, missense, and nonsense mutations. Most of these mutations lead to haploinsufficiency [3], whereas others have weak dominant negative activity [4]. The mutations with dominant negative effects tend to have higher frequency of leukemia progression [5]. Varying risks of progression to MDS/AML and other hematologic neoplasms in germline *RUNX1* mutation carriers may reflect the required additional mutations for disease progression and/or variable mutations that disrupt different domains within the protein. Studies have reported additional somatic mutations in *CDC25 C* [6]; loss of function mutation in second *RUNX1* allele; and acquired mutations in *TET2*, *DNMT3A*, *PDS5B*, and *PHF6* in patients who progressed to AML [7–9]. In asymptomatic individuals, clonal hematopoiesis was detected in much earlier age compared with general population [8], indicating accelerated secondary mutations in these germline *RUNX1* mutation carriers. Defects in DNA repair pathways could contribute to the increased accumulation of mutations in *RUNX1* mutant

cells. The *RUNX1* mutation carriers may also have elevated inflammatory bone marrow environment, which provides a selective pressure for HSCs that acquire additional mutations [10]. Somatic sequence variation in *RUNX1* also occurs in sporadic MDS/AML, but in this context they are usually not the initiating events but secondary events that drive disease progression [11,12]. These mutations show a worse prognosis, which is distinct from chromosomal translocations involving *RUNX1* [13–15] in AML.

Pathology and clinical findings

The platelet counts are mild-to-moderately reduced in most cases (20–130 × 10^9/L). The mean platelet volume is normal. Platelets have normal morphology or lack alpha granules, which render them a gray appearance. The bone marrow is mostly normocellular and eosinophils are often increased. The megakaryocyte count may be variable and morphologically are abnormal with scant cytoplasm, nuclear hypolobation with micromegakaryocytes even in the absence of MDS. Trilineage dysplasia becomes evident with progression to MDS. Fibrosis is not a constant feature and reticulin stain is negative for fibrosis. Platelet aggregation studies are abnormal on collagen, adenosine diphosphate, and epinephrine [16–18].

MDS/AMLs are the most common hematologic malignancies in germline *RUNX1* mutation carriers with an 11% to 100% lifetime risk (median ~44%). Other hematologic neoplasms, including T-cell acute lymphoblastic leukemia and rarely hairy cell leukemia, have been reported [19]. The age of onset of hematologic malignancies ranges widely (5–79 years) with a median of 33 years [20]. *RUNX1* mutations are unique for each familial platelet defect/AML and this makes detection of the mutation rather difficult. Sequencing of all *RUNX1* coding exons and copy number analysis for deletions may help capture most of the mutations.

Myeloid Neoplasms with Germline ANKRD26 Mutation

This entity was first described in two families, one from Italy and the other in United States [21,22]. In both these cases, the site of the aberration was linked to the same locus in the short arm of chromosome 10 (10p11.1-p12) and was later proven to be in the *ANKRD26* gene with the hot spot being a highly conserved region of the 19 bp sequence located in the 5′ untranslated region [23]. *ANKRD26* encodes for a 19-kd protein containing N-terminal ankyrin repeat domains and C-terminal spectrin helices [24]. The role of mutation in *ANKRD26* leading to thrombocytopenia

TABLE 1
World Health Organization Classification of Myeloid Neoplasms with Germline Predisposition

Category	Inheritance Patterns and Genes	Hematologic Neoplasms	Clinical Features
Myeloid neoplasms with germline predisposition without a preexisting disorder or organ dysfunction			
AML with germline CEBPA mutation	AD: CEBPA	AML	AML in children or young adults; favorable prognosis
Myeloid neoplasms with germline DDX41 mutation	AD: DDX41	MDS, AML, CML, CMML, and lymphoma	Associated with long latency and development of high-grade myeloid neoplasms; poor prognosis
Myeloid neoplasms with germline predisposition and preexisting platelet disorders			
Myeloid neoplasms with germline RUNX1 mutation	AD: RUNX1	MDS, AML, CMML, T-ALL/LBL, (rarely) B-cell neoplasms	Variable presentation with most having a mild to moderate bleeding tendency
Myeloid neoplasms with germline ANKRD26 mutation	AD: ANKRD26	MDS, AML, CML, CMML, CLL	Normal hemostasis or mild bleeding tendency
Myeloid neoplasms with germline ETV6 mutation	AD: ETV6	MDS, AML, CMML, B-ALL, PCM	Mild-to-moderate bleeding tendency; nonhematologic neoplasms
Myeloid neoplasms with germline predisposition and other organ dysfunction			
Myeloid neoplasms with germline GATA2 mutation	AD: GATA2	MDS, AML	MonoMAC syndrome; dendritic cell, monocyte, B- and NK-cell deficiency; lymphedema
JMML associated with NF, Noonan syndrome, or Noonan syndrome–like disorders	NF1, PTPN11, KRAS, NRAS, CBL	JMML, AML	Constitutional symptoms; evidence of infection; hepatosplenomegaly
Myeloid neoplasms associated with Down syndrome	Trisomy 21, mostly de novo	AML with megakaryocytic features, ALL	Constitutional features; TAM
Myeloid neoplasm associated with bone marrow failure syndromes and telomere biology disorders			

Abbreviations: B-ALL, B-lymphoblastic leukemia; CLL, chronic lymphocytic leukemia; CML, chronic myeloid leukemia; CMML, chronic myelomonocytic leukemia; JMML, juvenile myelomonocytic leukemia; MonoMAC, monocytopenia mycobacterial infection; NF, neurofibromatosis; NK, natural killer cell; PCM, plasma cell myeloma; T-ALL/LBL, T-lymphoblastic leukemia/lymphoma; TAM, transient abnormal myelopoiesis.

has been linked to its binding with *RUNX1* and *FLI1*, which are key transcription factors that control platelet production. The role of *ANKRD26* in platelet pathology has been linked to the disrupted assembly of *FLI1* and *RUNX1* on the *ANKRD26* promoter in the 5′ untranslated region, which would normally lead to the downregulation of the *ANKRD26* during megakaryocyte maturation and platelet production [21,22]. Impaired interaction with the mutated *ANKRD26* results in persistent expression of *ANKRD26* that leads to increased signaling via the thrombopoietin/*MPL* pathway and overactivation of the *JAK/STAT, PI3K,* and *MAPK/ERK* pathways [25,26]. Although increased *MPL* signaling is typically associated with platelet overproduction, EPHB2/MAPK inhibition reverses the proplatelet defect in vitro, implicating the MAPK pathway in the impaired platelet production [19].

Pathology and clinical findings
ANKRD26-related thrombocytopenia (*ANKRD26*-RT), also called thrombocytopenia 2, has an autosomal-dominant mode of inheritance and is considered one of the most frequent forms of familial thrombocytopenia. Patients usually present with moderate

TABLE 2
Myeloid Neoplasm Associated with Inherited Bone Marrow Failure Syndromes and Telomere Biology Disorders

Syndrome	Genes	Characteristic Hematologic Neoplasms	Lifetime Risk of Myeloid Neoplasm (%)	Usual Initial Hematologic Presentations
Selected bone marrow failure syndromes				
Diamond-Blackfan anemia	*RPS19, RPS17, RPS24, RPL35 A, RPL5, RPL11, RPS7, RPS26, RPS10, GATA1*	MDS, AML, ALL	~5	Anemia, BM erythroid hypoplasia
Fanconi anemia	*FANCA, FANCB, FANCC, FANCD1, FANCD2, FANCE, FANCF, FANCG, FANCI, FANCJ, FANCL, FANCM, FANCN, RAD51 C, SLX4*	MDS, AML	~10	BM failure
Shwachman-Diamond syndrome	SBDS	MDS, AML, ALL	5–24	Neutropenia
Severe congenital neutropenia	*ELANE, CSF3R, GFI1, HAX1, G6PC3, WAS*	MDS, AML	21–40	Neutropenia
Telomere biology disorders	*DKC1, TERT, TERC, TINF2, RTEL1, NOP10, NHP2, WRAP53, CTC1*	MDS, AML	2–30	BM failure

Abbreviations: ALL, acute lymphoblastic leukemia; BM, bone marrow.

thrombocytopenia (platelets 50–$150 \times 10^9/L$) with normal hemostasis or occasional mild bleeding tendency. Bone marrow reveals increased cellularity with an increase in dysplastic megakaryocytes showing small forms with hypolobated nuclei. Progression to MDS is often heralded by multilineage dysplasia. On electron microscopy, platelet showed decreased α granules and increased canalicular system [27].

Patients with *ANKRD26* have an increased predisposition to myeloid and lymphoid malignancies. In a published report, Noris and colleagues [28] have reported that 10% of patients developed hematologic malignancies including MDS, AML, and CLL. Transformation to chronic myelomonocytic leukemia (CMML) was reported in one patient with history of thrombocytopenia after acquisition of additional somatic mutations in *ASXL1* and *KRAS* [27].

Myeloid Neoplasms with Germline ETV6 Mutation

ETV6-related thrombocytopenia and its association with hematologic malignancies was first described by Zhang and colleagues [29] in 2015. *ETV6* (previously known at *TEL1*) is one of the most commonly rearranged genes in myeloid and lymphoid leukemias. *ETV6* is located on chromosome 12p13.2 and belongs to the ETS family of transcriptional regulators. In *ETV6* knockout mice, the hematopoietic progenitor cells fail to colonize the bone marrow showing that *ETV6* is vital for early hematopoiesis [29]. There is clustering of the germline mutations in the ETS domain, leading to inhibition of the activity of other ETS domain containing transcription factors critical in megakaryocyte development, such as *FLI1* [30]. *ETV6* typically shows nuclear localization, and mutation can result in abnormal localization of the protein within the cytoplasm and abnormal transcriptional changes with dominant negative effect of the mutant over the wild-type *ETV6*. In vitro studies have shown the crucial role of *ETV6* in platelet formation and differentiation [31].

Pathology and clinical findings

ETV6-related thrombocytopenia is a highly penetrant form of familial thrombocytopenia with an autosomal-dominant mode of inheritance [32]. Patients present with mild thrombocytopenia and are often asymptomatic, although some may have a mild bleeding diathesis. Platelets are normal in size and platelet aggregation studies have not shown major defects in platelet adhesion or platelet aggregation. Red cells showed macrocytosis in a small subset of patients in one study [33]. Bone marrow reveals trilineage hematopoiesis with mild dysplastic features in all lineages. These patients are predisposed to myeloid and lymphoid neoplasms and they include MDS, AML, CMML, and B-lymphoblastic leukemia [31–34]. Solid cancers have also been reported in these families [35].

MYELOID NEOPLASMS WITH GERMLINE PREDISPOSITION WITHOUT A PREEXISTING DISORDER OR ORGAN DYSFUNCTION
Acute Myeloid Leukemia with Germline CEBPA Mutation

First reported in 2004, AML with germline *CEBPA* mutation is a well-defined entity with clinical and pathologic features reminiscent of sporadic *CEBPA* mutation acquired AML. The CCAAT enhancer binding protein α (*CEBPA*) gene encodes a protein that belongs to the leucine zipper family of transcription factors. Most patients with AML have biallelic mutation with a frameshift mutation on the N-terminus and an in-frame mutation on the C-terminus. Families with the germline *CEBPA* mutations inherit an N-terminal nonsense or frameshift mutation that predisposes them to acquire a second somatic *CEBPA* mutation in the C-terminal domain on the other allele [36]. Families with the *CEBPA* mutations are rare and have been reported in only about 20 pedigrees. This disorder has near complete penetrance for development of AML. AML with biallelic mutation of *CEBPA* is seen in only 4% to 9% of children and young adult AML cases. It has also been found to constitute 8% to 13% of the subset of AML cases with "normal karyotype" and of these 7% to 11% of cases have the germline mutation [36,37].

Pathology and clinical findings

The onset of AML in these patients is much earlier with a median age at diagnosis of 24.5 years in contrast to 65 years in sporadic AML [38]. Morphologically these AMLs present with minimal differentiation and often express aberrant CD7. In general, bialleleic mutations of *CEBPA* in the presence of a normal karyotype have shown to have a better prognosis [39]. Germline *CEBPA* mutation associated AMLs may recur with a different *CEBPA* somatic mutation during relapse suggesting that relapses are triggered by independent clones. These patients, however, have a durable response to therapy and achieve a favorable long-term outcome [33]. The somatic *CEBPA* mutated AML, however, continues to harbor the same mutation throughout the course with minimal relapses [40]. Because of the variability of mutations, sequencing the entire *CEBPA* gene as a single gene assay is recommended.

Myeloid Neoplasms with Germline DDX41 Mutation

DEAD-box RNA helicase 41 (*DDX41*) is a recently described gene with predisposition to mainly develop MDS/AML, though development of lymphoid malignancies has also uncommonly been reported [36]. *DDX41* is located on chromosome 5q35.3. It codes for a probable ATP-dependent RNA helicase and may be involved in pre-mRNA splicing and alteration of RNA secondary structures. Somatic mutations in *DDX41* can also occur. In a study of 1045 myeloid neoplasms, *DDX41* variants were present in 2.6% (27 cases) of which 14 were germline mutations [41]. The most common germline mutations in *DDX41* are N-terminal frameshifts, such as c.415_418 dupGATG (p.D140Gfs*2) [41], which confer loss of function. In contrast to other myeloid neoplasms with germline mutation, those associated with *DDX41* have a long latency of onset. Just as in AML with germline *CEBPA* mutation, germline mutation in *DDX41* predisposes for a second somatic *DDX41* mutation on the other allele. Hence, presence of a biallelic mutation in *DDX41* is strongly indicative of a germline mutation.

Pathology and clinical findings

Patients with *DDX41* mutations are predisposed to myeloid malignancies. However, the mean age of diagnosis is in the sixth decade and the long latency before disease onset makes it difficult to identify individual patients who should be screened for germline mutations. Patients often present with leukopenia, macrocytosis, and the bone marrow is hypocellular with pronounced erythroid dysplasia. The karyotype is often normal and most of these patients carry a poor prognosis [36].

MYELOID NEOPLASMS WITH GERMLINE PREDISPOSITION AND OTHER ORGAN DYSFUNCTION

Myeloid Neoplasms with Germline GATA2 Mutation

GATA2 encodes for a zinc-finger transcription factor that regulates the expression of multiple target genes, playing an essential role in the development of hematopoietic and endocrine cell lineages. There were originally four clinical syndromes that were later associated with heterozygous mutations in GATA2, including (1) monocytopenia mycobacterial infection syndrome; (2) dendritic-cell, monocyte, B-, and NK-lymphoid deficiency with vulnerability to viral infections; (3) familial MDS/AML; and (4) Emberger syndrome [1,42]. Because of the considerable phenotypic overlap in the affected patients, these are now considered a spectrum of manifestations in the same disorder [43].

The human GATA2 gene localizes to chromosome 3q21.3 and has eight exons. Germline GATA2 mutations are located in the coding and noncoding region. Of note, more than 100 different germline mutations are present throughout the gene. They are monoallelic and include missense, null, and regulatory alterations. Significant germline GATA2 mutations result in a loss of function with resultant haploinsufficiency. Conversely, somatic mutations in GATA2 identified in adult myeloid malignancies are described as gain of function mutations.

GATA2 is highly expressed in immature hematopoietic cells, playing a crucial role in the proliferation and maintenance of HSCs by complex interactions between transcription factors RUNX1, MYB, PU.1, and FLI1 [44]. Two-thirds of patients with GATA2 disorders develop myeloid neoplasia; however, the drivers of myeloid transformation are not entirely known. Concurrent ASXL1 mutation has been postulated to be a collaborating event in GATA2-related MDS but this theory has not been completely elucidated. In addition, the most common karyotypic abnormality in these patients is the monosomy 7 [44]. Other studies have reported monosomy 7 as an early event in the pathogenesis of MDS in these patients, followed by acquisition of ASXL1 and SETBP1 mutations. No significant association between clinical manifestations and genotype has been identified.

Pathology and clinical findings

The median age at presentation was 20 years (5 months to 78 years) with 64% presenting with infections, 21% with MDS/AML, and 9% with lymphedema [45]. The three main hematologic malignancies that patients develop include AML, high-risk MDS, and CMML. Classic morphologic features include bone marrow hypocellularity with increased fibrosis and multilineage dysplasia. Dysplasia was most prominent in the megakaryocyte series displaying micromegakaryocytes with separate nuclear lobes. Review of literature shows numerous cytogenetic abnormalities including monosomy 7, trisomy 8, and trisomy 21.

Flow cytometry findings are characteristic with decreased monocyte count, abnormal granulocytic maturation, and reduced B- and NK-cells. Other reports have noted increased T-cell large granular lymphocyte populations [46]. In myeloid neoplasms, the presence of a germline GATA2 is associated with an aggressive course and warrants early intervention with stem cell transplant.

Myeloid Neoplasms Associated with Bone Marrow Failure Syndromes and Telomere Biology Disorders

A detailed description on the genetics and clinical feature of these entities is beyond the scope of this article. Briefly, this category encompasses familial MDS/AML that arises in the setting of inherited bone marrow failure syndromes characterized by cytopenias and genetic alterations with predisposition to solid tumors. These are well known disorders of childhood and are often diagnosed in childhood because of the classic phenotypic abnormalities as shown in Table 2. The inherited bone marrow failure syndromes include Diamond-Blackfan anemia, Fanconi anemia, Shwachman-Diamond syndrome, and severe congenital neutropenia. Fanconi anemia is characterized by classic limb abnormalities, short stature, microphthalmia, and bone abnormalities. Because the risk of MDS/AML is increased 600- to 800-fold, these are often the presenting features in some individuals [47–49].

The telomere biology disorders, such as dyskeratosis congenita, can result from mutations in one of several genes and their biology and inheritance patterns are complex. The two main players include the TERT and TERC genes, and these can lead to hematologic and solid cancers [50]. Early identification of these individuals is important for genetic counseling and treatment strategies including early stem cell transplantation.

RATIONALE FOR UNIVERSAL GENETIC TESTING FOR GERMLINE PREDISPOSITION TO ACUTE MYELOID LEUKEMIAS/ MYELODYSPLASTIC SYNDROME

According to the guidelines published by American Society of Clinical Oncology, inherited genetic testing is recommended when (1) the individual has personal or family history suggestive of a genetic cancer susceptibility condition, (2) the test can be adequately interpreted, and (3) the results will aid in the diagnosis or influence the medical or surgical management of the patients or family members at hereditary risk of cancer [51].

SIGNIFICANCE OF THE KNOWLEDGE OF GERMLINE PREDISPOSITION TO MYELOID NEOPLASMS IN DIAGNOSIS AND MANAGEMENT

Germline predisposition should be in the differential diagnosis especially in young patients presenting with cytopenias. Thorough clinical and family history is pertinent in the evaluation of cytopenias and bone marrow failure. A history of childhood infections or of a bleeding diathesis should prompt evaluation for genetic mutations in GATA2 and germline mutations with platelet disorders, respectively.

With the increasing usage of next-generation sequencing in newly diagnosed MDS and AML, it is now easier to recognize those patients with genetic predisposition syndromes. Such patients should undergo additional confirmatory testing on uninvolved tissue, such as buccal swab, skin biopsy, or cultured mesenchymal cells. The presence of significant mutations in a patient with MDS should warrant prompt evaluation for bleeding propensity, especially if younger aged at diagnosis. Clinicians should be notified of the possibility of genetic predisposition early on to avoid unnecessary treatment. For instance, presence of RUNX1, ANKRD26, or ETV6 in a patient with thrombocytopenia should preclude the use of steroids or splenectomy in clinical management. HSC transplant is a treatment of choice often offered to patients with AML and MDS. Knowledge of the inherited predisposition guides in the management of these patients for proper donor selection (to avoid use of related donors carrying the same mutation) and early transplantation of patients with germline mutations with an aggressive clinical course, such as GATA2 mutation.

With the advent of increasing use of gene sequencing for clinical and research setting, the recognition of these mutations will immensely help to study the many diverse pathways that are involved in leukemogenesis. A more robust strategy to detect these patients is critical to guide appropriate treatment and guide future research.

DISCLOSURE

The authors have nothing to disclose.

REFERENCES

[1] Peterson LC, Bloomfield CD, Niemeyer CM, et al. Myeloid neoplasms with germline predisposition. In: WHO Classification of Tumours of Haematopoietic and Lymphoid Tissues. 4th ed. Lyon, France: International Agency for Research on Cancer; 2017:122–8.

[2] Ichikawa M, Asai T, Saito T, et al. AML-1 is required for megakaryocytic maturation and lymphocytic differentiation, but not for maintenance of hematopoietic stem cells in adult hematopoiesis. Nat Med 2004;10(3): 299–304.

[3] Song WJ, Sullivan MG, Legare RD, et al. Haploinsufficiency of CBFA2 causes familial thrombocytopenia with propensity to develop acute myelogenous leukaemia. Nat Genet 1999;23(2):166–75.

[4] Matheny CJ, Speck ME, Cushing PR, et al. Disease mutations in RUNX1 and RUNX2 create nonfunctional, dominant-negative, or hypomorphic alleles. EMBO J 2007;26(4):1163–75.

[5] Michaud J, Wu F, Osato M, et al. In vitro analyses of known and novel RUNX1/AML1 mutations in dominant familial platelet disorder with predisposition to acute myelogenous leukemia: implications for mechanisms of pathogenesis. Blood 2002;99(4):1364–72.

[6] Yoshimi A, Toya T, Kawazu M, et al. Recurrent CDC25C mutations drive malignant transformation in FPD/AML. Nat Commun 2014;5:4770.

[7] Antony-Debre I, Duployez N, Bucci M, et al. Somatic mutations associated with leukemic progression of familial platelet disorder with predisposition to acute myeloid leukemia. Leukemia 2016;30(4):999–1002.

[8] Churpek JE, Pyrtel K, Kanchi K-L, et al. Genomic analysis of germ line and somatic variants in familial myelodysplasia/acute myeloid leukemia. Blood 2015;126(22): 2484–90.

[9] Manchev VT, Bouzid H, Antony-Debre I, et al. Acquired TET2 mutation in one patient with familial platelet disorder with predisposition to AML led to the development of pre-leukaemic clone resulting in T2-ALL and AML-M0. J Cell Mol Med 2017;21(6):1237–42.

[10] Bellissimo DC, Speck NA. RUNX1 mutations in inherited and sporadic leukemia. Front Cell Dev Biol 2017;5:111.

[11] Hirsch P, Zhang Y, Tang R, et al. Genetic hierarchy and temporal variegation in the clonal history of acute myeloid leukaemia. Nat Commun 2016;7:12475.

[12] Papaemmanuil E, Gerstung M, Bullinger L, et al. Genomic classification and prognosis in acute myeloid leukemia. N Engl J Med 2016;374(23):2209–21.

[13] Bejar R, Stevenson K, Abdel-Wahab O, et al. Clinical effect of point mutations in myelodysplastic syndromes. N Engl J Med 2011;364(26):2496–506.

[14] Steensma DP, Gibbons RJ, Mesa RA, et al. Somatic point mutations in RUNX1/CBFA2/AML1 are common in high-risk myelodysplastic syndrome, but not in myelofibrosis with myeloid metaplasia. Eur J Haematol 2005; 74(1):47–53.

[15] Gaidzik VI, Teleanu V, Papaemmanuil E, et al. RUNX1 mutations in acute myeloid leukemia are associated with distinct clinico-pathologic and genetic features. Leukemia 2016;30(11):2160–8.

[16] Gerrard JM, Israels ED, Bishop AJ, et al. Inherited platelet-storage pool deficiency associated with a high incidence of acute myeloid leukaemia. Br J Haematol 1991;79(2):246–55.

[17] Sun L, Mao G, Rao AK. Association of CBFA2 mutation with decreased platelet PKC-theta and impaired receptor-mediated activation of GPIIb-IIIa and pleckstrin phosphorylation: proteins regulated by CBFA2 play a role in GPIIb-IIIa activation. Blood 2004;103(3):948–54.

[18] Bluteau D, Glembotsky AC, Raimbault A, et al. Dysmegakaryopoiesis of FPD/AML pedigrees with constitutional RUNX1 mutations is linked to myosin II deregulated expression. Blood 2012;120(13):2708–18.

[19] Godley LA. Inherited predisposition to acute myeloid leukemia. Semin Hematol 2014;51(4):306–21.

[20] Liew E, Owen C. Familial myelodysplastic syndromes: a review of the literature. Haematologica 2011;96(10): 1536–42.

[21] Savoia A, Del Vecchio M, Totaro A, et al. An autosomal dominant thrombocytopenia gene maps to chromosomal region 10p. Am J Hum Genet 1999;65(5):1401–5.

[22] Drachman JG, Jarvik GP, Mehaffey MG. Autosomal dominant thrombocytopenia: incomplete megakaryocyte differentiation and linkage to human chromosome 10. Blood 2000;96(1):118–25.

[23] Pippucci T, Savoia A, Perrotta S, et al. Mutations in the 5′ UTR of ANKRD26, the ankirin repeat domain 26 gene, cause an autosomal-dominant form of inherited thrombocytopenia, THC2. Am J Hum Genet 2011;88(1): 115–20.

[24] Hahn Y, Bera TK, Pastan IH, et al. Duplication and extensive remodeling shaped POTE family genes encoding proteins containing ankyrin repeat and coiled coil domains. Gene 2006;366(2):238–45.

[25] Bluteau D, Balduini A, Balayn N, et al. Thrombocytopenia-associated mutations in the ANKRD26 regulatory region induce MAPK hyperactivation. J Clin Invest 2014;124(2):580–91.

[26] Marconi C, Canobbio I, Bozzi V, et al. 5′UTR point substitutions and N-terminal truncating mutations of ANKRD26 in acute myeloid leukemia. J Hematol Oncol 2017;10(1):18.

[27] Perez Botero J, Chen D, He R, et al. Clinical and laboratory characteristics in congenital ANKRD26 mutation-associated thrombocytopenia: a detailed phenotypic study of a family. Platelets 2016;27(7):712–5.

[28] Noris P, Biino G, Pecci A, et al. Platelet diameters in inherited thrombocytopenias: analysis of 376 patients with all known disorders. Blood 2014;124(6):e4–10.

[29] Zhang MY, Churpek JE, Keel SB, et al. Germline ETV6 mutations in familial thrombocytopenia and hematologic malignancy. Nat Genet 2015;47(2):180–5.

[30] Kwiatkowski BA, Bastian LS, Bauer TRJ, et al. The ets family member Tel binds to the Fli-1 oncoprotein and inhibits its transcriptional activity. J Biol Chem 1998; 273(28):17525–30.

[31] Poggi M, Canault M, Favier M, et al. Germline variants in ETV6 underlie reduced platelet formation, platelet dysfunction and increased levels of circulating CD34+ progenitors. Haematologica 2017;102(2):282–94.

[32] Feurstein S, Godley LA. Germline ETV6 mutations and predisposition to hematological malignancies. Int J Hematol 2017;106(2):189–95.

[33] Melazzini F, Palombo F, Balduini A, et al. Clinical and pathogenic features of ETV6-related thrombocytopenia with predisposition to acute lymphoblastic leukemia. Haematologica 2016;101(11):1333–42.

[34] Topka S, Vijai J, Walsh MF, et al. Germline ETV6 mutations confer susceptibility to acute lymphoblastic leukemia and thrombocytopenia. PLoS Genet 2015;11(6): e1005262.

[35] Noetzli L, Lo RW, Lee-Sherick AB, et al. Germline mutations in ETV6 are associated with thrombocytopenia, red cell macrocytosis and predisposition to lymphoblastic leukemia. Nat Genet 2015;47(5):535–8.

[36] Pabst T, Eyholzer M, Haefliger S, et al. Somatic CEBPA mutations are a frequent second event in families with germline CEBPA mutations and familial acute myeloid leukemia. J Clin Oncol 2008;26(31):5088–93.

[37] Preudhomme C, Sagot C, Boissel N, et al. Favorable prognostic significance of CEBPA mutations in patients with de novo acute myeloid leukemia: a study from the Acute Leukemia French Association (ALFA). Blood 2002;100(8):2717–23.

[38] Tawana K, Wang J, Renneville A, et al. Disease evolution and outcomes in familial AML with germline CEBPA mutations. Blood 2015;126(10):1214–23.

[39] Dufour A, Schneider F, Metzeler KH, et al. Acute myeloid leukemia with biallelic CEBPA gene mutations and normal karyotype represents a distinct genetic entity associated with a favorable clinical outcome. J Clin Oncol 2010;28(4):570–7.

[40] Tiesmeier J, Czwalinna A, Müller-Tidow C, et al. Evidence for allelic evolution of C/EBPalpha mutations in acute myeloid leukaemia. Br J Haematol 2003;123(3): 413–9.

[41] Polprasert C, Schulze I, Sekeres MA, et al. Inherited and somatic defects in DDX41 in myeloid neoplasms. Cancer Cell 2015;27(5):658–70.

[42] Fasan A, Eder C, Haferlach C, et al. GATA2 mutations are frequent in intermediate-risk karyotype AML with biallelic CEBPA mutations and are associated with favorable prognosis. Leukemia 2013;27(2):482–5.

[43] Grossmann V, Haferlach C, Nadarajah N, et al. CEBPA double-mutated acute myeloid leukaemia harbours concomitant molecular mutations in 76·8% of cases with TET2 and GATA2 alterations impacting prognosis. Br J Haematol 2013;161(5):649–58.

[44] Wlodarski MW, Collin M, Horwitz MS. GATA2 deficiency and related myeloid neoplasms. Semin Hematol 2017; 54(2):81–6.

[45] Spinner MA, Sanchez LA, Hsu AP, et al. GATA2 deficiency: a protean disorder of hematopoiesis, lymphatics, and immunity. Blood 2014;123(6):809–21.

[46] Calvo KR, Vinh DC, Maric I, et al. Myelodysplasia in autosomal dominant and sporadic monocytopenia immunodeficiency syndrome: diagnostic features and clinical implications. Haematologica 2011;96(8): 1221–5.

[47] Armanios M. Syndromes of telomere shortening. Annu Rev Genomics Hum Genet 2009;10:45–61.

[48] Soulier J. Fanconi anemia. Hematology Am Soc Hematol Educ Program 2011;2011:492–7.

[49] Parry EM, Alder JK, Qi X, et al. Syndrome complex of bone marrow failure and pulmonary fibrosis predicts germline defects in telomerase. Blood 2011;117(21): 5607–11.

[50] Heiss NS, Knight SW, Vulliamy TJ, et al. X-linked dyskeratosis congenita is caused by mutations in a highly conserved gene with putative nucleolar functions. Nat Genet 1998;19(1):32–8.

[51] American Society of Clinical Oncology. American Society of Clinical Oncology policy statement update: genetic testing for cancer susceptibility. J Clin Oncol 2003; 21(12):2397–406.

Infectious Disease

/

Molecular Diagnosis of Drug Resistance in *Mycobacterium tuberculosis*

Perspectives from a Tuberculosis-Endemic Developing Country

Priti Kambli[a], Camilla Rodrigues, MD[b],*

[a]Microbiology Section, P.D. Hinduja Hospital, Mumbai, India; [b]Microbiology Section, P.D. Hinduja National Hospital and Medical Research centre, Veer savarkar Marg, Mahim Mumbai-400016, India

---

KEYWORDS

- Drug-resistant tuberculosis • Nucleic acid–based assays • *Mycobacterium tuberculosis* • Resource-poor countries

KEY POINTS

- Drug susceptibility testing (DST), the gold standard for detection of drug-resistant tuberculosis, is time consuming and technically challenging, especially in low- and middle-income countries.
- Molecular tests are available with varying sensitivity and specificity for detection of gene mutations associated with resistance to drugs.
- Sequencing offers the final answer for drug-resistant SNPs compared with other molecular tests, but currently still not poised to replace the rapid molecular tests that are being implemented in primary health care settings.

INTRODUCTION

To reduce tuberculosis (TB) transmission worldwide, early case detection and treatment with appropriate drugs is key and considered to be most effective in managing this disease [1].

For several decades, the World Health Organization (WHO) standard for defining drug resistance in clinical *Mycobacterium tuberculosis* (MTB) isolates was culture-based drug susceptibility testing (DST). However, the qualitative phenotypic DST results, which can sometimes take up to 6 to 9 weeks, not only warrants skilled expertise but also requires sophisticated biosafety infrastructure that is not easily available in several developing countries [2].

Introduction of molecular diagnostic tests, such as line probe assays (LPA) and the GeneXpert System (Cepheid, Sunnyvale, CA), has considerably modified the MTB DST landscape by enabling much faster detection of common mutations related to resistance for first-line anti-TB drugs [3,4]. However, these technologies have restricted DST capabilities because they are designed to cover limited genomic mutations [5]. The beginning of high throughput technologies, such as pyrosequencing (PSQ) and next-generation sequencing (NGS) methods in the mid-2000s, offered more comprehensive detection of mutations related to drug-resistant (DR) TB (DR-TB) [6].

NGS not only solely determines the presence or absence of mutations, but offers additional sequence knowledge, that allows users to differentiate mutations conferring different levels of resistance from silent mutations [7,8]. Today NGS platforms offer attractive possibilities for detection and characterization of DR-TB with clinically relevant gene regions or whole genomes

---

*Corresponding author, *E-mail address:* dr_crodrigues@hindujahospital.com

https://doi.org/10.1016/j.yamp.2020.07.008
2589-4080/20/

of interest that will enable comprehensive and faster molecular DSTs, reducing the necessity for phenotypic DST for DR-TB diagnosis, particularly for drugs regarded as phenotypically unreliable.

SIGNIFICANCE

The risk of the patient developing resistance to antibiotics is significantly reduced if the right medication is administered from the start of treatment. Ultimately, this can improve the cure rates for patients with DR-TB and limit the spread of the disease in the community.

Comparative genomics of MTB isolates from infected patients are used to understand disease transmission and tracking transmission chains within the community. The effectiveness of public health interventions is aimed at controlling and preventing the spread of TB, rapidly detecting TB outbreaks, and defining transmission patterns accurately [8]. However, the complex and high cost of these sequencing tests is currently an issue.

DIAGNOSIS IMPLEMENTATION

A modified plan for a laboratory initiative model TB diagnostic algorithm with the NGS approach is shown in Fig. 1 [9].

MOLECULAR DIAGNOSIS

Diagnostic laboratory tests used in low- and middle-income countries are as follows:
1. GeneXpert MTB/RIF and Xpert MTB/RIF Ultra
2. TrueNat TB
3. LPAs
4. Sequencing

GeneXpert MTB/RIF
Xpert MTB/RIF
Background
The Xpert MTB/RIF (Cepheid) is a rapid molecular assay for the detection of the MTB complex and recurrent implantation failure (RIF) resistance screening in suspected cases [4].

Description of methods
This assay employs semiquantitative nested real-time polymerase chain reaction (PCR) to amplify a fragment containing the 81-bp hotspot region of the *rpoB* gene

(codons 507–533) that is then hybridized to five molecular beacon probes [10]. Each probe is specific for a different location in the gene sequence and is labeled with a fluorescent dye. To minimize cross-contamination between samples the whole experiment is done in a self-contained cartridge, like a mini-laboratory. With the detection time of RIF resistance decreased from 4 to 8 weeks (culture and DST) to 2 hours, this is a game changer for detection of multidrug-resistant (MDR)-TB. High accuracy of the assay increases the detection rate of MTB by 23% among culture-confirmed cases related with smear microscopy [11]. Specific detection of MTB also prevents the misdiagnosis between MTB and nontuberculous mycobacteria (NTM).

Sensitivity and specificity
Sensitivity and specificity for smear-positive samples can reach 100% and 99%, respectively, and for smear-negative samples 67% and 99%, respectively, compared with the standard culture-based DST. False-positive results caused by silent mutations (eg, at codon 514 of *rpo*B), and false-negative results because of the inability to detect RIF-resistance mutations outside the hotspot region (eg, mutations at codon 572) [10,12].

Limitations
In Eswatini (previously Swaziland) more than 30% of patients with resistance to rifampicin (RR)-TB carried the I572 F mutation not included in the *rpo*B target and were missed by Xpert [12]. Additionally, it uses RIF resistance as a proxy for MDR-TB detection because it does not detect mutations in genes associated with isoniazid (INH) resistance, resulting in misdiagnosis of INH monoresistant TB cases [13]. INH resistance arises before RIF resistance in all lineages, geographic regions, and time periods. Hence, being unable to identify INH monoresistance is a limitation.

World Health Organization recommendation
GeneXpert MTB/RIF was first recommended by the WHO in 2010 for the diagnosis of pulmonary TB in adults from sputum specimens [14]. It has been also validated for the diagnosis of TB in children and for some specific forms of extrapulmonary TB since 2013.

Xpert MTB/RIF Ultra
Background
Recently, a larger amplification chamber to increase the amount of sputum and two additional targets (IS1081 and IS6110) to identify MTB, the next-generation Xpert MTB/RIF Ultra system (Cepheid), has enhanced

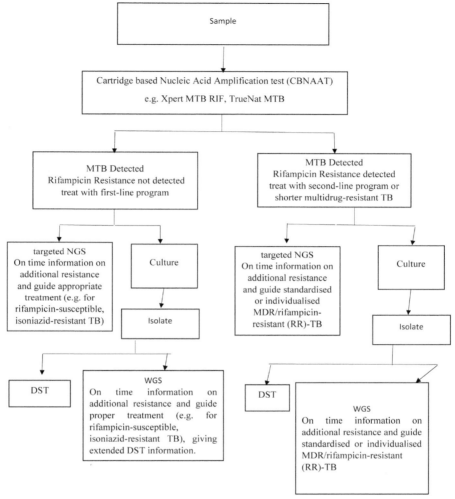

FIG. 1 Workflow of next-generation sequencing implementation. MDR, multidrug resistant; WGS, whole genome sequencing.

sensitivity of MTB detection [15]. By excluding *rpoB* mutations at Q513Q and F514 F, some silent mutation calls have been avoided.

Sensitivity and specificity

The Xpert MTB/RIF Ultra assay has increased the analytical sensitivity for the detection of MTB, by more than 10 times. MTB screening in specimens with low numbers of bacilli, such as sputum samples from children and from patients coinfected by human immunodeficiency virus, and in difficult-to-diagnose cases, such as smear-negative pulmonary and extrapulmonary TB with its higher MTB detection sensitivity (16 bacilli/

mL compared with 131 bacilli/mL for the current Xpert MTB/RIF cartridge), has expanded the utility of the assay [15]. Because of the higher sensitivity, the inevitable trade-off with the Xpert Ultra is specificity for MTB detection, which is lower than that of Xpert MTB/RIF [15]. RR-TB detection accuracy is similar for both cartridge types.

World Health Organization recommendations

Recently, WHO recommended using the Ultra cartridge as the initial diagnostic test for all adults and children with signs and symptoms of TB, and also for screening some extrapulmonary specimens, such as cerebrospinal fluid, lymph node, and tissue samples [16].

Xpert XDR-TB

For the detection of extensively drug-resistant (XDR)-TB, Xpert XDR cartridge is in development. The Xpert MTB/XDR assay will be evaluated for INH and second-line resistance detection, and the recommendation is to use it in diverse clinical settings.

Disadvantages

Uninterrupted electricity, temperature dependency, and cost have been cited as limitations of the Xpert equipment, particularly in resource-limited settings [17–19]. Annual recalibration of instruments is also required. Only 15 of the 48 (ie, 10% of all estimated TB cases globally in 2015) high TB-burden countries have used the Xpert tests for all suspected TB cases according to a 2016 WHO report.

TrueNat TB Test
Background

TB diagnosis within an hour and reflex testing for RR is possible with this chip-based technology. The TrueNat MTB and MTB Plus assays (Molbio Diagnostics, Chennai, India) also show comparable accuracy to the TB-LAMP assay as a replacement test for sputum smear microscopy. Compared with GeneXpert, TrueNat is more of a point-of-care test, but it is not fully automated. It is intended for situations where there might not be electricity and it can be deployed in areas where single testing is required and low RR is prevalent [20].

Description of methods

Using PCR, TrueNat works by the rapid detection of TB on a microchip. Any RR is detected by doing a second PCR. Automated battery-operated devices are used for the extraction of DNA (Trueprep Auto device, Molbio Diagnostics), amplification (TrueNat MTB chip, Molbio Diagnostics), and reading the presence of specific genomic sequences (Truelab PCR analyzer, Molbio Diagnostics).

Sensitivity and specificity

In 2013, TrueNat was found to have more than 91% sensitivity and 100% specificity [20].

World Health Organization recommendations

In December 2019, WHO validated the latest evidence on the use of the TrueNat MTB/RIF test and found it adequate in comparison with Xpert MTB Ultra [21].

LINE PROBE ASSAYS
Background

LPAs use multiple probes that allow the simultaneous detection of different mutations, and it is basically a DNA-DNA hybridization assay.

Description of Methods

LPA includes three-step DNA extraction, PCR (target amplification), and reverse hybridization [22]. Amplicons are hybridized to specific oligonucleotide probes that are complementary to the target sequences and are immobilized on the surface of a strip. The amplicon-probe hybrids are visualized by eye by presence or absence of bands on the strip, after several post-hybridization washes to remove nonspecific binding, and the turnaround time of the whole assay is 5 to 7 hours [22].

Several LPAs have been established that detect the hotspot regions of drug resistance and different genes are targeted by different assays. For example, only the *rpo*B hotspot region (codon 509 to codon 534; Asp516Val, His526Tyr, His526Asp, and Ser531Leu mutations) for MTB identification and RIF resistance is performed by the INNO-LiPA Rif TB LPA (Innogenetics, Zwijndrecht, Belgium). Three modules to detect first-line and second-line anti-TB drug resistance in culture and clinical specimens is possible by the AID TB Resistance LPA as follows [23].

Sensitivity and Specificity

High sensitivity and specificity for the detection of RIF, INH, Streptomycin (STR), Fluoroquinolones (FQs), and second-line injectable resistance (between 90% and 100%) has been observed [23]. However, uninterpretable results have been reported in up to 8.3% of smear-positive and 65% of smear-negative samples [24]. Good accuracy for the detection of MDR isolates in smear-positive specimens (sensitivity between 83.3% and 96.4%; specificity between 98.6% and 100%) has been observed by GenoType MTBDR*plus* VER2.0 [25]. High specificity (between 97% and 100%) for INH and RIF resistance screening is seen in cultured isolates and clinical (sputum) samples, but sensitivity varies between studies (from 50% to 95%) [26]. GenoType MTBDR*sl* VER 2.0 shows good sensitivity and specificity (between 91% and 100%) for detecting FQ resistance, but different sensitivity and specificity for the screening of resistance to second-line injectable drugs [27]. Thus, for detecting XDR isolates the overall Genotype MTBDRsl VER 2.0 specificity (between 59% and 100 %) and sensitivity (between

83% and 87%) differs among various studies [28]. Additionally, in sputum specimens, especially smear-negative samples, uninterpretable results were reported for drug resistance screening [28]. Some synonymous and nonsynonymous mutations (ie, that do not and that do change the encoded amino acid, respectively) in the gyrA gene prevent the hybridization of either the wild-type or mutant probe, leading to false-resistance results when GenoType MTBDRsl (VER1.0 and VER2.0) is used for FQ resistance screening [28]. In some regions even though these mutations (T80 A + A90 G, gcG/gcA A90 A, and atC/atT I92I) are not common, they account for around 7% of all MDR-TB strains [21].

World Health Organization Recommendations

Presently, WHO has recommended LPAs for the initial drug resistance screening of sputum smear-positive samples, which includes GenoType MTBDRplus, Geno-Type MTBDRsl (Hain LifeScience GmbH, Nehren, Germany), and Nipro NTM + MDR-TB (Nipro Co, Osaka, Japan) [18]. RIF and INH resistance detection by screening mutations in rpoB, katG, and the inhA promoter has been done by GenoType MTBDRplus VER2.0. MTB complex and its resistance to FQs, Ethambutol (EMB), and aminoglycosides/cyclic peptides by analyzing the gyrA, gyrB, rrs, embB, and eis genes is performed by GenoType MTBDRsl VER1.0 and VER2.0 [28]. This is used as the initial test for patients with confirmed RR-TB or MDR-TB. Four important Mycobacterium species (MTB, Mycobacterium avium, Mycobacterium intracellulare, and Mycobacterium kansasii) that cause the human disease are differentiated by Nipro NTM + MDR-TB, which also detects MDR-TB cases by targeting rpoB, katG, and inhA [28].

Disadvantages

These technologies require expertise and good laboratory infrastructure. The limitation of LPA target coverage is for the main DR mutations. Also, uninterpretable results need to be assessed. Finally, their sensitivity and specificity vary based on the mutation prevalence in the area under study.

SEQUENCING

Current molecular sequencing techniques have limitations because only a few genomic loci can be investigated simultaneously. The complexity and high sequencing cost of Sanger DNA sequencing developed in 1970s has remained a constraint [5].The advent of PSQ and then subsequently NGS in mid-2000s has somewhat ameliorated the cost with increase in sequencing output.

Pyrosequencing

The PyroMark (Qiagen, Hilden, Germany), which sequences short segments (<100 bp) of genomic DNA, is suitable for rapid detection of mutations with simple data handling [29]. Detection of drug resistance in MTB from culture isolates or directly from clinical specimens has been developed. PCR amplification of target sequences, capture of single-stranded DNA, and real-time sequencing are the three essential steps of PSQ. The deoxyribonucleotide triphosphate (dNTP) dispensation order is as follows: when the dNTP being dispensed is complementary to the first available base in the DNA template, hybridization occurs and pyrophosphate is generated. The end result of emission of light occurs when the pyrophosphate triggers a cascade of chemical reactions involving enzymes (adenosine triphosphate sulfurylase and luciferase) and substrates (adenosine 5'-phosphosulfate and luciferin). dNTP incorporated is proportional to the light generated. Representation of the bases sequenced is by the identity of dNTP incorporated. Sequence identities, wild-type or mutant, with high reproducibility and accuracy comparable with that of Sanger sequencing are results of PSQ. The sensitivity of PSQ ranged from 89% to 98% for the detection of phenotypic resistance to INH, RIF, FQ, and second-line injectables with high specificity of 94% to 100% [29].

Next-Generation Sequencing

Revolutionary changes have been seen in clinical microbiology practice by introduction of NGS technologies [30]. This technology allows for genotyping, outbreak investigation, and determination of known sequence variants involved in antimicrobial resistance and organism evolution [31]. Currently, there are several NGS-based technologies for targeted sequencing for DR-TB screening. For example, to detect first- and second-line drug resistance for full-length MTB gene analysis, eight genes (rpoB, katG, inhA, pncA, gyrA, eis, embB, and rpsL) are amplified and sequenced using Ion Torrent Personal Genome Machine (Thermo Fisher Scientific Inc, Waltham, MA) [32]. With varying sensitivity and specificity there are several NGS platforms on Illumina Inc (San Diego, CA; MiniSeq and MiSeq, or high-throughput [NextSeq 500, HiSeq 2500, and Novaseq]), Thermo Fisher Scientific Inc "benchtop" (Personal Genome Machine and S5) and high-throughput (Ion Proton), and RSII and Sequel (Pacific Biosciences of California Inc, Menlo Park, CA). MinION (Oxford Nanopore

Technologies Limited, Oxford, UK) offers similar workflow DNA extraction; library preparation through enzymatic or mechanical fragmentation, barcoding, and PCR amplification; and clustering and automated single and paired end sequencing [28]. The main advantage of WGS is that it covers the genome, provides epidemiologic information, and newer DR mechanisms for current and new drugs. However, it is best performed on culture isolates because it requires high quality and quantity of DNA [33].

Targeted Next-Generation Sequencing

Sequencing of large targets with a greater depth of sequence coverage, targeted NGS is implemented through either an amplicon-based assay or a hybridization/capture-based assay. High confidence mutation detection and detection of mixed populations, or compound resistance, within a sample can be assessed. This technology has been successfully implemented for the detection of TB drug resistance in clinical TB specimens. For DR-TB detection direct from sputum, two amplicon-based technologies are currently available, including the Next GenRDST assay (Translational Genomics Research Institute, Phoenix, AZ), which detects mutations in various MTBC gene regions associated with resistance to at least seven drugs [34], and the Deeplex-MycTB assay (GenoScreen, Lille, France), which is applied for identification of mycobacterial species and prediction of MTBC drug resistance through targeted NGS of 18 resistance-associated gene targets in a 24-plexed amplicon mix [35–37]. Reduction in the time and cost associated with TB culture makes these technologies an attractive option for DR-TB diagnosis in resource-limited settings.

Whole Genome Sequencing for Mycobacteria

WGS of mycobacteria has two main overlapping uses in clinical microbiology and public health. Both of these have direct patient benefits [38].

i. Prediction of DR phenotype is done by identification of genotype.
ii. Identification of transmission chains in potential outbreak scenarios is done by the determination of genetic relatedness. The advantages of WGS in the TB diagnostic workflow are clear when compared with standard DST; results are returned several weeks earlier and, in the future, this will only become faster and cheaper. Until WGS is routinely performed on sputum, results will lag by 1 to 2 weeks [38]. Nevertheless, the vastly increased resolution of WGS results means a more accurate

and comprehensive picture of resistance prediction than is currently possible.

Whole Genome Sequencing in Drug Resistance

For distinguishing between reinfection and persistent infection in isolates taken at different times from a single patient, WGS is a promising tool [39]. WGS has been used to demonstrate reinfection and persistent infection in MDR-TB based on the number of single-nucleotide polymorphisms: two single-nucleotide polymorphisms within 8 months for persistent infection versus greater than 60 single-nucleotide polymorphisms within 2 years for reinfection.

Direct DNA from Sputum and Whole Genome Sequencing

Attempts to use sputum as the direct source for WGS have been described. One of these include DNA sequence capture with biotinylated RNA bait oligonucleotides, spanning the entire MTB genome, followed by amplification and sequencing of the captured DNA [40]. This was applied to 24 TB sputum specimens and showed good on-target reads and depth of coverage for 23 samples with associated accurate prediction of drug resistance mutations. The genome sequence was able to identify a mixed infection with two strains in a single sample [39].

WGS has the potential to improve detection sensitivity for drugs, such as INH, over the currently available molecular tests. Interpretation of whole genome analysis is faster than current phenotypic testing methods mainly because of the ability to analyze raw sequence data and extract clinically relevant information in a few minutes [41]. A rapid and comprehensive view of the genotype of the organism, which enables reliable prediction of the drug susceptibility phenotype within a clinically acceptable time frame, is provided by WGS [39]. WGS of MTB provides resolution superior to that of current methods, such as spoligotyping and mycobacterial interspersed repetitive-unit–variable-number tandem repeat analysis for strain genotyping, and its usefulness in defining outbreaks has been demonstrated in earlier studies.

Targeted Next-Generation Sequencing Versus Whole Genome Sequencing

In the near future laboratories need to optimize their sequencing workflows for targeted NGS applications to directly sequence TB sputum samples. However, for epidemiologic investigations and various research applications WGS workflows may be preferred. Even for resource-limited settings, regardless of whether targeted NGS or WGS applications are implemented, these technologies will likely be available primarily at national reference laboratories, because these laboratories process a larger number of clinical specimens, making NGS applications more cost-effective than phenotypic methods. Additionally, if incorporated with workflows for the diagnosis of other MDR organisms and diseases, these applications become even more cost-effective [33]. Interpretation of mutations as predictors of MTB phenotypes and grading them as high confidence is paramount in understanding and extending these technologies as decision support tools. The Reseq TB platform is one such effort in this direction [42].

FUTURE DIRECTIONS

Implementing NGS or WGS in laboratories is complex, requires well-trained staff and training, adequate infrastructure, reliable power supply, a network with high-band Internet connections, computing capacity, and staff with adequate knowledge of bioinformatics. Having all these parameters in place is challenging, particularly for laboratories in resource-limited settings. Educational programs to train and certify technologists in these complex technologies have to be developed. These should assess performance, accuracy and reproducibility, quality control steps, quality thresholds use of standards and development of standard operating procedures, impact on turnaround times, and clinical management [30,43]. Microbiology laboratories introducing these technologies will need to undergo external proficiency testing programs that are already implemented in TB for molecular testing. Simple but comprehensive clinical reports are crucial to help clinicians arrive at the best decisions in the management of TB cases. A report should at least give information on sequencing quality and identification of mutations to infer genotyping and drug resistance profiles, and provide details on the exact nucleotide changes and standardized prediction of resistance levels. The future standard for DST and epidemiologic investigation in TB seems to be rooted in WGS and targeted NGS approaches [44,45]. Additional work is needed to address the feasibility of WGS from clinical specimens, to standardize and automate the laboratory procedures and postsequencing analyses, and to implement the NGS platforms in low-resource, high-burden settings.

SUMMARY

The progressive increase of DR-TB cases emphasizes the vital need for accurate and rapid diagnostic tools for their detection. The main current molecular techniques in low- and middle-income countries are cartridge-based nucleic acid tests, LPA, and sequencing. For the development and application of such tests/systems, cost, shelf-life, sample throughput, and accuracy are key factors. Target capacity and the personnel skills required for running the test are other factors that should be considered. Also, to have an actual impact, molecular diagnostic tests should be cheap for resource-poor countries, where TB and DR-TB are major problems, with a rapid turnaround time to quickly prescribe the adapted treatment to patients. Because the epidemiology of DR-TB is associated with mutations in different genes in different regions, an ideal test should simultaneously detect all known mutations in one reaction. A simple testing algorithm will increase the test accessibility at different laboratory levels.

DISCLOSURE

Dr.C.Rodrigues has received speaker honoraria from Pfizer, Cipla, Sanofi, Astrazeneca, Novartis.

REFERENCES

[1] World Health Organization (WHO). Guidelines for the programmatic management of drug-resistant tuberculosis, 2011 update. Geneva (Switzerland): World Health Organization; 2011.

[2] Kim SJ. Drug-susceptibility testing in tuberculosis: methods and reliability of results. Eur Respir J 2005;25: 564–9.

[3] WHO. Molecular line probe assays for rapid screening of patients at risk of multi-drug resistant tuberculosis 2008. Available at: http://www.who.int/tb/dots/%20laboratory/lpa_policy.pdf. Accessed November 18, 2009.

[4] WHO. Road map for rolling out Xpert MTB/RIF for rapid diagnosis of TB and MDR-TB. 2010. Available at: http://www.who.int/tb/dots/laboratory/roadmap_xpert_mtb-rif.pdf.

[5] Besser J, Carleton HA, Gerner-Smidt P, et al. Next-generation sequencing technologies and their application to the study and control of bacterial infections. Clin Microbiol Infect 2018;24:335–41.

[6] Goldberg B, Sichtig H, Geyer C, et al. Making the leap from research laboratory to clinic: challenges and opportunities for next-generation sequencing in infectious disease diagnostics. MBio 2015;6:e01888-15.

[7] Ajbani K, Lin SY, Rodrigues C, et al. Evaluation of pyrosequencing for detecting extensively drug-resistant *Mycobacterium tuberculosis* among clinical isolates from four

high-burden countries. Antimicrob Agents Chemother 2014;59(1):414–20.

[8] Available at: http://www.stoptb.org/wg/new_diagnostics/assets/documents/NGS%20Factsheet_EN_WEB.pdf.

[9] Global Laboratory Initiative (GLI), Stop TB Partnership. GLI Model TB diagnostic algorithms. 2018. Available at: www.stoptb.org/wg/gli/assets/documents/GLI_algorithms.pdf.

[10] Bunsow E, Ruiz-Serrano MJ, López Roa P, et al. Evaluation of GeneXpert MTB/RIF for the detection of Mycobacterium tuberculosis and resistance to rifampin in clinical specimens. J Infect 2014;68:338–43.

[11] Steingart KR, Schiller I, Horne DJ, et al. Xpert R MTB/RIF assay for pulmonary tuberculosis and rifampicin resistance in adults. Cochrane Database Syst Rev 2014;(1): CD009593.

[12] Sanchez-Padilla E, Merker M, Beckert P, et al. Detection of drug-resistant tuberculosis by Xpert MTB/RIF in Swaziland. N Engl J Med 2015;372:1181–2.

[13] Manson AL, Cohen KA, Abeel T, et al. Genomic analysis of globally diverse Mycobacterium tuberculosis strains provides insights into the emergence and spread of multidrug resistance. Nat Genet 2017;49:395–402.

[14] WHO endorses new rapid tuberculosis test". Geneva (Switzerland): WHO; 2010. Available at: www.who.int/mediacentre/news/releases/2010/.

[15] Chakravorty S, Simmons M, Rowneki M, et al. The new xpert MTB/RIF ultra: improving detection of Mycobacterium tuberculosis and resistance to rifampin in an assay suitable for point-of-care testing. mBio 2017;8: e00812–7.

[16] WHO. Global tuberculosis report 2017. Geneva (Switzerland): WHO; 2017.

[17] Walzl G, McNerney R, du Plessis N, et al. Tuberculosis: advances and challenges in development of new diagnostics and biomarkers. Lancet Infect Dis 2018;18: E199–210.

[18] WHO. Global tuberculosis report 2016. Geneva (Switzerland): WHO; 2017.

[19] Trébucq A, Enarson DA, Chiang CY, et al. Xpert® MTB/RIF for national tuberculosis programmes in low-income countries: when, where and how? Int J Tuberc Lung Dis 2011; 15(12):1567–72. https://doi.org/10.5588/ijtld.11.0392.

[20] Nikam C, Jagannath M, Narayanan MM. Rapid diagnosis of Mycobacterium tuberculosis with TrueNat MTB: a near-care approach. PLoS One 2013;8(1):e51121. Available at: http://journals.plos.org/.

[21] Guideline development Group meeting. 2019. Available at: https://www.who.int/tb/areas-of-work/laboratory/en/. Accessed 3-6 December 2019.

[22] Makinen J, Marttila HJ, Marjama M, et al. Comparison of two commercially available DNA line probe assays for detection of multidrug-resistant Mycobacterium tuberculosis. J Clin Microbiol 2006;44:350–2.

[23] Molina-Moya B, Lacoma A, Prat C, et al. AID TB resistance line probe assay for rapid detection of resistant Mycobacterium tuberculosis in clinical samples. J Infect 2014;70:400–8.

[24] Deggim-Messmer V, Bloemberg GV, Ritter C, et al. Diagnostic molecular mycobacteriology in regions with low tuberculosis endemicity: combining real-time PCR assays for detection of multiple mycobacterial pathogens with line probe assays for identification of resistance mutations. EBioMedicine 2016;9:228–37.

[25] Bai Y, Wang Y, Shao C, et al. GenoType MTBDRplus assay for rapid detection of multidrug resistance in Mycobacterium tuberculosis: a meta-analysis. PLoS One 2016; 11:e0150321.

[26] Mitarai S, Kato S, Ogata H, et al. Comprehensive multicenter evaluation of a new line probe assay kit for identification of Mycobacterium species and detection of drug-resistant Mycobacterium tuberculosis. J Clin Microbiol 2012;50:884–90.

[27] Bang D, Andersen SR, Vasiliauskienë E, et al. Performance of the GenoType MTBDRplus assay (v2.0) and a new extended GenoType MTBDRsl assay (v2.0) for the molecular detection of multi- and extensively drug-resistant Mycobacterium tuberculosis on isolates primarily from Lithuania. Diagn Microbiol Infect Dis 2016;86:377–81.

[28] Available at: https://www.frontiersin.org/articles/10.3389/fmicb.2019.00794/full#B14. Accessed April 16, 2019.

[29] Georghiou SB, Seifert M, Lin SY, et al. Shedding light on the performance of a pyrosequencing assay for drug-resistant tuberculosis diagnosis. BMC Infect Dis 2016; 16(1):458.

[30] Rossen JWA, Friedrich AW, Moran-Gilad J, et al. Practical issues in implementing whole-genome-sequencing in routine diagnostic microbiology. Clin Microbiol Infect 2018;24:355–60.

[31] Cabibbe AM, Walker TM, Niemann S, et al. Whole genome sequencing of Mycobacterium tuberculosis. Eur Respir J 2018;52:1801163.

[32] Daum LT, Rodriguez JD, Worthy SA, et al. Next-generation ion torrent sequencing of drug resistance mutations in Mycobacterium tuberculosis strains. J Clin Microbiol 2012;50:3831–7.

[33] WHO. The use of next-generation sequencing technologies for the detection of mutations associated with drug resistance in Mycobacterium tuberculosis complex: technical guide. Geneva (Switzerland): World Health Organization; 2018.

[34] Colman RE, Anderson J, Lemmer D, et al. Rapid drug susceptibility testing of drug-resistant Mycobacterium tuberculosis isolates directly from clinical samples by use of amplicon sequencing: a proof-of-concept study. J Clin Microbiol 2016;54(8):2058–67.

[35] Tagliani E, Hassan MO, Waberi Y, et al. Culture and next-generation sequencing-based drug susceptibility testing unveil high levels of drug-resistant-TB in Djibouti: results from the first national survey. Sci Rep 2017;7(1):17672.

[36] Mycobacterium tuberculosis prediction of drug resistance on clinical samples by deep sequencing. Available at:

https://www.genoscreen.fr/images/genoscreen/pla-quette/DEEPLEX-MycTBSOLUTION—GenoScreen.pdf. Accessed May 10.

[37] Ritter C, Lucke K, Sirgel FA, et al. Evaluation of the AID TB resistance line probe assay for rapid detection of genetic alterations associated with drug resistance in *Mycobacterium tuberculosis* strains. J Clin Microbiol 2014;52: 940–6.

[38] Witney AA, Cosgrove CA, Arnold A, et al. Clinical use of whole genome sequencing for *Mycobacterium tuberculosis*. BMC Med 2016;14:46.

[39] Faksri K, Tan JH, Disratthakit A, et al. Whole-genome sequencing analysis of serially isolated multi-drug and extensively drug resistant *Mycobacterium tuberculosis* from Thai patients. PLoS One 2016;11(8):e0160992.

[40] Brown AC, Bryant JM, Einer-Jensen K, et al. Rapid whole-genome sequencing of *Mycobacterium tuberculosis* isolates directly from clinical samples. J Clin Microbiol 2015; 53(7):2230–7.

[41] Coll F, McNerney R, Preston MD, et al. Rapid determination of anti-tuberculosis drug resistance from whole-genome sequences. Genome Med 2015;7:51.

[42] Miotto P, Tessema B, Tagliani E, et al. A standardised method for interpreting the association between mutations and phenotypic drug resistance in *Mycobacterium tuberculosis*. Eur Respir J 2017;50:170135.

[43] Kozyreva VK, Truong CL, Greninger AL, et al. Validation and implementation of clinical laboratory improvements act-compliant whole-genome sequencing in the public health microbiology laboratory. J Clin Microbiol 2017; 55:2502–20.

[44] Ellington MJ, Ekelund O, Aarestrup FM, et al. The role of whole genome sequencing in antimicrobial susceptibility testing of bacteria: report from the EUCAST Subcommittee. Clin Microbiol Infect 2017;23:2–22.

[45] Lee RS, Pai M. Real-time sequencing of *Mycobacterium tuberculosis*: are we there yet? J Clin Microbiol 2017;55: 1249–54.

Advances in Molecular Pathology 3 (2020) 97–105

ADVANCES IN MOLECULAR PATHOLOGY

The Role of Human Immunodeficiency Virus Molecular Diagnostics in Ending the Epidemic

Justin Laracy, MD[a], Jason Zucker, MD[b],*

[a]NewYork-Presbyterian Hospital/Columbia University Irving Medical Center, New York, NY, USA; [b]Department of Medicine, Division of Infectious Diseases, Columbia University Irving Medical Center, 622 West 168th Street, 8th Floor, New York, NY 10032, USA

KEYWORDS
- HIV • Viral load • Molecular diagnostics • EtE

KEY POINTS
- Since the discovery and identification of the human immunodeficiency virus (HIV) virus in the early 1980s, the HIV/AIDS pandemic has spread to all corners of the globe.
- Over the subsequent decades, HIV diagnostic techniques have transformed the landscape of patient care.
- As the technologies have evolved, HIV molecular assays have allowed for large-scale population surveillance and individual patient diagnosis and management.
- This article aims to summarize the relevance of molecular testing in HIV diagnosis and to review the role of molecular diagnostics in primary and secondary prevention, with a special focus on algorithms for large-scale population testing.
- Lastly, this article discusses novel prevention efforts utilizing molecular epidemiology to characterize transmission networks across populations.

MOLECULAR DIAGNOSTICS TO END THE HUMAN IMMUNODEFICIENCY EPIDEMIC

Tremendous progress has been made over the past decades with respect to the understanding of the immunopathogenesis of human immunodeficiency virus (HIV)/AIDS. This progress has transformed the HIV epidemic from an unprecedented human catastrophe to a potentially manageable chronic disease for individuals with access to appropriate medical care. In 2014, the Joint United Nations Programme on HIV and AIDS (UNAIDS) announced an ambitious treatment target, with the aim of ending the AIDS epidemic, the "90-90-90: Treatment For All" program. The objective of the program is that by 2020, 90% of all people living with HIV will know their HIV status, 90% of all people diagnosed with HIV infection will receive sustained antiretroviral therapy (ART), and 90% of all people receiving ART will have viral suppression [1]. The benefits of HIV viral suppression are multifold but include individual patients benefits and treatment as prevention to limit transmission of the virus to HIV-negative individuals.

Despite these advances and hopeful ambitions, HIV infection continues to present major diagnostic and management challenges on a global scale. According the most recent statistics from the Centers for Disease Control and Prevention (CDC), in 2018, there were 37.9 million people living with HIV around the world and 770,000 deaths from AIDS-related illnesses, with sub-Saharan Africa, which bears the heaviest burden of HIV and AIDS worldwide, accounting for 61% of all new HIV infections [2]. The third objective of the

---

*Corresponding author, E-mail address: JZ2700@cumc.columbia.edu

https://doi.org/10.1016/j.yamp.2020.07.009
2589-4080/20/

90-90-90 goal—that 90% of all individuals with HIV achieve viral suppression—reflects the critical role molecular diagnostics plays in the struggle to end the epidemic.

A detailed understanding of the time course of viremia, antigen detectability, and antibody seroconversion during acute HIV infection is essential for optimizing screening and diagnostic algorithms. Primary infection, a period of rapid viral replication and infection of CD4 cells, is characterized by an exponential rise in viral titers to extraordinary levels in the plasma [3]. By approximately 6 months, plasma viremia declines to a set point, coinciding with the emergence of HIV-1–specific cytotoxic T lymphocytes [4].

Despite the introduction of newer-generation antigen/antibody screening tests capable of earlier HIV infection, molecular diagnostic techniques continue to play a central role in the diagnosis of HIV. Modern fourth-generation enzyme-linked immunoassays (which test for both IgM and IgG antibodies and p24 antigen) can detect HIV infection 13 days to 42 days after infection [5]. Nucleic acid amplification testing (NAAT) of HIV-1 RNA allows for the diagnosis of acute infection in the window period before fourth-generation HIV antigen/antibody combination immunoassay turns positive, closing the gap by an additional 7 days. Early detection of acute HIV using molecular diagnostics allows for linkage to care and rapid initiation of ART, which now is recognized to facilitate immune function, limit the size of the viral reservoir, and reduce the risk of onward transmission during a time of high viremia characteristic of acute infection [6].

THE ROLE OF MOLECULAR DIAGNOSTICS IN PRIMARY PREVENTION
The Role of Molecular Diagnostics in Patients Adherent to Pre-exposure Prophylaxis

Pre-exposure prophylaxis (PrEP) is an important tool in efforts to end the HIV epidemic. The current CDC testing algorithm begins with an initial fourth-generation HIV antigen/antibody combination immunoassay followed by an HIV-1/HIV-2 differentiation immunoassay if positive and an NAAT if indeterminate or inconclusive [7]. There has been no consensus interpretation on how PrEP could have an impact on diagnosis of acute HIV infection, and the challenge of screening with current algorithms is highlighted by the statement from the Association of Public Health Laboratories stating that more data are needed to assess

the likelihood of false-negative results in individuals on PrEP [8].

In the Partners PrEP study, a randomized placebo-controlled trial conducted in Kenya and Uganda to investigate whether PrEP alters timing and patterns of seroconversion after HIV infection, it was found that PrEP delayed the time to seroconversion [9]. Using the Fiebig classification schema of sequential assay reactivity in primary HIV-1 infection [10], the study found a consistent pattern of relative increase in time to reach each Fiebig stage in individuals taking PrEP. The study concluded that the delay in progression of seroconversion was likely the result of PrEP's suppression of viral replication, a claim supported by the finding that plasma HIV RNA levels were approximately 0.75 log lower compared with those taking placebo [9].

There now are several case reports of individuals seroconverting while taking PrEP and, in many, the diagnosis was challenging due to a low or undetectable viral load. A recent report demonstrates the importance of sensitive viral load testing in patients adherent to PrEP [11]. In this case, a patient was started on PrEP 7 days after testing negative with a third-generation rapid HIV and HIV-1 RNA qualitative polymerase chain reaction (PCR). A fourth-generation HIV test was negative on the day of initiation. Twenty-eight days later he returned to clinic where a fourth-generation test was positive, but the supplemental HIV-1/HIV-2 confirmation assay was negative. A qualitative HIV-1 RNA sent to the state Department of Health for analysis. Four days later, the fourth-generation test was repeated and a DNR/RNA qualitative PCR Abbott Combo antigen/antibody screen and a qualitative DNR/RNA PCR (COBAS-Qualitative, AmpliPrep/TaqMan HIV-1 Qual Test) were negative. An HIV-1 RNA quantitative PCR was sent this same day, and viral RNA was detected but below the lower limit of detection. The RNA PCR sent to the Department of Health ultimately returned with detectable viremia 18 days later. Because of the delayed seroconversion secondary to PrEP adherence during acute infection, providers should consider using viral load testing in high risk individuals.

Serologic testing in populations with a low incidence of HIV represents another potential shortcoming of antigen/antibody assays. In settings with effective HIV prevention strategies, rapid HIV assays are the mainstay of HIV diagnosis. When HIV prevalence or incidence falls due to effective HIV prevention strategies, the proportion of HIV assays that are falsely positive will rise. In a study assessing the frequency of true-positive and false-positive rapid HIV assay results in the Partners PrEP study, among individuals receiving PrEP the number of false-positive results was greater than the number of true-positive results [12].

These studies highlight the unique potential advantages of HIV molecular diagnostics for the diagnosis of HIV in low prevalence settings or populations or individuals with potential delayed seroconversion due to PrEP.

The Role of Molecular Diagnostics in Pooled Sampling

Acute HIV-1 infection is a time of rapid viral turnover, with peak plasma HIV-1 RNA levels up to 10 [6] copies/mL [13]. For many individuals, this dynamic phase of high viral replication is accompanied by a nonspecific mononucleosis-like syndrome that can be undiagnosed or misdiagnosed [14]. Diagnosis at the early stages of HIV infection is critical for patient counseling and intervention. Early diagnosis allows for the counseling of patients regarding behavior modification during this highly infectious acute period. The probability of transmitting HIV is closely correlated with the viral burden in plasma. In a rhesus macaque model, plasma from animals with acute infection was up to 750 as infectious, on a per virion basis, as plasma from animals with chronic infection [15]. Although models used to estimate the role of acute infections in the spread of HIV have produced varied results [16], acute infection continues to be a primary focus of public health prevention efforts to limit the spread of HIV. Current guidelines strongly encourage early initiation of effective ART therapy given the benefits early treatment found in the START and TEMPRANO trials [17–19]. With an estimated 1.7 million new HIV infections in 2018 [20], the need for population-level testing strategies to improve early detection of HIV is critically important.

The pooling of individual serum samples as a cost-saving technique to diagnose infectious processes first was used successfully for syphilis [21] and still is used by the American Red Cross to screen millions of blood donations per year [22]. The use of algorithms for testing of pooled specimens has been proposed as a method to make HIV NAAT accurate and cost effective [23]. The use of pooled testing using NAAT prior to seroconversion is being investigated as a tool to test en masse for acute HIV infection. Because of the high viral load typical of acute infection, plasma can be diluted for the purposes of pooled sampling and still yield a positive test for HIV RNA [24]. In contrast, the dynamic curve of p24 antigen in serum during acute infection does not allow for an individual's serum to be diluted into a pool and still yield a positive result.

In an older study of 700 seronegative patients in India, a multistage pooling algorithm for HIV RNA was more sensitive and 5-fold less expensive than individual p24 antigen testing [24]. One study investigated the use of pooled HIV RNA testing in a large urban medical center in the United States, where it was found to increase HIV case detection by 3.5% [25].

In a more recent 12-month observational study conducted in North Carolina, the diagnostic performance of standard HIV antibody tests was compared with an algorithm whereby serum from individuals who tested negative by standard testing were tested again by pooled nucleic acid amplification. Of 606 total HIV-positive results, 23 acutely infected persons were identified only with the use of the NAAT [26]. In a prospective, multi-site study of 5 community-based programs in New York, California, and North Carolina, participants were screened with a rapid point-of-care supplemental HIV-1/HIV-2 antibody test [27]. Participants who screened negative then were tested with a fourth-generation HIV antigen/antibody combination immunoassay and with pooled HIV RNA testing in an attempt to diagnose acute HIV infection. Of the 86,836 participants who were tested, 168 participants were diagnosed with acute HIV. Of the 168 cases of acute infection, the combination assay detected 134 cases versus the 164 cases detected by the pooled HIV RNA testing strategy. These values equate to an increase in sensitivity from 79.8% to 97.6% when using the HIV antigen/antibody testing versus pooled HIV RNA testing, respectively, with an increase in relative diagnostic yield of 2.6% [27].

Although additional research is needed to evaluate the utility and cost effectiveness of pooled testing strategies for HIV RNA across high-incidence and low-incidence populations, 1 study showed that pooled NAAT testing in men who have sex with men and injection drug users in the United States may be cost effective, given the sufficiently high prevalence of HIV in these populations [28].

THE ROLE OF MOLECULAR DIAGNOSTICS IN SECONDARY PREVENTION
Treatment as Prevention

In 2016, the Prevention Access Campaign launched the treatment as prevention slogan "Undetectable = Untransmittable", or U = U, to signify that individuals with HIV on effective ART therapy who have achieved and maintained an undetectable viral load cannot sexually transmit the virus to others [29].

The concept of U = U has broad implications for the treatment of HIV infection from a scientific and public health standpoint and also for the self-esteem of individuals living with the stigma associated with HIV. Because of the promise of U = U, achieving and maintaining an undetectable viral load have become aspirational goals and offer hope to providers and patients alike in the fight against HIV [30].

The use of molecular diagnostic viral load testing has been fundamental to the body of research that has generated the U = U concept. The first declaration of U = U came from a 2008 article published by the Swiss Federal Commission for HIV/AIDS [31]. It was not until several years later, however, with the support of evidence provided by randomized clinical trials that U = U was embraced more universally. The HIV Prevention Trials Network 052 study published in 2011, comparing early versus delayed ART therapy in HIV-discordant couples, found a 96% relative reduction in HIV transmission in the early ART group [32]. After an additional 5 years of follow-up to the 052 study, in which there were no linked transmissions when viral load was suppressed by ART, the protective effect of early ART in maintaining viral suppression and preventing HIV transmissions was further validated [33]. Building on these studies, the PARTNER 1 study showed that in HIV-discordant couples, in which the HIV-positive partner was on ART and had maintained viral suppression, there were no HIV transmissions [34]. The Opposites Attract study showed that in HIV-discordant men who have sex with men, when the HIV-positive partner was adherent to ARVs and had viral loads consistently less than 200 copies/mL, there were no phylogenetically linked transmissions [35]. Similarly, the PARTNER 2 study showed that in HIV-discordant men who have sex with men, there were no transmissions across 2072 couple-years of follow-up and 76,088 condomless sex acts, if the partner with HIV was on ART and had achieved viral suppression [36]. A systematic review of 12 recent studies concluded that there was minimal to no risk of HIV sexual transmission among HIV-discordant couples when the partner with HIV adheres to ART and maintains a suppressed viral load of less than 200 copies/mL, measured routinely every 4 months to 6 months [37]. These findings have culminated with the CDC endorsing that a person with HIV who has achieved viral suppression with ART "has effectively no risk of sexually transmitting HIV to HIV-negative partners" [38]. Achieving viral load suppression for at least 6 months while continuing to remain adherent to ARVs is when U = U becomes applicable [39,40]. For HIV-positive patients adherent to ART, viral load testing is the most important indicator of initial and sustained response to ART. Much as viral load suppression is used to determine efficacy of a patient's ART regimen and the attainment of U = U status, failure to achieve viral suppression is the first sign to providers that viral resistance should be considered [17].

Medical providers should routinely communicate the concept of U = U to all their patients living with HIV, because the benefits of informing patients with HIV about U = U are substantial. Awareness of U = U incentivizes attainment and maintenance of viral suppression, thus strengthening patients motivation to initiate and adhere to ART therapy. Beyond that, education surrounding U = U offers psychosocial benefits by alleviating the stigma of being HIV positive and relieving the guilt surrounding potential transmission. Widespread dissemination of treatment as prevention messaging has the potential to shift public discourse away from HIV-positive individuals as vectors of transmission and may lead to changes in legal and public health policies that represent structural forms of HIV stigma [41]. Despite the robust scientific evidence in support of U = U and the positive implications of public awareness, widespread misinformation surrounding U = U persists. In a recent international survey of more than 1000 providers, it was found that only 77% of infectious disease specialists and 42% of primary care physicians communicated the message of U = U to patients when sharing the news of their undetectable viral load [42]. In another United States–based study among men who have sex with men, it was found that even among HIV-positive men, nearly one-third of the participants viewed the slogan "Undetectable = Untransmittable" as somewhat or completely inaccurate [43]. Targeted education campaigns to more widely disseminate and promote the concept of U = U to the general public are needed.

There also is evidence to suggest that some providers of HIV care may doubt the concept of U = U. One study based in Africa found that many providers lacked confidence in U = U and continued to counsel condom use even after viral suppression was achieved, and others reported that they did not counsel patients about the reduced risk of transmission after viral suppression for fear of being blamed if HIV transmission did occur [44]. Similarly, a United States–based study of HIV practitioners found that only 51% accepted the evidence of the efficacy of treatment as prevention and would not recommend the safety of condomless sex [45]. The use of point-of-care HIV RNA viral load testing may have an important role to play in assuring providers, patients, and partners that the patient has achieved viral suppression and there is no risk of transmission [46]. Pooled data from the PARTNER, Opposites Attract, and PARTNER 2 studies produces a combined transmission risk estimate for condomless less among heterosexual or men who have sex with men couples of 0.00 per 100 couple-years [47].

CD4 Versus Viral Load Testing and Low-Income and Middle-Income Countries

Global shifts in the HIV treatment response in low-income and middle-income countries (LMICs) have driven rapid changes in the prioritization of CD4 and viral load testing. The 2003 World Health Organization (WHO) global HIV treatment guidelines did not recommend viral load monitoring for LMICs due to the requirements for transportation, limited assay availability, and relatively high cost of viral load monitoring. Instead, clinical monitoring and CD4 count measurements were used to detect treatment failure [48]. In the years following the initial WHO HIV treatment guidelines, advances in molecular diagnostic testing and new management guidelines challenged the initial recommendation not to use viral load testing to monitor the outcome of HIV treatment. The "third 90" of the 2014 UNAIDS 90-90-90 campaign promotes the goal of 90% viral suppression by 2030, further emphasizing the need for global viral load testing. Perhaps most critical to the transition away from CD4 testing has been the WHO 2016 recommendation to treat all HIV-positive individuals regardless of immune status [49], because this led to the loss of one of the primary indications for CD4 testing.

Although CD4 testing continues to serve an important role in the management of HIV-positive individuals in LMICs, the scale-up of viral load monitoring has absorbed most of the resources dedicated to laboratory services. This reflects primarily the shift toward starting ART irrespective of CD4 count and using viral load for routine monitoring of immunologic response to ART [50]. A 2018 study forecasting the global demand for HIV monitoring and diagnostic tests predicted a gradual decline in the number of CD4 tests with a concomitant rise in viral load testing [51]. The scaling up of HIV viral load testing capabilities in LMICs represents a massive public health undertaking, and lessons learned from large-scale CD4 testing programs can inform more effective scale-up of viral load testing [52]. One potential solution that has emerged is the adoption of existing platforms that are already established in LMICs. For example, the GeneXpert technology, used for tuberculosis diagnosis, has been shown efficacious in viral load testing in countries, such as South Africa and India [53,54].

Increasing viral load monitoring for patients on ART therapy requires lowering costs associated with testing and improving access in LMICs. Certainly, all stakeholders are concerned about the financial strain that large-scale testing changes may have on their already limited health care resources. A diagnostic access initiative launched in 2014 by UNAIDS challenged the global community to work with manufacturers to provide reasonably priced viral load testing [55]. Several older studies concluded that routine viral load monitoring is cost effective in LMICs [56,57]. More recent studies have concluded that the cost effectiveness of viral load monitoring in LMICs depends on the context and manner in which it is delivered. One study found that that the 3 main factors that will make viral load testing in LMICs cost effective are the use of lower-cost testing strategies, ensuring that viral load results are acted on, and using viral load results to facilitate differentiated care [58]. A pooled testing strategy of HIV-positive patients adherent to ART holds promise as a method of reducing costs of viral load testing in LMICs. The utility of pooled viral load testing to diagnose acute/early HIV infection is discussed previously. There is a body of literature examining the efficacy of pooled viral load testing of HIV-infected patient on ART to assess for virologic failure. One study found that an algorithm for pooled viral load testing of HIV-infected children in Kenya on ART was efficient at detecting virologic failure, had a high negative predictive value, and offered substantial cost savings [59]. Another study of HIV-positive adults in South Africa on ART with a low pretest probability of virologic failure found that pooled viral load testing could reduce the cost of virologic monitoring without compromising accuracy [60].

Viral load monitoring is the preferred method of immunologic monitoring of HIV-infected patients on ART because it allows earlier and more accurate detection of treatment failure than any other testing strategy. In order to achieve the ambitious targets set forth by the UNAIDS 90-90-90 initiative, viral load testing for HIV-infected patients must become more widely available in LMICs. Of the estimated 19.5 million people in LMICs on ART, fewer than 40% have routine access to VL testing [61]. Continued efforts to scale-up viral load testing in LMICs will be a crucial and necessary step in the fight to end the HIV epidemic.

The Role of Molecular Diagnostics in Tracing Human Immunodeficiency Across Populations

The connectivity of infectious disease transmission networks can have implications for the design and targeting of public health intervention practices. Molecular techniques have been used to evaluate transmission clusters of infectious diseases, such as tuberculosis and syphilis, dating from the 1990s [62,63]. Molecular techniques to monitor HIV transmission dynamics within populations are being investigated as new methods of identifying high-risk clusters, with the ultimate goal of being able to interrupt HIV transmission.

HIV genetic sequence data can provide valuable insight into viral transmission dynamics. The genetic profile of HIV within a person is determined by numerous factors, including the genetic background of the infecting virus, the high mutation rate of the virus, the target cell availability of the host, and the potential pressures of ART [64–67]. As a result of the genetic heterogeneity of HIV between individuals, the genetic composition of HIV is relatively unique to each infected person. By comparing the degree of HIV genetic relatedness between individuals, viral sequencing analysis can be used to investigate HIV transmission networks to better inform public health prevention interventions. Molecular techniques have been used to trace HIV transmission across various network types. In a 1992 study, molecular biologic analysis using PCR of the HIV proviral envelope gene was used to demonstrate that a HIV-positive dentist transmitted the virus to 5 patients who had undergone an invasive dental procedures [68]. In a 2004 study focused on the Los Angeles adult entertainment industry, genetic sequencing data of the *env* and *gag* genes was able to show that an acutely HIV-infected man had transmitted the virus to 2 women during the production of adult films [69]. Molecular epidemiology approaches have been used to evaluate other variables in HIV transmission networks that may help to inform public health interventions. One United Kingdom–based study constructed dated phylogenies based on *pol* gene sequences to conclude that a small proportion of self-reported heterosexual men diagnosed with HIV could have been infected homosexually [69]. International transmission routes also have been evaluated using molecular testing. Phylogenetic network analysis on HIV-infected individuals at the San Diego, California –Tijuana, Mexico, border found evidence of bidirectional cross-border transmission, thus highlighting the border region as a melting pot of high-risk groups [70]. ART resistance transmission dynamics also have been characterized using molecular phylogenetic analysis [71].

HIV transmission network analyses using routinely collected HIV resistance genotypes can be implemented to direct public health resources toward transmission hotspots. In a 2016 study, an automated phylogenetic system monitoring database using routinely collected HIV genotypes was used to detect an HIV outbreak to support an ensuing public health response. Their approach was cost effective, attained near real-time monitoring of new cases, and can be implemented in all settings where HIV genotyping is the standard of care [72]. A recent study based out of New York City (NYC) sought to investigate whether HIV transmission network dynamics could identify individuals and clusters of individuals most like to transmit HIV [73]. In this study, *Pro/RT* gene sequencing from an NYC surveillance registry of more than 65,000 genotyped individuals was used to identify correlates of cluster growth. It was found that by interrogating the history of past cluster growth, the clusters with the greatest potential future growth could be identified. Another NYC-based study found that genetic linkage may provide more reliable evidence of identifying potential transmission partners than partner naming [74]. HIV molecular epidemiology has been coupled with partner contact tracing with the ultimately goal of being able to interrupt HIV transmission. One study based out of San Diego, California, used phylogenetic clustering to identify individuals within highly related HIV transmission groups, and then contact tracing was used to define transmission clusters [75].

Novel public health interventions to understand transmission dynamics within populations are needed to better develop interventions aimed at the interruption of viral transmission. As discussed in this article, molecular testing can be used to track the spread HIV within and across populations. In this way, molecular testing may become another instrument in the fight to end the HIV epidemic.

In 2018, more than 37,000 new cases of HIV were diagnosed in the United States, with 1.7 million new cases worldwide [20,76]. There is no doubt that enormous progress has been made in regard to understanding of HIV and in regard to the diagnosis and management of individuals living with HIV. The concept of U = U is testament to this progress, and the "90-90-90: Treatment For All" program reflects current ambitions to end the HIV epidemic. The contribution of molecular diagnostics toward this progress cannot be overstated. Without molecular testing to assess transmission risk in individuals with viral suppression, the very idea of U = U could not be proved and the 90-90-90 program could not exist. This article describes the critical role of HIV molecular diagnostics in ending the epidemic. The use of viral load testing in patients adherent to PrEP, pooled sampling of patient plasma for viral load testing, the role of molecular diagnostics in the concept of treatment as prevention, the evolution of viral load testing in LMICs, and the use of molecular diagnostics in tracking HIV across populations are reviewed.

DISCLOSURE

The authors have nothing to disclose.

REFERENCES

[1] 90-90-90: treatment for all | UNAIDS. Available at: https://www.unaids.org/en/resources/909090. Accessed May 13, 2020.

[2] Basic Statistics | HIV Basics | HIV/AIDS | CDC. Available at: https://www.cdc.gov/hiv/basics/statistics.html. Accessed May 13, 2020.

[3] Clark SJ, Saag MS, Decker WD, et al. High titers of cytopathic virus in plasma of patients with symptomatic primary HIV-1 infection. N Engl J Med 1991;324(14):954–60.

[4] Koup RA, Safrit JT, Cao Y, et al. Temporal association of cellular immune responses with the initial control of viremia in primary human immunodeficiency virus type 1 syndrome. J Virol 1994;68(7):4650–5.

[5] HIV Testing Overview | HIV.gov. Available at: https://www.hiv.gov/hiv-basics/hiv-testing/learn-about-hiv-testing/hiv-testing-overview. Accessed May 13, 2020.

[6] Smith MK, Rutstein SE, Powers KA, et al. The detection and management of early HIV infection: A clinical and public health emergency. J Acquir Immune Defic Syndr 2013;63(SUPPL. 2):S187.

[7] Branson BM, Owen SM, Wesolowski LG, et al. Laboratory testing for the diagnosis of HIV infection : updated recommendations - guidelines and Recommendations. Centers for disease control and prevention; 2014. p. 4–7. https://doi.org/10.15620/cdc.23447.

[8] Association of Public Health Laboratories. Suggested Reporting Language for the Diagnostic Testing Algorithm. 2013;(November):1-8. Available at: https://www.aphl.org/aboutAPHL/publications/Documents/ID_2017Apr-HIV-Lab-Test-Suggested-Reporting-Language.pdf Accessed May 11, 2020.

[9] Donnell D, Ramos E, Celum C, et al. The effect of oral preexposure prophylaxis on the progression of HIV-1 seroconversion. AIDS 2017;31(14):2007–16.

[10] Fiebig E, Wright D, Rawal B, et al. Dynamics of HIV viremia and antibody seroconversion in plasma donors: implications for diagnosis and staging of primary HIV infection. AIDS 2003;17(August 2002):1871–9.

[11] Zucker J, Carnevale C, Rai AJ, et al. Positive or Not, That is the Question: HIV Testing for Individuals on Pre-Exposure Prophylaxis (PrEP). J Acquir Immune Defic Syndr 2018. https://doi.org/10.1097/QAI.0000000000001665.

[12] Ndase P, Celum C, Kidoguchi L, et al. Frequency of false positive rapid HIV serologic tests in African men and women receiving PrEP for HIV prevention: Implications for programmatic roll-out of biomedical interventions. PLoS One 2015;10(4):1–8.

[13] Lavreys L, Baeten JM, Overbaugh J, et al. Virus Load during Primary Human Immunodeficiency Virus (HIV) Type 1 Infection Is Related to the Severity of Acute HIV Illness in Kenyan Women. Clin Infect Dis 2002;35(1):77–81.

[14] Bollinger RC. Risk factors and clinical presentation of acute primary HIV infection in India. JAMA 1997; 278(23):2085.

[15] Ma Z-M, Stone M, Piatak M, et al. High specific infectivity of plasma virus from the pre-ramp-up and ramp-up stages of acute simian immunodeficiency virus infection. J Virol 2009;83(7):3288–97.

16 Cohen MS, Shaw GM, McMichael AJ, et al. Acute HIV-1 infection. New England Journal of Medicine 2011;364(20): 1943–54. https://doi.org/10.1056/NEJMra1011874.

[17] Panel on Antiretroviral Guidelines for Adults and Adolescents. Guidelines for the use of antiretroviral agents in adults and adolescents with HIV. Department of Health and Human Services; 2018. p. 298. Available at: https://aidsinfo.nih.gov/contentfiles/lvguidelines/adultandadolescentgl.pdf.

[18] Danel C, Moh R, Gabillard D, et al. A trial of early antiretrovirals and isoniazid preventive therapy in Africa. N Engl J Med 2015;373(9):808–22.

[19] Lundgren JD, Babiker AG, Gordin F, et al. Initiation of antiretroviral therapy in early asymptomatic HIV infection. N Engl J Med 2015;373(9):795–807.

[20] Global Statistics | HIV.gov. Available at: https://www.hiv.gov/hiv-basics/overview/data-and-trends/global-statistics. Accessed May 13, 2020.

[21] Dorfman R. The Detection of Defective Members of Large Populations. Ann Math Stat 1943;14(4):436–40.

[22] Blood Donation Process Explained | Red Cross Blood Services. Available at: https://www.redcrossblood.org/donate-blood/blood-donation-process/donation-process-overview.html. Accessed May 13, 2020.

[23] Pilcher CD, McPherson JT, Leone PA, et al. Real-time, universal screening for acute HIV infection in a routine HIV counseling and testing population. J Am Med Assoc 2002;288(2):216–21.

[24] Quinn TC, Brookmeyer R, Kline R, et al. Feasibility of pooling sera for HIV-1 viral RNA to diagnose acute primary HIV-1 infection and estimate HIV incidence. Aids 2000;14(17):2751–7.

[25] Christopoulos KA, Zetola NM, Klausner JD, et al. Leveraging a rapid, round-the-clock HIV testing system to screen for acute HIV infection in a large urban public medical center. J Acquir Immune Defic Syndr 2013; 62(2):1–16.

[26] Pilcher CD, Fiscus SA, Nguyen TQ, et al. Detection of acute infections during HIV testing in North Carolina. N Engl J Med 2005;352(18):1873–83.

[27] Peters PJ, Westheimer E, Cohen S, et al. Screening yield of HIV antigen/antibody combination and pooled HIV RNA testing for acute HIV infection in a high-prevalence population. JAMA 2016;315(7):682–90.

[28] Long EF. HIV screening via fourth-generation immunoassay or nucleic acid amplification test in the united states: A cost-effectiveness analysis. PLoS One 2011;6(11). https://doi.org/10.1371/journal.pone.0027625.

[29] U=U | United States | Prevention Access Campaign. Available at: https://www.preventionaccess.org/. Accessed May 13, 2020.

[30] Eisinger RW, Dieffenbach CW, Fauci AS. HIV viral load and transmissibility of HIV infection undetectable equals untransmittable. JAMA 2019;321(5):451–2.

[31] Vernazza P, Hirschel B, Bernasconi E, et al. Les personnes séropositives ne souffrant d'aucune autre MST et suivant un traitement antirétroviral efficace ne transmettent pas le VIH par voie sexuelle. Bulletin des Médecins Suisses 2008;89(05):165–9.

[32] Cohen MS, Chen YQ, McCauley M, et al. Prevention of HIV-1 Infection with Early Antiretroviral Therapy. N Engl J Med 2011;6:493–505.

[33] Cohen MS, Chen YQ, McCauley M, et al. Antiretroviral therapy for the prevention of HIV-1 transmission. N Engl J Med 2016;375(9):830–9.

[34] Rodger AJ, Cambiano V, Bruun T, et al. Sexual activity without condoms and risk of HIV transmission in serodifferent couples when the HIV-positive partner is using suppressive antiretroviral therapy. JAMA 2016;316(2):171–81.

[35] Bavinton BR, Pinto AN, Phanuphak N, et al. Viral suppression and HIV transmission in serodiscordant male couples: an international, prospective, observational, cohort study. Lancet HIV 2018;5(8):e438–47.

[36] Rodger AJ, Cambiano V, Phillips AN, et al. Risk of HIV transmission through condomless sex in serodifferent gay couples with the HIV-positive partner taking suppressive antiretroviral therapy (PARTNER): final results of a multicentre, prospective, observational study. Lancet 2019;393(10189):2428–38.

[37] LeMessurier J, Traversy G, Varsaneux O, et al. Risk of sexual transmission of human immunodeficiency virus with antiretroviral therapy, suppressed viral load and condom use: A systematic review. CMAJ 2018;190(46):E1350–60.

[38] HIV Treatment as Prevention | HIV Risk and Prevention | HIV/AIDS | CDC. Available at: https://www.cdc.gov/hiv/risk/art/index.html. Accessed May 13, 2020.

[39] U=U Frequently Asked Questions. Available at: https://www.health.ny.gov/diseases/aids/ending_the_epidemic/faq.htm. Accessed June 6, 2020.

[40] FAQ | United States | Prevention Access Compaign. Available at: https://www.preventionaccess.org/faq. Accessed June 6, 2020.

[41] Chaudoir SR. Stigma mechanism measures. AIDS Behav 2015;13(6):1160–77.

[42] U = U – A Destigmatizing Message Inconsistently Communicated by Clinicians to PLHIV. (Abstract 223). Available at: https://www.iapac.org/AdherenceConference/presentations/ADH2018_OA223.pdf. Accessed June 6, 2020.

[43] Rendina HJ, Parsons JT. Factors associated with perceived accuracy of the Undetectable = Untransmittable slogan among men who have sex with men: Implications for messaging scale-up and implementation: Implications. J Int AIDS Soc 2018;21(1):1–10.

[44] Ngure K, Ongolly F, Dolla A, et al. "I just believe there is a risk" understanding of undetectable equals untransmissible (U = U) among health providers and HIV-negative partners in serodiscordant relationships in Kenya. J Int AIDS Soc 2020;23(3):1–6.

[45] Schreier T, Sherer R, Sayles H, et al. US Human Immunodeficiency Virus (HIV) practitioners' recommendations regarding condomless sex in the era of HIV pre-exposure prophylaxis and treatment as prevention. Open Forum Infect Dis 2019;6(3). https://doi.org/10.1093/ofid/ofz082.

[46] Agutu CA, Ngetsa CJ, Price MA, et al. Systematic review of the performance and clinical utility of point of care HIV-1 RNA testing for diagnosis and care. PLoS One 2019;14(6):1–25.

[47] Evidence of HIV Treatment and Viral Suppression in Preventing the Sexual Transmission of HIVTransmission | HIV Risk and Prevention | HIV/AIDS | CDC. Available at: https://www.cdc.gov/hiv/risk/art/evidence-of-hiv-treatment.html. Accessed August 6, 2020.

[48] World Health Organisation. Scaling up antiretroviral therapy in resource-limited settings: treatment guidelines for 2003 revision. Geneva (Switzerland): World Health Organisation; 2004. p. 1–68.

[49] The Use of Antiretroviral Drugs for Treating and Preventing HIV Infection. 2016. Available at: https://apps.who.int/iris/bitstream/handle/10665/208825/9789241549684_eng.pdf;jsessionid=5616E5674843EE885681FB0D86B3EA92?sequence=1. Accessed May 13, 2020.

[50] Carmona S, Peter T, Berrie L. HIV viral load scale-up: Multiple interventions to meet the HIV treatment cascade. Curr Opin HIV AIDS 2017;12(2):157–64.

[51] Habiyambere V, Dongmo Nguimfack B, Vojnov L, et al. Forecasting the global demand for HIV monitoring and diagnostic tests: A 2016-2021 analysis. PLoS One 2018;13(9):1–14.

[52] Peter T, Zeh C, Katz Z, et al. Scaling up HIV viral load - Lessons from the large-scale implementation of HIV early infant diagnosis and CD4 testing. J Int AIDS Soc 2017;20:9–15.

[53] Nash M, Ramapuram J, Kaiya R, et al. Use of the GeneXpert tuberculosis system for HIV viral load testing in India. Lancet Glob Health 2017;5(8):e754–5.

[54] O'connor. Diagnostic accurace of the Point-of-care Xpert® HIV-1 viral load assay in a South African HIV clinic. Physiol Behav 2016;176(1):139–48.

[55] UNAIDS and partners launch initiative to improve HIV diagnostics | UNAIDS. Available at: https://www.unaids. org/en/resources/presscentre/press-releaseandstatementarchive/2014/july/20140723dai. Accessed May 13, 2020.

[56] Walensky RP, Ciaranello AL, Park J, et al. Cost-effectiveness of laboratory monitoring in Sub-Saharan Africa: a review of the current literature. Clin Infect Dis 2010; 51(1):85–92.

[57] Hamers RL, Sawyer AW, Tuohy M, et al. Cost-effectiveness of laboratory monitoring for management of HIV treatment in sub-Saharan Africa: A model-based analysis. Aids 2012;26(13):1663–72.

[58] Barnabas Rv, Revill P, Tan N, et al. Cost-effectiveness of routine viral load monitoring in low- and middle-income countries: A systematic review. J Int AIDS Soc 2017;20:50–61.

[59] Lakhani CM, Manrai AK, Jian Yang PMV, et al. Pooled HIV-1 RNA Viral Load Testing for Detection of Antiretroviral Treatment Failure in Kenyan children. Physiol Behav 2019;176(3):139–48.

[60] van Zyl GU, Preiser W, Potschka S, et al. Pooling strategies to reduce the cost of HIV-1 RNA load monitoring in a resource-limited setting. Clin Infect Dis 2011; 52(2):264–70.

[61] Report T, Medicines A, Service D. Hiv diagnostic tests in low-and middle-income countries: Forecasts of global demand for 2014-2018 aids Medicines and diagnostics Service. 2015. 2015. Available at: http://apps.who.int/iris/bitstream/handle/10665/179864/9789241509169_eng.pdf;jsessionid=A5E-F2E34E02B8368101F56AA5AD79E69?sequence=1. Accessed May 18, 2020.

[62] Sutton MY, Liu H, Steiner B, et al. Molecular Subtyping of Treponema pallidum in an Arizona County with Increasing Syphilis Morbidity: Use of Specimens from Ulcers and Blood. J Infect Dis 2001;183(11):1601–6.

[63] van Deutekom H, Gerritsen JJJ, van Soolingen D, et al. A Molecular Epidemiological Approach to Studying the Transmission of Tuberculosis in Amsterdam. Clin Infect Dis 1997;25(5):1071–7.

[64] Overbaugh J, Bangham CRM. Selection forces and constraints on retroviral sequence variation. Science 2001; 292(5519):1106–9.

[65] Robertson D, Sharp P, McCutchan F, et al. Recombination in HIV-1. Nature 1995;374(6518):124–6.

[66] Frost SDW, Günthard HF, Wong JK, et al. Evidence for positive selection driving the evolution of HIV-1 env under potent antiviral therapy. Virology 2001;284(2): 250–8.

[67] Burger H, Weiser B, Flaherty K, et al. Evolution of human immunodeficiency virus type 1 nucleotide sequence diversity among close contacts. Proc Natl Acad Sci U S A 1991;88(24):11236–40.

[68] Ou CY, Ciesielski CA, Myers G, et al. Molecular epidemiology of HIV transmission in a dental practice. Science 1992;256(5060):1165–71.

[69] Brooksa JT, Robbinsb KE, Youngpairojb AS, et al. Molecular analysis of HIV strains from a cluster of worker infections in the adult film industry, Los Angeles 2004. Physiol Behav 2018;176(1):139–48.

[70] Mehta SR, Wertheim JO, Brouwer KC, et al. HIV Transmission Networks in the San Diego-Tijuana Border Region. EBioMedicine 2015;2(10):1456–63.

[71] Hué S, Gifford RJ, Dunn D, et al. Demonstration of Sustained Drug-Resistant Human Immunodeficiency Virus Type 1 Lineages Circulating among Treatment-Naïve Individuals. J Virol 2009;83(6):2645–54.

[72] Poon AFY, Gustafson R, Daly P, et al. Near real-time monitoring of HIV transmission hotspots from routine HIV genotyping: an implementation case study. Lancet HIV 2017;3(5):1–15.

[73] Wertheim JO, Murrell B, Mehta SR, et al. Growth of HIV-1 molecular transmission clusters in New York City. J Infect Dis 2018;218(12):1943–53.

[74] Wertheim JO, Kosakovsky Pond SL, Forgione LA, et al. Social and genetic networks of HIV-1 Transmission in New York City. PLoS Pathog 2017;13(1):1–19.

[75] Smith DM, May SJ, Tweeten S, et al. A public health model for the molecular surveillance of HIV transmission in San Diego, California. AIDS 2009;23:225–32.

[76] Statistics Overview | Statistics Center | HIV/AIDS | CDC. Available at: https://www.cdc.gov/hiv/statistics/overview/index.html. Accessed May 13, 2020.

Pharmacogenomics

Advances in Molecular Pathology 3 (2020) 107–115

ADVANCES IN MOLECULAR PATHOLOGY

Pharmacogenomics of Drug-Induced Liver Injury

Ann K. Daly, PhD

Translational and Clinical Research Institute, Faculty of Medical Sciences, Newcastle University, Framlington Place, Newcastle upon Tyne NE2 4HH, UK

KEYWORDS

• Pharmacogenomics • Drug-induced liver injury • HLA gene • Adverse drug reaction

KEY POINTS

• Drug-induced liver injury is a rare but serious consequence of drug treatment and can occur with a range of licensed drugs. It also is an important cause of attrition during drug development.

• Genetic factors predicting susceptibility to drug-induced liver injury have been investigated for approximately 30 years with evidence for a role for HLA serotype or genotype for liver injury due to several different causative drugs reported from the 1980s onwards.

• Genome-wide association studies on drug-induced liver injury have led to increased understanding of the importance of HLA genotype in predicting individual susceptibility, with strong associations reported for particular HLA genotypes with specific drugs, including for flucloxacillin-induced liver injury with *HLA-B*57:01*.

• Genotype for non-HLA immunogenes, such as *PTPN22*, also may predict risk of drug-induced liver injury.

• There appears to be a limited role for genetic polymorphisms that affect drug disposition in susceptibility to drug-induced liver injury but an association between genotype for N-acetyltransferase 2 (*NAT2*) and isoniazid-induced liver injury is well established.

INTRODUCTION

Drug-induced liver injury (DILI) is a relatively rare but potentially very serious complication of treatment with several widely used licensed drugs. In addition, identification of a liability to induce DILI is one of the more frequent causes of drug attrition on grounds of risk of adverse drug reaction [1]. When evidence of potential to cause DILI is detected during clinical trials, it is likely to lead to cessation of the development program for a new drug, but there are numerous examples of licensed drugs where DILI occasionally arises (see Thakkar and colleagues [2] for specific examples). For many of these drugs, their therapeutic advantages outweigh the risk of DILI and, therefore, although hepatotoxicity may be listed as a possible adverse event in the prescribing information, they continue to be used widely. The possibility that some individuals are at risk of developing DILI due to their genetics has received considerable attention, and there is increasing evidence that certain genetic profiles are associated with risk, although this is dependent mainly on the individual drug, with the overall relationship between genetics and DILI complex. There is some potential for using genetic data to predict risk of DILI in individual patients but up to the present the associations reported have limited positive predictive value. This is in contrast to certain other types of adverse drug reactions, such as abacavir-induced hypersensitivity and serious skin

---

E-mail address: a.k.daly@ncl.ac.uk

https://doi.org/10.1016/j.yamp.2020.07.010
2589-4080/20/

rash induced by carbamazepine, where genetic testing prior to drug prescription has been implemented widely (for review, see Alfirevic and Pirmohamed [3]).

This article is concerned with genetic susceptibility to idiosyncratic DILI, where DILI develops when the drug is used at the recommended dose and toxicity generally is not dependent on plasma levels. DILI also may result when certain drugs (eg, acetaminophen) are used at higher than recommended levels, but this type of DILI is not discussed, because in general genetic risk factors are less important than in idiosyncratic DILI, although they may be of some relevance (see Athersuch and colleagues [4] for further discussion of this aspect).

HISTORICAL PERSPECTIVE

DILI has been recognized as an important clinical problem since the 1950s. Interest in the possibility that genetic factors might predict susceptibility developed from 2 perspectives, pharmacogenetic and immunogenetic (HLA). The pharmacogenetic perspective came first from studies on isoniazid. It has been well known for many years that isoniazid causes DILI in 1% to 5% of patients undergoing treatment [5]. Isoniazid metabolism also has been well studied, mainly because the N-acetyltransferase polymorphism (now known as $NAT2$ polymorphism) was first detected in the 1950s, when this drug first was used to treat tuberculosis, with acetylation shown to be a key step in its metabolism [6]. Approximately 50% of Europeans are fast acetylators and metabolize isoniazid more rapidly than the remaining 50%, who are described as slow acetylators. This polymorphism has relevance to overall response to isoniazid treatment because it affects plasma levels of the parent drug, and this aspect was well studied during the 1950s and 1960s. In the 1970s, DILI due to isoniazid started to receive more attention, and the possibility that acetylator status might be a predictor of this toxicity was investigated in detail for the first time, although the early studies did not yield clear-cut findings [7,8]. As discussed in more detail later, these issues continue up to the present. Another early pharmacogenetic study relevant to DILI concerned the debrisoquine polymorphism (now referred to as the $CYP2D6$ polymorphism), where patients who had suffered hepatotoxicity due to the antianginal drug perhexiline appeared more likely to be debrisoquine poor metabolizers [9].

In parallel with pharmacogenetic studies, HLA serotype also was investigated as a determinant of DILI susceptibility, because susceptibility to other liver diseases, such as autoimmune hepatitis, showed HLA associations and at least some DILI cases showed hypersensitivity features, such as rash, fever, and eosinophilia. Initial studies on a possible HLA association generally were negative [10]. There also were reports, however, which suggested an association between the HLA serotype DR2 and halothane-related DILI [11], and a study of DILI cases associated with several different drugs, including nitrofurantoin [12], found an apparent increased incidence in frequency of the HLA class II serotypes HLA-DR2 and HLA-DR6 among cases. Another larger study also involving several different causative drugs found a trend toward significance for the class I serotype HLA-A11 in DILI associated with tricyclic antidepressants and diclofenac and for the class II serotype HLA-DR6 with DILI due to chlorpromazine [13]. All these early reports on immunogenetic associations are quite limited, reflecting particularly the difficulties of HLA serotyping, which captures overall diversity less well than modern genotyping. Interest in genetic risk factors for DILI has continued and this has been facilitated by increased understanding of the human genome, development of improved approaches, such as use of genome-wide association studies (GWASs), which enable a more open approach to genetic risk factors, and collaborative studies, which enable larger numbers of DILI cases to be collected for genetic studies.

HLA GENOTYPE AS A RISK FACTOR FOR DRUG-INDUCED LIVER INJURY

More recently, HLA associations with DILI have been studied directly by genotyping. The first genotyping studies were on amoxicillin-clavulanate–related DILI. Two independent studies reported an identical association with the $HLA-DRB1*15:01$ allele [14,15]. This corresponds to the DR2 serotype already reported as a risk factor for DILI due to halothane [11]. Most subsequent studies on HLA associations with DILI GWASs, which sometimes also included direct HLA typing. It is now possible to impute HLA genotypes directly from GWAS data with a high level of accuracy [16], so in general there is a trend away from direct HLA typing. A large number of HLA associations for DILI due to particular drugs have now been reported and in most cases replicated (Table 1 for summary). This list continues to grow.

The first association of an HLA allele with DILI to be detected by GWAS related to DILI due to the antimicrobial flucloxacillin [17]. This finding showing an association with $HLA-B*57:01$ has been replicated and studied in more detail subsequently [18] and appears

TABLE 1
HLA Risk Factors for Drug-Induced Liver Injury

Allele	Drug	Odds Ratio (Allelic)	P Value	Reference
HLA class I				
A*02:01	Amoxicillin-clavulanate	2.3 (1.8–2.9)	1.8×10^{-10}	Lucena et al. [20], 2011
A*31:01	Carbamazepine	7.3 (2.5–23.7)	.0004	Nicoletti et al. [57], 2019
A*33:01	Terbinafine	40.5 (12.5–131.4)	6.7×10^{-10}	Nicoletti et al. [22], 2017
	Fenofibrate	58.7 (12.3–279.8)	3.2×10^{-7}	Nicoletti et al. [22], 2017
	Ticlopidine	163.1 (16.2–1642)	.00002	Nicoletti et al. [22], 2017
A*33:03	Ticlopidine	13.0 (4.4–38.6)	1.2×10^{-5}	Hirata et al. [23], 2008
B*14:01-C*08:02	Trimethoprim-sulfamethoxazole	8.7 (3.2–19.5)	2.3×10^{-4}	Li et al. [58], 2019
B*35:02	Minocycline	29.6 (7.8–89.8)	2.57×10^{-8}	Urban et al. [29], 2017
B*57:01	Flucloxacillin	36.6 (26.1–51.3)	2.6×10^{-97}	Nicoletti et al. [18], 2019
	Pazopanib	2.1 (1.3–3.6)	.0058	Xu et al. [59], 2016
B*57:02 & B*57:03	Anti-HIV and anti-TB combination	30.1 (3.4–263.1)	.002	Petros et al. [60], 2017
B*57:03	Flucloxacillin	19.8 (3.37–116.1)	.001	Nicoletti et al. [18], 2019
B*39:01	Infliximab	43.6 (2.8-inf)	.001	Bruno et al. [25], 2020
C*03:02	Methimazole	14.9 (2.4–182.9)	.03	Li et al. [61], 2019
HLA class II				
DRB1*07:01	Ximelagatran	4.4 (2.2–8.9)	6×10^{-6}	Kindmark et al. [62], 2008
	Lapatinib	2.9 (1.3–6.6)	.007	Parham et al. [63], 2016
DRB1*15:01	Lumiracoxib	5.0 (3.6–7.0)	6.8×10^{-25}	Singer et al. [21], 2010
	Amoxicillin-clavulanate	2.8 (2.1–3.8)	3.5×10^{-11}	Lucena et al. [20], 2011
DRB1*16:01	Flupirtine	18.7 (2.5–140.5)	.002	Nicoletti et al. [64], 2016

Abbreviation: TB, tuberculosis.

to represent the strongest HLA association reported to date for any type of DILI on the basis of a high odds ratio (approximately 40) and very low P value. There are some limitations despite the strong association. Approximately 20% of confirmed flucloxacillin DILI cases are not positive for HLA-B*57:01 or the related B*57:03 allele [18]. Despite the strong association with B*57:01, the facts that only approximately 1 in 500 patients positive for B*57:01 develops clinically detectable DILI when prescribed flucloxacillin and that approximately 20% of flucloxacillin-DILI cases are not positive for B*57 alleles mean that clinical implementation is unlikely currently. Data suggesting an increased susceptibility to flucloxacillin DILI in those aged 70 and older, however, point to the possibility that there still may be a place for preprescription genotyping in this group [19]. In addition, individual HLA

genotypes may be available in the future via patient medical records and also could inform prescribing decisions.

As discussed previously, early genotyping studies on HLA associations in amoxicillin-clavulanate DILI showed that the HLA class II allele DRB1*15:01 was a risk factor, although the overall effect size was more modest (odds ratio approximately 2.5) than that reported for B*57:01 as a factor for flucloxacillin DILI [14,15]. The genetic basis of DILI due to amoxicillin-clavulanate was studied further by GWAS more recently. This confirmed the DRB1*15:01 association but showed a second independent association with a class I HLA allele A*02:01 [20] (Fig. 1, see Table 1). This second HLA association was associated with a risk of DILI of the same order of magnitude as the DRB1*15:01 risk (odds ratio approximately 2.5), but there was evidence

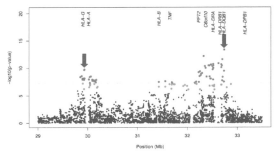

FIG. 1 Manhattan plot for the major histocompatibility complex region of chromosome 6 from a GWAS of 201 amoxicillin-clavulanate DILI cases and 532 population controls. The X axis shows the chromosomal position in megabases and the Y axis the negative log of the P value for the frequency difference between cases and controls for the allelic variants (SNPs). SNPs with P values less than 10^{-6} and less than 10^{-7} are highlighted in green and red, respectively. P values for other SNPs are shown in blue. The positions of the most significant SNPs within the HLA-A and HLA-DRB1 loci are indicated by arrows. (*Adapted from* Lucena MI, Molokhia M, Shen Y, et al. Susceptibility to amoxicillin-clavulanate-induced liver injury is influenced by multiple HLA class I and II alleles. Gastroenterology. 2011;141(1):342; with permission.). TNF, tumor necrosis factor.

of a genetic interaction between the 2 alleles, which resulted in a greater than additive increase in DILI risk if an individual was positive for both variants.

Table 1 lists several examples of HLA variants associated with risk of DILI with more than 1 drug. These drugs are structurally unrelated. In cases of *DRB1*15:01*, this allele is a risk factor for DILI due to the nonsteroidal anti-inflammatory drug lumiracoxib, in addition to amoxicillin-clavulanate [21]. Increased risk of lumiracoxib DILI does not appear to extend to any other HLA alleles. In addition, the phenotype of lumiracoxib DILI is almost entirely hepatocellular whereas amoxicillin-clavulanate DILI typically is either mixed or cholestatic. Underlying mechanisms for HLA associations are considered in more detail later, but the reason for this variation in phenotype still is not clear. Another association seen for a particular HLA allele with DILI due to unrelated drugs is with the class I allele, *A*33:01*. This association was relevant to DILI due to several unrelated drugs, including terbinafine, ticlopidine, sertraline, and fenofibrate [22]. Another allele with an almost identical sequence to *A*33:01*, *A*33:03* also has been reported to be a risk factor for ticlopidine DILI [23]. The finding that several closely related HLA alleles could be risk factors for DILI due to the same drug also extends to both flucloxacillin

and amoxicillin-clavulanate DILI. A rare B*57 allele, *B*57:03* is a risk factor for flucloxacillin DILI in addition to *B*57:01* [18], and *DRB1*15:02* also appears to be a risk factor for amoxicillin-clavulanate DILI in addition to *DRB1*15:01* [24].

A vast majority of DILI causes listed in Table 1 are small molecule drugs but 1 recent study of DILI due to a biologic, infliximab, which is a chimeric human-mouse IgG monoclonal antibody, has shown an association with the HLA class I allele *B*39:01* [25]. Although several other biologics also have been shown to induce DILI [26,27], the findings of an HLA association as a susceptibility factor is unexpected, as discussed later. The emphasis in Table 1 is on DILI due to licensed drugs, but HLA associations also have been reported with liver injury caused by herbal medicines (HILIs). For example, there is a recent report that *B*35:01* is a risk factor for liver injury due to *Polygonum multiflorum*, which is used widely in China [28]. There are some limitations with studying HILIs because these herbal preparations are complex mixtures, making data interpretation difficult, but in this case it is interesting that a closely related HLA allele, *B*35:02*, is associated with risk of DILI due to minocycline [29].

NON-HLA IMMUNOGENETIC RISK FACTORS

A majority of immunogenetic associations in DILI relate to HLA genes but a few additional genes have been reported as risk factors (Table 2). The first report from GWAS data relates to DILI due to the biologic interferon beta. A genome-wide significant signal from a single nucleotide polymorphism (SNP) that is known to affect levels of *IRF6*, which encodes interferon regulatory factor 6, was detected and replicated [26]. This protein has a role in craniofacial development and also may contribute to wound healing [30], which might explain, at least in part, its relevance to liver injury. There also is a recent report that mice lacking *IRF6* are more susceptible to development of liver steatosis with overexpression resulting in protection [31].

The largest GWAS to date on DILI, which involved 2048 cases of DILI due to any prescribed drug and 12,429 population controls, detected a genome-wide significant signal on chromosome 1 in addition to the expected signal in the HLA region on chromosome 6 [32]. The chromosome 1 signal related to a nonsynonymous polymorphism in the *PTPN22* gene rs2476601, with the variant allele associated with an approximately 1.4-fold increase in risk. This SNP already was well established as a risk factor of a similar magnitude for certain autoimmune diseases, including type 1 diabetes

TABLE 2
Non-HLA Immunogenetic Risk Factors for Drug-Induced Liver Injury

Gene	Variant	Drug	Odds Ratio (95% Confidence Interval)	P Value	Reference
IRF6	rs2205986	Interferon beta	8.3 (3.6–19.2)	2.3×10^{-8}	Kowalec et al. [26], 2018
PNPN22	rs2476601	Amoxicillin-clavulanate and others	1.44 (1.28–1.62)	1.2×10^{-9}	Cirulli et al. [32], 2019
ERAP2	rs1363907	Amoxicillin-clavulanate, amoxicillin	Not calculated	4.5×10^{-6}	Nicoletti et al. [35], 2019

mellitus, rheumatoid arthritis, and systemic lupus erythematosis. It is believed that the phosphatase enzyme encoded by PTPN22 contributes to both T-cell and B-cell immune responses and possibly also to function of other immune cells [33]. The overall effect of the amino acid change at codon 620 (W to R) still is not understood fully but carriers of the variant form are at increased risk of developing autoimmune disease as well as DILI. The GWAS which discovered and replicated the PTPN22 association also found that the association was particularly with DILI cases where the causative drug was amoxicillin-clavulanate but there was also an association with DILI cases due to certain other drug causes, including some which also showed HLA associations, and several such as methotrexate and valproate where no HLA association with DILI has been reported [32]. This suggests that immune mechanisms independent of HLA and possibly T-cell responses could be relevant to some forms of DILI.

Finally, a further immunogenetic risk factor has emerged from studies using a novel approach to GWASs, known as PrediXcan analysis [34]. This approach allows differentially expressed genes in liver to be selected and used for a new GWAS analysis, which have significance thresholds different from those used normally in GWASs due to a smaller gene set being studied. Applying this analysis to amoxicillin-clavulanate DILI cases resulted in identification of a signal within the endoplasmatic reticulum aminopeptidase 2 (ERAP2) gene [35]. An SNP associated with low ERAP2 expression (rs1363907) was found to be a risk factor for this form of DILI. The odds ratio for the low expression variant among amoxicillin-clavulanate DILI cases generally is approximately 1.4, with a genome-wide significant P value. When individuals positive for the 2 HLA risk factors and the rare PTPN22 variant are considered alone, the odds ratio for the ERAP2 variant rises to 18.5 ($P = 2 \times 10^{-23}$), although this needs to be treated with caution because only 5% of

amoxicillin-clavulanate DILI cases are positive for all 4 variants compared with less than 1% of population controls. The association appears to relate to the role for ERAP2 in processing of peptides for antigen presentation to T cells [36] although why DILI susceptibility is associated with a decreased expression variant is unclear. ERAP2 associations with autoimmune disease have been reported previously but generally higher gene expression is associated with increased risk [36].

MECHANISM FOR IMMUNOGENETIC ASSOCIATIONS IN DRUG-INDUCED LIVER INJURY

The large number of reported HLA associations with DILI due to a variety of drugs provides a basis for understanding the underlying mechanism for the injury. As discussed in detail recently [37], however, overall understanding remains limited despite efforts made to understand the underlying mechanisms using a variety of different approaches. When DILI shows an HLA association, this would seem to provide evidence that the immune system is contributing to the underlying toxicity mechanism. As summarized in Table 1, DILI due to a wide range of drugs shows an association with HLA genotype. There also are several examples of drugs that are well-established causes of DILI where no HLA association has been detected. These include diclofenac, where genetic risk factors for DILI have been studied using both genome-wide and candidate gene approaches with no evidence of HLA association [22,38,39], and isoniazid, where some evidence of a limited role for HLA genotype [40] has been suggested although not confirmed in a recent GWAS [41]. Both isoniazid and diclofenac are subject to extensive metabolism in the liver and may form reactive metabolites that bind to hepatocyte components [42,43]. It is possible that the formation of adducts of this type provokes an innate immune response and that this may result in cellular effects with similarity to those observed in the adaptive immune response. Limited data involving increased frequency of *PTPN22* variants in cases of DILI, which do not show HLA associations (eg, due to valproate), also would be consistent with a role for innate immunity in at least some forms of DILI that are not HLA dependent.

In vitro studies on the underlying mechanism for some of the HLA associations with DILI have been reported and provide some further understanding of the basis for the associations, summarized in Table 1. The *HLA-B*57:01* association with flucloxacillin DILI is relatively well studied due to both the strength of the association and existing knowledge on the association of another adverse drug reaction, hypersensitivity induced by abacavir, with the same HLA allele. The underlying mechanism for abacavir hypersensitivity involves direct interaction of abacavir or a metabolite with the B*57:01 protein. This binding induces a conformational change that results in the protein presenting self-peptides inappropriately to T cells, which induces a strong T-cell response at several sites [44]. Using broadly similar in vitro approaches, studies to determine whether flucloxacillin induces T-cell responses by a similar mechanism were conducted. The overall findings suggested that T-cell responses to flucloxacillin could be induced in cells derived from B*57:01 individuals but that covalent binding to cellular proteins to generate modified peptides (haptens) was required prior to induction of cell proliferation [45]. Support for absence of direct interaction of flucloxacillin with the B*57:01 protein has been obtained from binding studies using recombinant protein [46]. Studies on in vitro responses to amoxicillin-clavulanate by T cells also have been performed. The relevance of HLA genotype (*HLA-A*02:01* and *HLA-DRB1*15:01*) was confirmed but, slightly unexpectedly, it was demonstrated that T-cell clones responsive to amoxicillin only and to clavulanic acid only could be isolated [47]. This suggests a role for both drug components in this type of DILI and, that similar to T-cell responses to flucloxacillin, covalent binding to protein is required.

More limited in vitro and molecular modeling studies on other forms of DILI provide some evidence that direct interaction of the drug or a metabolite with the HLA protein may occur with some drugs. For ticlopidine, evidence that the drug may bind directly to *HLA-A*33:03* has been reported [48], whereas for minocycline, molecular modeling suggests direct binding of the drug to *HLA-B*35:02* occurs [29]. It seems possible that there is no universal mechanism for DILI where HLA associations have been reported, with considerable

dependence of individual drug structure on whether the HLA protein can bind the drug. It is clear, however, that only a very small minority of those positive for the particular HLA risk factor develop DILI if exposed to the causative drug. The basis for susceptibility remains unclear, although, as discussed previously for flucloxacillin DILI, nongenetic factors, including age and drug dose, also contribute [19]. It is likely that both these factors may cause high levels of drug to be present within the liver. It is possible that to develop DILI involving an inappropriate T-cell response, the liver needs to be already stressed prior to drug exposure, with increased levels of immune cells present compared with a healthy liver.

DRUG DISPOSITION GENOTYPES AS RISK FACTORS

It generally is considered that genetic polymorphisms affecting drug disposition should affect risk of idiosyncratic DILI but any strong associations are limited. Probably the most consistent data relate to isoniazid, which is a common cause of DILI. As discussed previously, the phase II enzyme NAT2 has a key role in isoniazid metabolism. The *NAT2* gene is subject to a well-studied genetic polymorphism, with approximately 50% of individuals from several different ethnic groups lacking this enzyme activity. Acetylhydrazine, an isoniazid metabolite, which can undergo metabolism by cytochrome P450 to a toxic metabolite or by NAT2 to the less toxic diacetylhydrazine, may be the cause of DILI, but the parent drug, which is seen at higher plasma levels in those with no NAT2 activity, also may contribute [49]. A recent GWAS based in Thailand ,involving 79 patients with tuberculosis who suffered DILI when treated with isoniazid-containing drug regimens together with controls who had not suffered DILI, found a signal on chromosome 8 close to *NAT2* and concluded that *NAT2* genotype is the most important genetic risk factor for isoniazid-related DILI, in general agreement with findings from previous candidate gene studies [41]. There also are reports that polymorphisms in other phase II metabolism genes, in particular the Uridine diphosphate-glucuronosyltransferases and the glutathione S-transferases, affect DILI risk but the literature on these generally is not conclusive and most observations are based on small sample numbers (for review, see Daly [50]).

Cytochrome P450 polymorphisms also seem plausible candidates for a contribution to DILI. There are few data suggesting *CYP2B6* genotype could be relevant to the risk of DILI induced by efavirenz [51] and by ticlopidine [52], but overall any P450 contribution to DILI currently seems unconvincing.

ABC transporters, especially *ABCB11* (BSEP), are an important component of strategies to investigate the potential of drugs to cause DILI (for review, see Weaver and colleagues [53]). The possibility that transporter polymorphisms could be relevant to DILI has been investigated widely (for review, see Daly [50]), but overall findings are negative with, for example, early positive reports in relation to *ABCB11* not confirmed by more detailed studies [54].

PRESENT RELEVANCE AND FUTURE AVENUES TO CONSIDER OR TO INVESTIGATE

GWASs on DILI have provided evidence of strong HLA associations, but, with a few recent exceptions [32,35], no other genetic associations. This almost certainly is due to limited statistical power. As was demonstrated recently in relation to *PTPN22*, a sufficiently large set of samples will lead to new signals [32]. *PTPN22* may be an exception, however, because the association is less drug-specific than most other genetic risk factors for DILI and, importantly, the GWAS that detected this signal found no evidence for additional non–drug-specific signals elsewhere on the genome. Another recent study involving an enlarged sample collection for DILI due to flucloxacillin also failed to detect non-HLA signals [18]. Although GWASs on complex diseases have shown clearly the advantage of increasing samples size to 10s of 1000s and more (for review, see Tam and colleagues [55]), it is not feasible to do this for DILI due to the rarity of the event. The alternative approach is more detailed genome analysis by whole-genome sequencing [56]. This will allow detection of rare variants relevant to disease and should improve understanding the underlying biology. It is unlikely, however, that rare variant genotyping will be of value at a population level as a means to predict DILI, even if strategies involving genetic risk scores can be developed.

SUMMARY

Considerable progress in understanding genetic risk factors for DILI has been made in approximately the past 12 years by GWASs. This has enabled the important role of HLA genes in these reactions to be established. In addition, some progress has been made on understanding the underlying mechanisms for the HLA associations. A few additional genes that contribute to

immune reactions have also emerged as risk factors, mainly where an HLA association also has been reported. Progress on identifying genes outside the immune system that cause DILI has been limited, although the role of *NAT2* genotype in determining susceptibility to isoniazid DILI now has been better established through GWAS approaches. The situation at present is that it is not possible to predict an individual's risk of DILI using genotyping but it may be possible to combine with additional nongenetic factors, as suggested recently [19].

DISCLOSURE

The author has nothing to disclose.

REFERENCES

[1] Wilke RA, Lin DW, Roden DM, et al. Identifying genetic risk factors for serious adverse drug reactions: current progress and challenges. Nat Rev Drug Discov 2007; 6(11):904–16.

[2] Thakkar S, Li T, Liu Z, et al. Drug-induced liver injury severity and toxicity (DILIst): binary classification of 1279 drugs by human hepatotoxicity. Drug Discov Today 2020;25(1):201–8.

[3] Alfirevic A, Pirmohamed M. Genomics of adverse drug reactions. Trends Pharmacol Sci 2017;38(1):100–9.

[4] Athersuch TJ, Antoine DJ, Boobis AR, et al. Paracetamol metabolism, hepatotoxicity, biomarkers and therapeutic interventions: a perspective. Toxicol Res (Camb) 2018; 7(3):347–57.

[5] Saukkonen JJ, Cohn DL, Jasmer RM, et al. An official ATS statement: hepatotoxicity of antituberculosis therapy. Am J Respir Crit Care Med 2006;174(8):935–52.

[6] Harris HW, Knight RA, Selin MJ. Comparison of isoniazid concentrations in the blood of people of Japanese and European descent; therapeutic and genetic implications. Am Rev Tuberc 1958;78(6):944–8.

[7] Mitchell JR, Thorgeirsson UP, Black M, et al. Increased incidence of isoniazid hepatitis in rapid acetylators: possible relation to hydranize metabolites. Clin Pharmacol Ther 1975;18(1):70–9.

[8] Gurumurthy P, Krishnamurthy MS, Nazareth O, et al. Lack of relationship between hepatic toxicity and acetylator phenotype in three thousand South Indian patients during treatment with isoniazid for tuberculosis. Am Rev Respir Dis 1984;129(1):58–61.

[9] Morgan MY, Reshef R, Shah RR, et al. Impaired oxidation of debrisoquine in patients with perhexiline liver injury. Gut 1984;25(10):1057–64.

[10] Eade OE, Grice D, Krawitt EL, et al. HLA A and B locus antigens in patients with unexplained hepatitis following halothane anaesthesia. Tissue Antigens 1981;17(4): 428–32.

[11] Otsuka S, Yamamoto M, Kasuya S, et al. HLA antigens in patients with unexplained hepatitis following halothane anesthesia. Acta Anaesthesiol Scand 1985;29(5): 497–501.

[12] Stricker BH, Blok AP, Claas FH, et al. Hepatic injury associated with the use of nitrofurans: a clinicopathological study of 52 reported cases. Hepatology 1988;8(3): 599–606.

[13] Berson A, Freneaux E, Larrey D, et al. Possible Role of Hla in Hepatotoxicity - an Exploratory-Study in 71 Patients with Drug-Induced Idiosyncratic Hepatitis. J Hepatol 1994;20(3):336–42.

[14] Hautekeete ML, Horsmans Y, van Waeyenberge C, et al. HLA association of amoxicillin-clavulanate-induced hepatitis. Gastroenterology 1999;117(5):1181–6.

[15] O'Donohue J, Oien KA, Donaldson P, et al. Co-amoxiclav jaundice: clinical and histological features and HLA class II association. Gut 2000;47(5):717–20.

[16] Zheng X, Shen J, Cox C, et al. HIBAG–HLA genotype imputation with attribute bagging. Pharmacogenomics J 2014;14(2):192–200.

[17] Daly AK, Donaldson PT, Bhatnagar P, et al. HLA-B*5701 genotype is a major determinant of drug-induced liver injury due to flucloxacillin. Nat Genet 2009;41:816–9.

[18] Nicoletti P, Aithal GP, Chamberlain TC, et al. Drug-induced liver injury due to flucloxacillin: relevance of multiple human leukocyte antigen alleles. Clin Pharmacol Ther 2019;106(1):245–53.

[19] Wing K, Bhaskaran K, Pealing L, et al. Quantification of the risk of liver injury associated with flucloxacillin: a UK population-based cohort study. J Antimicrob Chemother 2017;72(9):2636–46.

[20] Lucena MI, Molokhia M, Shen Y, et al. Susceptibility to amoxicillin-clavulanate-induced liver injury is influenced by multiple HLA class I and II alleles. Gastroenterology 2011;141(1):338–47.

[21] Singer JB, Lewitzky S, Leroy E, et al. A genome-wide study identifies HLA alleles associated with lumiracoxib-related liver injury. Nat Genet 2010;42:711–4.

[22] Nicoletti P, Aithal GP, Bjornsson ES, et al. Association of liver injury from specific drugs, or groups of drugs, with polymorphisms in HLA and other genes in a genome-wide association study. Gastroenterology 2017;152(5): 1078–89.

[23] Hirata K, Takagi H, Yamamoto M, et al. Ticlopidine-induced hepatotoxicity is associated with specific human leukocyte antigen genomic subtypes in Japanese patients: a preliminary case-control study. Pharmacogenomics J 2008;8(1):29–33.

[24] Kaliyaperumal K, Grove JI, Delahay RM, et al. Pharmacogenomics of drug-induced liver injury (DILI): Molecular biology to clinical applications. J Hepatol 2018;69(4): 948–57.

[25] Bruno CD, Fremd B, Church RJ, et al. HLA associations with infliximab-induced liver injury. Pharmacogenomics J 2020. https://doi.org/10.1038/s41397-020-0159-0.

[26] Kowalec K, Wright GEB, Drogemoller BI, et al. Common variation near IRF6 is associated with IFN-beta-induced liver injury in multiple sclerosis. Nat Genet 2018;50(8): 1081–5.

[27] Bjornsson ES, Bergmann OM, Bjornsson HK, et al. Incidence, presentation, and outcomes in patients with drug-induced liver injury in the general population of Iceland. Gastroenterology 2013;144(7):1419–25, 1425.e1-3; [quiz: e1419–20].

[28] Li C, Rao T, Chen X, et al. HLA-B*35:01 allele is a potential biomarker for predicting polygonum multiflorum-induced liver injury in humans. Hepatology 2019; 70(1):346–57.

[29] Urban TJ, Nicoletti P, Chalasani N, et al. Minocycline hepatotoxicity: Clinical characterization and identification of HLA-B *35:02 as a risk factor. J Hepatol 2017; 67(1):137–44.

[30] Rhea L, Canady FJ, Le M, et al. Interferon regulatory factor 6 is required for proper wound healing in vivo. Dev Dyn 2020;249(4):509–22.

[31] Tong J, Han CJ, Zhang JZ, et al. Hepatic interferon regulatory factor 6 alleviates liver steatosis and metabolic disorder by transcriptionally suppressing peroxisome proliferator-activated receptor gamma in mice. Hepatology 2019;69(6):2471–88.

[32] Cirulli ET, Nicoletti P, Abramson K, et al. A missense variant in PTPN22 is a risk factor for drug-induced liver injury. Gastroenterology 2019;156(6): 1707–16.e2.

[33] Mustelin T, Bottini N, Stanford SM. The contribution of PTPN22 to rheumatic disease. Arthritis Rheumatol 2019;71(4):486–95.

[34] Gamazon ER, Wheeler HE, Shah KP, et al. A gene-based association method for mapping traits using reference transcriptome data. Nat Genet 2015;47(9):1091–8.

[35] Nicoletti P, Innocenti F, Etheridge A, et al. Discovery of ERAP2 gene expression as a risk factor for drug-induced liver injury due to amoxicillin-clavulanic acid. Hepatology 2019;70:137A–8A.

[36] de Castro JAL, Stratikos E. Intracellular antigen processing by ERAP2: Molecular mechanism and roles in health and disease. Hum Immunol 2019;80(5):310–7.

[37] Uetrecht J. Mechanistic studies of idiosyncratic DILI: clinical implications. Front Pharmacol 2019;10:837.

[38] Daly AK, Aithal GP, Leathart JB, et al. Genetic susceptibility to diclofenac-induced hepatotoxicity: contribution of UGT2B7, CYP2C8, and ABCC2 genotypes. Gastroenterology 2007;132(1):272–81.

[39] Urban TJ, Shen Y, Stolz A, et al. Limited contribution of common genetic variants to risk for liver injury due to a variety of drugs. Pharmacogenet Genomics 2012;22(11): 784–95.

[40] Sharma SK, Balamurugan A, Saha PK, et al. Evaluation of clinical and immunogenetic risk factors for the development of hepatotoxicity during antituberculosis treatment. Am J Respir Crit Care Med 2002;166(7): 916–9.

[41] Suvichapanich S, Wattanapokayakit S, Mushiroda T, et al. Genomewide association study confirming the association of nat2 with susceptibility to antituberculosis drug-induced liver injury in thai patients. Antimicrob Agents Chemother 2019;63(8):e02692-18.

[42] Iwamura A, Nakajima M, Oda S, et al. Toxicological potential of acyl glucuronides and its assessment. Drug Metab Pharmacokinet 2017;32(1):2–11.

[43] Wang P, Pradhan K, Zhong XB, et al. Isoniazid metabolism and hepatotoxicity. Acta Pharm Sin B 2016; 6(5):384–92.

[44] Illing PT, Vivian JP, Dudek NL, et al. Immune self-reactivity triggered by drug-modified HLA-peptide repertoire. Nature 2012;486(7404):554–8.

[45] Monshi MM, Faulkner L, Gibson A, et al. Human leukocyte antigen (HLA)-B*57:01-restricted activation of drug-specific T cells provides the immunological basis for flucloxacillin-induced liver injury. Hepatology 2013; 57(2):727–39.

[46] Norcross MA, Luo S, Lu L, et al. Abacavir induces loading of novel self-peptides into HLA-B*57: 01: an autoimmune model for HLA-associated drug hypersensitivity. AIDS 2012;26(11):F21–9.

[47] Kim SH, Saide K, Farrell J, et al. Characterization of amoxicillin- and clavulanic acid-specific T cells in patients with amoxicillin-clavulanate-induced liver injury. Hepatology 2015;62(3):887–99.

[48] Usui T, Tailor A, Faulkner L, et al. HLA-A*33:03-restricted activation of ticlopidine-specific T-cells from human donors. Chem Res Toxicol 2018;31(10):1022–4.

[49] Metushi IG, Cai P, Zhu X, et al. A fresh look at the mechanism of isoniazid-induced hepatotoxicity. Clin Pharmacol Ther 2011;89(6):911–4.

[50] Daly AK. Are polymorphisms in genes relevant to drug disposition predictors of susceptibility to drug-induced liver injury? Pharm Res 2017;34(8):1564–9.

[51] Yimer G, Amogne W, Habtewold A, et al. High plasma efavirenz level and CYP2B6*6 are associated with efavirenz-based HAART-induced liver injury in the treatment of naive HIV patients from Ethiopia: a prospective cohort study. Pharmacogenomics J 2012;12(6):499–506.

[52] Ariyoshi N, Iga Y, Hirata K, et al. Enhanced susceptibility of HLA-mediated ticlopidine-induced idiosyncratic hepatotoxicity by CYP2B6 polymorphism in Japanese. Drug Metab Pharmacokinet 2010;25(3):298–306.

[53] Weaver RJ, Blomme EA, Chadwick AE, et al. Managing the challenge of drug-induced liver injury: a roadmap for the development and deployment of preclinical predictive models. Nat Rev Drug Discov 2020;19(2): 131–48.

[54] Ali I, Khalid S, Stieger B, et al. Effect of a common genetic variant (p.V444A) in the bile salt export pump on the inhibition of bile acid transport by cholestatic medications. Mol Pharm 2019;16(3):1406–11.

[55] Tam V, Patel N, Turcotte M, et al. Benefits and limitations of genome-wide association studies. Nat Rev Genet 2019;20(8):467–84.

[56] Lappalainen T, Scott AJ, Brandt M, et al. Genomic analysis in the age of human genome sequencing. Cell 2019;177(1):70–84.

[57] Nicoletti P, Barrett S, McEvoy L, et al. Shared genetic risk factors across carbamazepine-induced hypersensitivity reactions. Clin Pharmacol Ther 2019;106(5):1028–36.

[58] Li YJ, Dellinger A, Nicoletti P, et al. HLA B*14:01 is associated with Trimethoprim-sulfamethoxazole induced liver injury. J Hepatol 2019;70:e419.

[59] Xu CF, Johnson T, Wang X, et al. HLA-B*57:01 confers susceptibility to pazopanib-associated liver injury in patients with cancer. Clin Cancer Res 2016;22(6):1371–7.

[60] Petros Z, Kishikawa J, Makonnen E, et al. HLA-B*57 allele is associated with concomitant anti-tuberculosis and antiretroviral drugs induced liver toxicity in ethiopians. Front Pharmacol 2017;8:90.

[61] Li X, Jin S, Fan Y, et al. Association of HLA-C*03:02 with methimazole-induced liver injury in Graves' disease patients. Biomed Pharmacother 2019;117:109095.

[62] Kindmark A, Jawaid A, Harbron CG, et al. Genome-wide pharmacogenetic investigation of a hepatic adverse event without clinical signs of immunopathology suggests an underlying immune pathogenesis. Pharmacogenomics J 2008;8:186–95.

[63] Parham LR, Briley LP, Li L, et al. Comprehensive genome-wide evaluation of lapatinib-induced liver injury yields a single genetic signal centered on known risk allele HLA-DRB1*07:01. Pharmacogenomics J 2016;16(2):180–5.

[64] Nicoletti P, Werk AN, Sawle A, et al. HLA-DRB1*16: 01-DQB1*05: 02 is a novel genetic risk factor for flupirtine-induced liver injury. Pharmacogenet Genomics 2016; 26(5):218–24.

Advances in Molecular Pathology 3 (2020) 117–129

ADVANCES IN MOLECULAR PATHOLOGY

Bringing Pharmacogenetics to Prescribers

Progress and Challenges

David L. Thacker, PharmD, Jessica Savieo, MPGx, Houda Hachad, PharmD, MRes*

Translational Software Inc, 12410 Southeast 32nd Street, Suite 250, Bellevue, WA 98005, USA

KEYWORDS
- Pharmacogenetics • Pharmacogenomics • Implementation • Challenges • Barriers • Reporting
- Precision medicine • Genomics

KEY POINTS
- Progress has been made in implementing pharmacogenetics programs.
- Resources are needed for reconciliation of pharmacogenetic knowledge.
- Community is self-organizing to obtain consensus for evidence quality metrics.
- Health care providers' uptake of pharmacogenetics information is encouraging.

INTRODUCTION

With the advent of the Precision Medicine Initiative, announced in 2015 [1], there was a reinvigoration in the promise of pharmacogenetics to help patients and providers improve overall health. In response, several initiatives launched to support the implementation of PGx programs. In 2000, the National Institutes of Health established the Pharmacogenomics Research Network (PGRN), which, in its current iteration, supports pharmacogenomics research and provides resources to advance the practice of PGx testing. The Electronic Medical Records and Genomics Network was created to facilitate the integration of genomic medicine into electronic health records (EHR) systems. Around the same time, several PGx clinical trials were under way as part of the Implementing Genomics in Practice Pragmatic Clinical Trials Network. This network funded institutions that implemented pilot PGx testing and provided an opportunity for multi-institutional collaboration, initiating the creation of a sufficient

real-world patient population to examine the impact of PGx testing on important clinical outcomes [2].

One of the promises of PGx testing is a reduction in adverse drug reactions. Despite recent advances in knowledge and publication of PGx guidelines, adverse drug reactions continue to be a significant impediment and burden to the health care system. According to the Centers for Disease Control and Prevention, approximately 1.3 million emergency room visits each year are attributable to adverse drug events, of which 350,000 patients need to be hospitalized [3]. Although both clinical effectiveness [4–7] and cost effectiveness [8,9] of PGx-guided treatment strategies have been shown in studies, implementers continue to explore ways to enhance utilization and reach consensus around optimal PGx program deployment models. One of the key facilitators for clinical applicability has been the publication of evidence-based practice guidelines for actionable gene-drug pairs by established expert groups, such as the Clinical Pharmacogenetics

---

*Corresponding author, *E-mail address:* Houda.Hachad@translationalsoftware.com

https://doi.org/10.1016/j.yamp.2020.07.011
2589-4080/20/

Implementation Consortium (CPIC) [10], the Dutch Pharmacogenetics Working Group (DPWG) [11], and the Canadian Pharmacogenomics Network for Drug Safety [12]. These expert guidelines are the cornerstone for operationalizing PGx knowledge into therapeutic strategies by health care providers (HCPs) from various medical specialties.

This article discusses the progress and challenges in interpreting and reporting PGx test results. The focus on the quality of the PGx information, the infrastructure required to implement a successful testing program, the regulatory framework encountered while implementing in a clinical setting, and the different deployments of PGx models.

NAVIGATING AN EXPANDING EVIDENTIARY LANDSCAPE
Collecting and Distilling Relevant Data Sets
Of concern to clinicians, regulators, researchers, and stakeholders is the quality of the PGx information used to make clinical decisions. The US Food and Drug Administration (FDA) has been troubled by the marketing of PGx tests to providers and consumers with dubious scientific claims. In particular, the agency mentioned its concern on marketing claims "that are not supported by recommendations in the FDA-approved drug labeling or other scientific evidence" [13]. It was recognized early on that high-quality evidence, evaluated by panels of experts, would be required for successful uptake of PGx-guided interventions by HCPs.

As such, the CPIC [10] was established in 2009 as a joint project between the PGRN and the Pharmacogenomics Knowledgebase (PharmGKB) [14]. CPIC has published 24 guidelines covering 20 genes and 61 drugs. CPIC's evidence-based practice guidelines provide clear, actionable, genotype-based prescribing recommendations for known gene-drug pairs. CPIC guidelines intend to help HCPs understand how a PGx test result can be used for prescribing decisions. They are not intended, however, to be a determinant of whether a test should be ordered or to whom it should be offered [10]. CPIC membership is composed of international volunteers and a staff who are interested in "facilitating the use of pharmacogenetic tests for patient care." An impediment to establishing PGx testing in a clinical setting is the complexity of translating laboratory research into actionable prescribing interventions. Hence, "CPIC's goal is to address this barrier to clinical implementation of pharmacogenetic tests

by creating, curating and posting freely available, peer-reviewed, evidence-based, updatable, and detailed gene/drug clinical practice guidelines" [15].

Another organization actively providing PGx recommendations is the DPWG [16]. Founded by the Royal Dutch Pharmacists Association in 2005, the DPWG has reviewed PGx evidence for numerous gene-drug pairs and issued key genotype-based therapeutic recommendations. The DPWG has developed recommendations for 97 drug-gene interactions. Along with drug regulatory agencies, both CPIC and DPWG now are recognized by the community as the leading expert entities for creating and disseminating up-to-date clinical PGx recommendations. The European Ubiquitous Pharmacogenomics (U-PGx), a consortium leading the clinical implementation efforts across Europe, adopted the DPWG recommendations [11]. Although the DPWG guidelines are available to HCPs in the Netherlands, the U-PGx goal is to encourage "wide-spread adoption" throughout the European community and has translated these guidelines into English, German, Spanish, Greek, Italian, and Slovene.

Reconciliating Information from Multiple Sources
An examination of the PGx data quality reviewed by the FDA or recognized expert groups CPIC and DPWG shows a wide range of heterogeneity. Although recommendations for some drug-gene pairs derive from multiple replicated and independent studies, others are formulated based on a class effect. For example, CPIC's guideline for tricyclics with CYP2D6 and CYP2C19 applies to 10 distinct medications: amitriptyline, nortriptyline, doxepin, clomipramine, desipramine, imipramine, maprotiline, protriptyline, amoxapine, and trimipramine; however, a vast majority of the supportive PGx findings pertain to amitriptyline and nortriptyline [17]. In the FDA-approved labeling of tricyclic medications, changes in systematic plasma concentrations are recognized in individuals harboring CYP2D6 abnormal phenotypes, but no corrective actions are proposed [18]. Given that tricyclic medications have been available for many decades, it is unlikely that new data will emerge from PGx studies, and it will be essential to use data in a real-world setting to confirm and validate the pharmacogene(s) associations for this therapeutic class.

The overall community views the recent effort by the FDA to share its perspective on what type of PGx information is available to HCPs from labels as beneficial because it opens a dialogue between the agency, testing laboratories, and evidence producers. In its current format, however, the list of PGx associations [18] is not consumable for HCPs and is insufficient for diagnostic partners. For example, with an established pharmacogene, such as *CYP2C9*, the table identifies 8 medications with variable outcomes in individuals with reduced CYP2C9 enzyme activity (intermediate or poor metabolizers). Although the information provided is valuable, a closer examination of the information within the labels shows some noticeable gaps. For example, in the FDA label for warfarin, guidance is provided for *CYP2C9* and *VKORC1* to provide dosing adjustments for different genotype groups; however, for *CYP2C9*, the only alleles mentioned in the label dosing table are *CYP2C9*1*, *CYP2C9*2*, and *CYP2C9*3*. *CYP2C9* alleles that are common among some African and African American populations, such as *CYP2C9*5*, *CYP2C9*6*, *CYP2C9*8*, and *CYP2C9*11* [19,20], are mentioned in the text of the label, but they are not accounted for in the dosing table and could lead to the potential of overdosing of individuals of these ethnicities. HCPs will not be able to rely on the label when a patient's result reveals the presence of a *CYP2C9* genotype that contains 1 of these *CYP2C9* alleles that are not covered in the dosing table in the FDA label. A similar example is siponimod, which is contraindicated for patients with a *CYP2C9*3/*3* genotype [21]. It is left to the end user to extrapolate the interpretation for *CYP2C9* genotypes that include other no-function alleles, such as *CYP2C9*6*.

Moreover, the interpretation of genotype results from laboratory developed tests on existing commercial platforms [22] is possible only if a laboratory can identify which allelic variants to test and how to translate a given genotype result into a likely phenotype. Neither of these steps is available from FDA labels. It then becomes crucial to rely on other vetted sources and experts, such as CPIC authors, who can assemble all the necessary data sets for a laboratory to make proper use of the FDA label information. This need can be filled by software vendors and companies specializing in interpretation, such as Translational Software [23], who have created a knowledge base of PGx information contained within FDA labels as well as other data sets from authoritative sources, such as CPIC and DPWG. The more sophisticated vendors provide a practical and complete process for tracing the source of the interpretation of a result, its supporting evidence, and quality. Maintenance of a knowledge base demands expertise and the establishment of standard operating procedures for data collection, representation, and updates.

Another factor that can affect the confidence in the data used for PGx recommendations is discrepancies between multiple sources. To cope with this discordance, it is essential to adhere to a rigorous evidence review process. Components of a quality evidence review process include not only a critical review of the FDA label but also any published clinical guidelines. These reviews can be enhanced further by data gathered from peer-reviewed literature. A useful implementation of a literature review is exemplified with the clopidogrel-*CYP2C19* interaction. The FDA label recognizes that an alternate therapy should be considered in CYP2C19 poor metabolizers, but it is silent regarding other CYP2C19 phenotypes. A clinical guideline by CPIC does address all of the CYP2C19 phenotypes but has not been updated since 2013, and new evidence indicates that CYP2C19 ultrarapid metabolizers may be at increased risk of bleeding events [24], which is not underscored by the CPIC guideline.

Recognizing Gaps of Knowledge and Limitations of Use

Many laboratories often are tempted to test for PGx genes and variants that b have been included in commercial assays or have been cataloged in PharmGKB but are not subject to a practice guideline. When these variants or genes are offered in existing testing panels, it becomes necessary to analyze the published associations and formulate an interpretation for the expected results, although actionability is limited. A good example is the association between the acylphosphatase 2 (*ACYP2*) rs1872328 variant and the risk of cisplatin-induced ototoxicity in white patients. This association has consistent findings from distinct groups [25–27] and can be used to identify individuals at higher risk, although the effective corrective actions are unclear. When evaluating the evidence used for PGx recommendations, it is important to provide the underlying references for the supportive data used. Another factor that can affect the confidence and quality of a PGx recommendation is whether the PGx effect is provided as data or as an interpretation. If it is an interpretation, it could introduce a bias into the recommendation. A controversy around PGx recommendations also exists when proprietary algorithms and combinatorial approaches are used to make extrapolated recommendations. Often the input and rules for existing PGx algorithms are obscured and not available for evaluation by the scientific community or the end user. Furthermore, to achieve these algorithms and combinations, some of the scored genetic variants still are in the exploratory stage and do not have indisputable evidence [28].

An additional issue that can affect the accuracy of a likely phenotype, based on genotype, is not factoring in other patient-specific variables, such as comedications that potentially could limit the phenotype assignment. For example, a genotype may predict a normal metabolizer phenotype for a particular enzyme, but in the presence of a coprescribed drug that is a strong inhibitor, the enzyme activity could be converted from that of a normal metabolizer to a poor metabolizer. This phenomenon is known as phenoconversion. It is important to acknowledge the possibility of phenoconversion, and, in certain circumstances, it should be called out more explicitly [29]. For instance, when comedications are taken into consideration with tamoxifen, the prediction of phenotype based on CYP2D6 activity score is improved [30,31]. PGx consultation by clinical pharmacists for polypharmacy patients or those with multiple conditions or comorbidities is necessary. The use of a PGx report alone in these patients is unlikely to capture all factors related to atypical drug responses [30].

CONTINUOUS AND EFFECTIVE USE OF PHARMACOGENETIC TEST RESULTS RELIES ON SYSTEMS AND EXPERTS
Tackling Heterogeneity in Testing Modalities
The effective use of PGx information relies on the accurate prediction of a drug-associated phenotype for the individual patient. It is important for HCPs to have access to this information from reliable testing. For many actionable pharmacogenes, testing is performed by genotyping for common variants that are prevalent in the general population, and many variants are sequence variations (ie, single nucleotide variants or small insertions and deletions) that easily can be assayed by various commercial and laboratory-developed platforms. For genes, such as CYP2D6, however, testing can be complex, requiring the analysis of both sequence variants and structural variations [32]. The criteria used by testing laboratories to select which variants to interrogate depends on the methodology they select, how familiar they are with its limitations, their understanding of the loci, and the patient population they serve. Test panels with a greater number of actionable variants (those associated with known functional effects) would likely be expected

to predict phenotype status more accurately. Recent efforts by the Association for Molecular Pathology (AMP) seek to provide a consensus minimum list of variants constituting a valid test for commonly tested pharmacogenes [33,34]. Adoption of these criteria by laboratories hopefully will reduce interlaboratory heterogeneity or discrepancies. Until a list is defined for required variants, it is essential for laboratory directors and commercial testing vendors to understand and document which results can be obtained accurately versus those that will be omitted by each testing panel. This is a continuous challenge because laboratories may use a wide variety of methods for PGx testing, change testing modalities over time, and face difficulties when targeting complex loci, such as CYP2D6. The authors' experience, as an interpretation partner, shows that despite the successful deployment of a fully automated system that takes raw results and calls haplotypes and diplotypes, it remains essential to provide expertise to laboratory directors who are not always familiar with unexpected or rare results. For example, access via PharmVar [35] to the growing catalog of hundreds of CYP2D6 alleles and suballeles may be overwhelming for a user who is not familiar with the complexities of this gene. As shown in the recent efforts to characterize CYP2D6 reference material samples, the choice of the testing technology is crucial to understanding what a test can or cannot detect [36].

Adopting New Knowledge and Executing Updates
A fundamental assumption of preemptive PGx is that results are useful over a patient's lifetime and, therefore, must be interpreted with new knowledge as scientific evidence arises. In past years, the CPIC, DPWG, and FDA have provided updates to existing PGx information within their recommendations. Table 1 shows examples of updated PGx knowledge for drug-gene pairs post-implementation. They include changes to the genotype to phenotype assignment rules for CYP2D6 [22] as well as changes to both functional effects of specific TPMT variants [37] and recommended interventions for specific DPYD genotypes or phenotypes [38]. In some cases, the nomenclature of a specific allele can change as well (eg, CYP2D6*14A was updated to CYP2D6*114) [35]. The adoption of these updates across institutions is challenging and requires both domain expertise and infrastructure. A small change, such as the change of an allele, name might seem minor, but it may become an issue if the retired name is stored in a patient's record. Meanwhile,

TABLE 1
Examples of Recent Updates in Pharmacogenetics Knowledge

Type of Update and Example	Description	Impact
Change in the variant/allele function change *TPMT*8*	Published studies showed limited evidence for the allele functionality. This resulted in CPIC changing the predicted allele function from "probable reduced function/decreased activity" to "unknown function."	• The *TPMT*8*, when found in a diplotype with a normal function allele (*TPMT*1*), leads to an unknown phenotype under the newest recommendations; previously, these diplotypes were given an intermediate metabolizer phenotype. When found with a no function allele (*2, *3A, *11), the *8 leads to a possible intermediate metabolizer phenotype. All phenotypes containing 2 unknown function alleles have unknown metabolizer status. • Changes in allele function frequently occur as the number of published findings on these alleles increases over time. Because these changes have a direct impact on patient phenotype, it is important to ensure that a patient record is updated accordingly. Additionally, care should be taken in dating any documents that cannot be easily updated (static PDFs, etc.).
Change in the genotype to phenotype assignment CYP2D6	A group of CYP2D6 experts collaborated to reach a consensus genotype to phenotype assignment for CYP2D6 to allow for consistent reporting across the PGx community. An activity scoring approach was maintained; however, the allele score assigned to the *CYP2D6*10* and the activity score ranges for each phenotype were modified.	• Genotype to phenotype updates are used to bring consensus and consistency to PGx reporting. These changes have a direct impact on patient phenotype; therefore, it is important to ensure that a patient record is updated accordingly. • For CYP2D6, a majority of the changes shifted patient phenotypes from normal to intermediate metabolizers, which can lead to a significant impact on clinical recommendations for some medications. The clinical impact of these updates is less evident, however, on other phenotypes, such as ultrarapid and poor metabolizers. • Although these phenotype updates do not invalidate the recommendations made at the time of reporting, updating phenotypes can play an important role in future prescribing decisions.

(continued on next page)

TABLE 1
(continued)

Type of Update and Example	Description	Impact
Change in the variant/allele name *CYP2D6*14A*	The *14A allele was separated from the *14B allele due to a key variant difference in the haplotype definition that resulted in a distinct allele function. The *14B then was given the *14 designation maintaining a decreased function status while the *14A became the *114 allele with a no function status.	• From a phenotypic and clinical implementation standpoint, there was no change for any diplotype containing either *14 suballele. Splitting the 2 alleles, however, can prevent phenotype mistakes that may occur if the suballele letter designation was missed or improperly assigned. • Because these changes have a direct impact on the genotype name that may be stored in a patient's record, it is important to update genotype name when used in post-test alerts triggers.
Change in the recommendation *DPYD*	In 2013, CPIC published a guideline for fluoropyrimidine dosing based on *DPYD* diplotypes. In 2017, CPIC updated the guideline using an activity scoring method to establish DPYD phenotype.	• The activity scoring method made a difference not only in the translation of variant results to phenotype terms but also in the granularity of the prescribing recommendations. When using activity score, the recommendations for the DPYD phenotype terms of intermediate and poor metabolizers were able to be broken down to the contributing activity scores. • By considering more detailed activity information, initial fluoropyrimidine dosing can be tailored closer to a patient's anticipated needs.
Change in the severity of a PGx issue *G6PD and quinine*	From acceptance, the FDA label for quinine (Qualaquin) stated a contraindication in patients with known G6PD deficiency. As of June 2019, the FDA removed the contraindication for these high-risk patients.	• Downgrades in severity may not have a negative clinical impact on patients but keeping up to date on this information is necessary to maintain clinical accountability. • Additionally, it highlights the importance of updating with transparency to establish legitimacy in clinical application of pharmacogenomics.

patients can change HCPs or leave the health care system where the test was conducted, creating challenges for implementers and laboratories that attempt to recontact them and update their health records. Having traceability of the historical records of changes in PGx data sets within the EHRs records adds complexity during deployment.

INFRASTRUCTURE FOR DELIVERING PHARMACOGENETIC INSIGHT
Focusing on Pharmacogenetic Interventions Rather than Results

The complexity of interpreting PGx test results and effectively transforming laboratory raw results into therapeutic interventions is a challenge faced by many laboratories. Software and interpretation companies, such as Translational Software, can provide the needed expertise and technology to laboratories with a variety of experience in PGx. When working with multiple laboratories, the authors recognized early that multiple strategies must be employed to receive results from distinct testing modalities and interpret and deliver them into existing clinician workflows. Efforts led to the deployment of PGx reports based on HCPs preferences, incorporating the use of established visual presentations and iconography, like the stoplight approach, along with the therapeutic implications and proposed corrective interventions. Unlike traditional genetic test reports aimed at disease susceptibility or diagnosis, which often are ordered by a limited number of physicians with some genetic training, the use of nonspecialized genetic terminology .and language became crucial to facilitate the comprehension of PGx reports by a diverse community of HCPs. When possible, PGx recommendations borrow language from other common drug recommendations, such as drug-drug interactions or drug-age recommendations, that are presented to physicians by drug information resources (Fig. 1). The adoption of more intuitive standard phenotype terms [39] provides a common vocabulary to enhance communication between PGx natives and non-natives. The genetic details of the results in terms of variant coordinates, genotypes, and methodology still are provided on the report but no longer are the focal point of the interpretation. Clear section headings establish a hierarchy that orders information from most to least clinically relevant (see Fig. 1).

The authors' experience delivering PGx interpretation within a report indicates that a lack of PGx knowledge by HCPs and laboratorians is one of the biggest challenges for uptake and best use of the report. Many surveys of HCPs show that although they are enthusiastic in employing testing strategies, they still struggle with how to best use recommendations in their therapeutic decisions [40–45]. Warning physicians about a potential genotype or phenotype-associated issue for an individual is insufficient and is likely to be ignored unless precise interventions or corrective actions are offered. This is supported further by AMP's position that a PGx report that has only genotype and predicted phenotypes will likely be underutilized if not entirely ignored.

Achieving Dynamic Integration of Pharmacogenetics Insight into Clinical Workflow

As indicated by different PGx implementers [46], PGx test reports became the first necessary step to presenting novel genotype-based therapeutic interventions to prescribers. The static nature of the data represented in these stand-alone documents, however, ultimately limited broader use and slowly is being replaced by the development of pop-up alerts at the point of care and within existing clinical workflows. Successful adoption of pharmacogenomics into routine clinical care requires a curated and machine-readable database of PGx knowledge suitable for use in an EHR with clinical decision support (CDS). Meanwhile, many EHR vendors do not provide a standard set of CDS functions for PGx knowledge. This opened an opportunity to create an EHR-agnostic resource for implementers.

Different examples of deployment of such CDS have been described by implementers in the United States and Europe [47,48]. As reported by implementers, the logistical needs grow significantly when an institution decides to go beyond the PDF report, requiring multidisciplinary teams to employ in-house expertise and infrastructure and, in some cases, third-party partnerships for successful implementation. The Sanford health PGx program is an example that leverages a combination of Translational Software technologies and in-house laboratory and expertise to support the delivery of PGx recommendations in both a PDF report and interruptive post-test result alerts [49]. Monitoring of prescription changes can be achieved by interfacing directly with the EHR, allowing the addition of other patient parameters to refine eligibility. The deployment of post-test result alerts can be achieved in a systematic manner where actionable results can be held in escrow until a medication is considered.

Many PGx programs began by offering reactive PGx testing at the time of medication prescribing, but, as PGx testing was embraced, interest in preemptive testing has begun to gain popularity. For preemptive testing, a question that often arises is, "Who to test?" There is no 1-size-fits-all solution, but possible scenarios include polypharmacy patients, high-risk patients, or those taking medications that have phenotype-specific dosing recommendations. In cases of patients on numerous drugs, the chances of adverse drug reactions are related directly to the number of medications the patient is taking [50,51]. A provider may order a preemptive PGx test to help prescribing or deprescribing, to minimize the chance of having an adverse effect. High-risk patients, such as the elderly or patients taking certain narrow therapeutic medications, also could benefit from PGx testing. Although clinical guidelines are available for defining what a test result means, the PGx community lacks tools that

A

Comprehensive Pharmacogenetic Report

Current Patient Medications

Metoprolol, Voriconazole, Codeine, Siponimod

⊗ **Voriconazole**
Vfend

Non-Response to Voriconazole (CYP2C19: Rapid Metabolizer)   ACTIONABLE

Voriconazole plasma concentrations are expected to be low if a standard dose is used, increasing the risk of loss of response and effectiveness and subsequent disease progression. Consider an alternative medication that is not dependent on CYP2C19 metabolism, such as isavuconazole, liposomal amphotericin B or posaconazole.
- Moriyama B, Obeng AO, Barbarino J, Penzak SR, Henning SA, Scott SA, Agúndez J, Wingard JR, McLeod HL, Klein TE, Cross SJ, Caudle KE, Walsh TJ. Clinical Pharmacogenetics Implementation Consortium (CPIC) Guidelines for CYP2C19 and Voriconazole Therapy. Clin Pharmacol Ther 2017 07;102(1)45-51.

⚠ **Codeine**
Codeine; Fioricet with Codeine

Possible Non-Response to Codeine (CYP2D6: Intermediate Metabolizer)   ACTIONABLE

Reduced morphine levels are anticipated, and the patient may or may not experience adequate pain relief with codeine. Codeine can be prescribed at standard label-recommended dosage and administration, with monitoring for symptoms of insufficient pain relief. Other opioids not metabolized by CYP2D6 may also be considered (i.e., morphine, oxymorphone, buprenorphine, fentanyl, methadone, and hydromorphone).
- Crews KR, Gaedigk A, Dunnenberger HM, Leeder JS, Klein TE, Caudle KE, Haidar CE, Shen DD, Callaghan JT, Sadhasivam S, Prows CA, Kharasch ED, Skaar TC, . Clinical Pharmacogenetics Implementation Consortium guidelines for cytochrome P450 2D6 genotype and codeine therapy: 2014 update. Clin Pharmacol Ther 2014 Apr;95(4):376-82.

⚠ **Metoprolol**
Lopressor

Increased Exposure to Metoprolol (CYP2D6: Intermediate Metabolizer)   ACTIONABLE

The patient's genotype may be associated with an increased metoprolol exposure following standard dosing. When compared to a normal metabolizer, an intermediate metabolizer may require a 50% dose reduction. If metoprolol is prescribed, be alert to adverse events (e.g., bradycardia or cold extremities).
- The Royal Dutch Pharmacists Association of the KNMP. (2019). Pharmacogenetic Recommendations 2019 [PDF file]. Retrieved from https://www.knmp.nl/downloads/pharmacogenetic-recommendations-august-2019.pdf (Accessed August 21, 2019).

✓ **Siponimod**
Mayzent

Normal Exposure to Siponimod (CYP2C9: Normal Metabolizer)   ACTIONABLE

The patient's genotype is associated with a normal siponimod clearance. Consider the following standard daily dosing regimen:

- Initiation and up-titration: d1–2: 0.25 mg - d 3: 0.50 mg - d 4: 0.75 mg - d 5: 1.25 mg
- Maintenance dose starting d 6 and after: 2 mg

Concomitant use of CYP2C9/3A4 dual inhibitor (e.g. fluconazole) or moderate CYP2C9 inhibitor concomitantly with a strong or moderate CYP3A4 inhibitor are not recommended. Caution should be exercised for concomitant use of moderate CYP2C9 inhibitors.

Concomitant use of strong CYP3A4/moderate CYP2C9 inducers (e.g. rifampicin or carbamazepine) is not recommended.
- Mayzent [package insert]. East Hanover, NJ: Novartis Pharmaceuticals Corporation: 2019.

B

Potentially Impacted Medications

CATEGORY	DRUG CLASS	STANDARD PRECAUTIONS	USE WITH CAUTION	CONSIDER ALTERNATIVES
Cardiovascular	Anticoagulants	Apixaban (Eliquis) Betrixaban (Bevyxxa) Dabigatran Etexilate (Pradaxa) Edoxaban (Savaysa) Fondaparinux (Arixtra) Rivaroxaban (Xarelto) Warfarin (Coumadin)		
	Antiplatelets	Prasugrel (Effient) Ticagrelor (Brilinta) Vorapaxar (Zontivity)	Clopidogrel (Plavix)	
	Beta Blockers	Atenolol (Tenormin) Bisoprolol (Zebeta) Carvedilol (Coreg) Labetalol (Normodyne, Trandate) Nebivolol (Bystolic) Propranolol (Inderal)	Metoprolol (Lopressor) Timolol (Timoptic)	
Infections	Antifungals	Amphotericin B (AmBisome, Abelcet) Anidulafungin (Eraxis) Caspofungin (Cancidas) Fluconazole (Diflucan) Isavuconazonium (Cresemba) Itraconazole (Sporanox) Micafungin (Mycamine) Posaconazole (Noxafil)		Voriconazole (Vfend)
	Anti-HIV Agents	Dolutegravir (Tivicay, Triumeq) Doravirine (Pifeltro) Efavirenz (Sustiva) Etravirine (Edurant) Raltegravir (Isentress, Dutrebis) Rilpivirine (Intelence)		

C
Dosing Guidance

⊗ **Amitriptyline**
Elavil

Decreased Amitriptyline Exposure (CYP2C19: Rapid Metabolizer)   INFORMATIVE

The patient's high CYP2C19 activity is likely to result in a significantly increased metabolism of amitriptyline to nortriptyline and a subsequent decrease in amitriptyline exposure leading to therapy failure or increased side effects.

Psychiatric Conditions: Consider an alternative medication. If amitriptyline is warranted, consider therapeutic drug monitoring to guide dose adjustments.

Neuropathic Pain: Consider an alternative medication. If amitriptyline is warranted titrate dose according to the patient's clinical response and tolerability.
- Hicks JK, Sangkuhl K, Swen JJ, Ellingrod VL, Müller DJ, Shimoda K, Bishop JR, Kharasch ED, Skaar TC, Gaedigk A, Dunnenberger HM, Klein TE, Caudle KE, Stingl JC. Clinical pharmacogenetics implementation consortium guideline (CPIC) for CYP2D6 and CYP2C19 genotypes and dosing of tricyclic antidepressants: 2016 update. Clin Pharmacol Ther 2017 07;102(1):37-44.

⊗ **Citalopram**
Celexa

Insufficient Response to Citalopram (CYP2C19: Rapid Metabolizer)   ACTIONABLE

At standard label-recommended dosage, citalopram plasma concentrations levels are expected to be low which may result in a loss of efficacy. Consider an alternative medication. If citalopram is warranted, consider increasing the dose to a maximum of 150% and titrate based on the clinical response and tolerability.
- Hicks JK, Bishop JR, Sangkuhl K, Müller DJ, Ji Y, Leckband SG, Leeder JS, Graham RL, Chiulli DL, LLerena A, Skaar TC, Scott SA, Stingl JC, Klein TE, Caudle KE, Gaedigk A . Clinical Pharmacogenetics Implementation Consortium (CPIC) Guideline for CYP2D6 and CYP2C19 Genotypes and Dosing of Selective Serotonin Reuptake Inhibitors. Clin Pharmacol Ther 2015 Aug;98(2):127-34.

⊗ **Clomipramine**
Anafranil

Decreased Clomipramine Exposure (CYP2C19: Rapid Metabolizer)   INFORMATIVE

The patient's high CYP2C19 activity is likely to result in a significantly increased metabolism of clomipramine to desmethyl clomipramine and a subsequent decrease in clomipramine exposure leading to therapy failure or increased side effects.

Psychiatric Conditions: Consider an alternative medication. If clomipramine is warranted, consider therapeutic drug monitoring to guide dose adjustments.
- Hicks JK, Sangkuhl K, Swen JJ, Ellingrod VL, Müller DJ, Shimoda K, Bishop JR, Kharasch ED, Skaar TC, Gaedigk A, Dunnenberger HM, Klein TE, Caudle KE, Stingl JC. Clinical pharmacogenetics implementation consortium guideline (CPIC) for CYP2D6 and CYP2C19 genotypes and dosing of tricyclic antidepressants: 2016 update. Clin Pharmacol Ther 2017 07;102(1):37-44.

⊗ **Doxepin**
Silenor

Decreased Doxepin Exposure (CYP2C19: Rapid Metabolizer)   INFORMATIVE

The patient's high CYP2C19 activity is likely to result in a significantly increased metabolism of doxepin to desmethyl doxepin and a subsequent decrease in doxepin exposure leading to therapy failure or increased side effects.

Psychiatric Conditions: Consider an alternative medication. If doxepin is warranted, consider therapeutic drug monitoring to guide dose adjustments.

Insomnia: Doxepin can be prescribed according to the standard recommended dosage and administration.
- Hicks JK, Sangkuhl K, Swen JJ, Ellingrod VL, Müller DJ, Shimoda K, Bishop JR, Kharasch ED, Skaar TC, Gaedigk A, Dunnenberger HM, Klein TE, Caudle KE, Stingl JC. Clinical pharmacogenetics implementation consortium guideline (CPIC) for CYP2D6 and CYP2C19 genotypes and dosing of tricyclic antidepressants: 2016 update. Clin Pharmacol Ther 2017 07;102(1):37-44.

⊗ **Escitalopram**
Lexapro

Insufficient Response to Escitalopram (CYP2C19: Rapid Metabolizer)   ACTIONABLE

At standard label-recommended dosage, escitalopram plasma concentrations levels are expected to be low which may result in a loss of efficacy. Consider an alternative medication. If escitalopram is warranted, consider increasing the dose to a maximum of 150% and titrate based on the clinical response and tolerability.
- Hicks JK, Bishop JR, Sangkuhl K, Müller DJ, Ji Y, Leckband SG, Leeder JS, Graham RL, Chiulli DL, LLerena A, Skaar TC, Scott SA, Stingl JC, Klein TE, Caudle KE, Gaedigk A . Clinical Pharmacogenetics Implementation Consortium (CPIC) Guideline for CYP2D6 and CYP2C19 Genotypes and Dosing of Selective Serotonin Reuptake Inhibitors. Clin Pharmacol Ther 2015 Aug;98(2):127-34.

D
Test Details

Gene	Genotype	Phenotype	Alleles Tested
CYP2B6	*1/*1	Normal Metabolizer	*16, *18, *22
CYP2C19	*1/*17	Rapid Metabolizer	*2, *3, *4A, *4B, *5, *6, *8, *10, *17
CYP2C9	*1/*1	Normal Metabolizer	*2, *3, *4, *5, *8, *11
CYP2D6	*5/*17	Intermediate Metabolizer	*2, *3, *4, *4M, *6, *8, *9, *10, *12, *114, *14, *17, *29, *41, *5 (gene deletion), XN (gene duplication)
CYP3A5	*1/*7	Intermediate Metabolizer	*2, *3, *6, *7, *8
SLCO1B1	521T>C T/T	Normal Function	521T>C
VKORC1	-1639G>A G/A	Intermediate Warfarin Sensitivity	2255C>T, 3730G>A, 1542G>C, -1639G>A, 1173C>T

FIG. 1 (*Continued*)

can help a non-PGx specialty provider and/or a health care organization prioritize who could benefit from a test. By simply analyzing the medications taken by a patient, the authors developed a PGx benefit index based on potential PGx associations with the patients' self-reported medications, the clinical significance of the gene-drug interaction, and the evidentiary quality of the PGx associations. Using an application programming interface, it is possible for a central PGx service to remotely and continuously monitor poly-medicated patients and detect if or when they would be most suitable for a PGx test.

Two recognized modalities for PGx testing have been used when deciding when and who to test. Reactive testing is conducted for a single gene after a medication has been selected but before initiation, whereas pre-emptive panel-based testing is performed on multiple genes before the HCP chooses a medication to prescribe. Both modalities take place only when a physician is considering a PGx-informed medication for the patient. The authors' experience working with laboratories and clinical organizations demonstrates they favor the preemptive panel-based approach because it allows multiple pharmacogenes to be tested and their results saved to be later used for subsequent prescriptions.

Although the creation and maintenance of point-of-care CDS for a single gene-test result is feasible, the retention of multiple PGx results records in the EHRs and their use to drive CDS requires continuous efforts and a solid and scalable infrastructure [52–56]. As more diverse genetic phenotypes are obtained for a patient, the lack of consensus in the community regarding where this information should be held in the patient's record can force important phenotype data to go unnoticed by the physician. Depending on the organization's preference and the EHR system, PGx information, such as phenotypes, may be stored under an allergies section or within a problem list section, and not necessarily in patient-facing consulting activities during medication reviews or it may reside in a separate dedicated pharmacogenomic section of the record.

Furthermore, in domains where there is no established guideline or best-practice model, the decision often is left to the laboratory or the provider who ordered the test. Reporting of incidental findings is one instance, and it occurs when an ordering HCP interested in a test for a specific medication receives results for additional medications that are pertinent to the patient. In many of these situations, providers are unclear on their responsibility in returning these secondary PGx findings to patients. In response, implementers have called for the development of guidelines documenting a standard practice [57]. Until such guidelines become available, the clinician and laboratory must decide whether or not to report incidental findings when a patient's medications are known at the time of the test order.

When offered to patients through their HCPs, PGx testing can serve as a catalyst to promote engagement by both parties. HCPs will use PGx knowledge as augmentative information about the individual patient to promote behavioral changes, while the patient's voice also is amplified during the interaction. The role of clinical pharmacists with PGx expertise will become crucial in facilitating this dialogue and offering support to both HCPs and patients. Pharmacists can undertake education roles for HCPs, who are increasingly expected to understand and interpret genetic test results while continuing to use clinical services and define treatment intervention aided by PGx testing [58]. Similarly, an effort by a group in the Netherlands has shown that a community pharmacist–led initiative was able to effectively identify patients requiring changes in their pharmacotherapy (24.2% of the subjects) based on preemptive PGx testing, in a primary care setting [59].

REGULATORY FRAMEWORK

When implementing a PGx program, not only the scientific intricacies and deployment hurdles need to be

---

FIG. 1 (**A**) Examples of recommendations provided for current patient medications. This section is placed at the beginning of a report to allow an HCP to direct immediate attention to the interpretations most relevant to the patient. (**B**) Example of a potentially impacted medications table. This table allows an HCP to make a quick comparison of medications in the same class and assess the safety of a medication as it pertains to a patient's PGx profile. (**C**) Example of a dosing guidance section. Detailing each PGx association and the resulting clinical recommendation for all medications evaluated, this section is the heart of the report and the main reference for the provider. (**D**) Example of a test details section, which lists the patient's results in genotype/diplotype and phenotype terms. The alleles tested list provides transparency to an HCP on which alleles were examined in the laboratory test.

considered but also the regulatory requirements from federal and state agencies. PGx testing is considered a laboratory-developed test of high complexity, and, although to date the FDA has exercised enforcement discretion, regulatory discussions are ongoing. Likewise, laboratories that perform PGx testing must be Clinical Laboratory Improvement Amendments of 1988 certified under the Centers for Medicare & Medicaid Services. Regional Medicare Administrative Contractors may approve only certain PGx panels for reimbursement, and an assortment of state regulations must be navigated for a laboratory to offer interstate services. The availability of an FDA-approved direct-to-consumer (DTC) PGx test in 2019 created domains of uncertainty surrounding the DTC test and its meaning. Although consumers may self-select to undergo this test, it is not clear whether these results are acceptable for clinical decision making. The lack of incorporation of these results in the patients' charts and their acceptance by an HCP who did not initiate testing is likely to limit their benefit.

More importantly, the recent launch of a new FDA table with selected drug-gene associations and labeling information [18] indicates that the agency is opening a path for implementation and is offering the community an additional resource that can be used to promote the value of PGx testing. Although many in the community still are unclear how regulators are weighing the evidence underlying PGx tests, FDA officials assure that they will work with the community to be more transparent. Some regulators suggest that because the FDA is still practicing enforcement discretion when it comes to laboratory-developed tests, the agency would allow laboratories to continue to offer PGx tests without its approval as long as they were making evidence-based claims. The FDA's new table cannot be considered a 1-stop resource for proper test result interpretation because it lacks many of the necessary steps for translating raw genotype results into therapeutic recommendations. For example, it will remain the responsibility of the implementer to gather the evidence to properly define which variants are actionable and to translate genotype signatures to known phenotypes. Because most of the supporting evidence for these steps already have been reviewed by experts within CPIC or DPWG, the community likely will consume this information in conjunction with the information provided by the FDA table of drug-gene associations or labels.

SUMMARY AND FUTURE DIRECTIONS

In the past years, the convergence of clinical genomics knowledge, informatics, and cost-efficient technologies has provided an opportunity for health care systems to embrace precision medicine. The establishment of a strong peer-reviewed clinical PGx evidence infrastructure through publicly available practice guidelines by expert groups, such as CPIC in the United States and DPWG in Europe, acted as the main catalysts for facilitating PGx testing into clinical care. The democratization of this clinical intervention and its deployment at a larger scale, however, still are lagging. Although several PGx initiatives have demonstrated the benefits of reactive PGx testing, preemptive testing is likely to be adopted as the best deployment approach to maximize the benefit of PGx. The development of innovative technologies that can help institutions qualify and prioritize patients for preemptive testing for pharmacogenes with potential clinical utility will help in the dissemination of genotype-guided strategies. The authors' experience indicates that although advances have been made in establishing standards for PGx testing and interpretation, implementers continue to require support for service expansion and sustainability. Organizations that successfully engage patients, their caretakers, and clinician champions will be able to demonstrate success for their pilot programs and scale operations effectively. Although large clinical organizations have in-house PGx expertise and informatics infrastructure to initiate and support a program, smaller institutions will rely on commercial partners to provide support for their clinical PGx service. Every PGx program will be reliant on a multidisciplinary team with expertise in laboratory operations, PGx knowledge, and information technology systems.

DISCLOSURE

All authors are employed by, receive wages from, and hold stocks for Translational Software Inc., a provider of pharmacogenomics content.

REFERENCES

[1] The White House. The Precision Medicine Initiative. 2015. Available at: https://obamawhitehouse.archives.gov/precision-medicine. Accessed March 11, 2020.

[2] GMKB and the IGNITE Network. IGNITE. 2012. Available at: https://gmkb.org/ignite/. Accessed March 11, 2020.

[3] Center for Disease Control (CDC). Adverse drug events in adults 2020. Available at: https://www.cdc.gov/medicationsafety/adult_adversedrugevents.html. Accessed February 13, 2020.

[4] Cavallari LH, Lee CR, Beitelshees AL, et al. Multisite investigation of outcomes with implementation of

CYP2C19 genotype-guided antiplatelet therapy after percutaneous coronary intervention. JACC Cardiovasc Interv 2018;11(2):181–91.

[5] Smith DM, Weitzel KW, Elsey AR, et al. CYP2D6-guided opioid therapy improves pain control in CYP2D6 intermediate and poor metabolizers: a pragmatic clinical trial. Genet Med 2019;21(8):1842–50.

[6] Henricks LM, Lunenburg CATC, de Man FM, et al. DPYD genotype-guided dose individualisation of fluoropyrimidine therapy in patients with cancer: a prospective safety analysis. Lancet Oncol 2018;19(11):1459–67.

[7] Walden LM, Brandl EJ, Tiwari AK, et al. Genetic testing for CYP2D6 and CYP2C19 suggests improved outcome for antidepressant and antipsychotic medication. Psychiatry Res 2018. https://doi.org/10.1016/j.psychres.2018.02.055.

[8] Limdi NA, Cavallari LH, Lee CR, et al. Cost-effectiveness of CYP2C19-guided antiplatelet therapy in patients with acute coronary syndrome and percutaneous coronary intervention informed by real-world data. Pharmacogenomics J 2020. https://doi.org/10.1038/s41397-020-0162-5.

[9] Henricks LM, Lunenburg CATC, de Man FM, et al. A cost analysis of upfront DPYD genotype-guided dose individualisation in fluoropyrimidine-based anticancer therapy. Eur J Cancer 2019;107:60–7.

[10] Relling MV, Klein TE. CPIC 2009. Available at: https://cpicpgx.org/. Accessed March 11, 2020.

[11] Guchelaar H. Ubiquitous Pharmacogenomics (U-PGx). 2005. Available at: http://upgx.eu/. Accessed March 11, 2020.

[12] CPNDS. Canadian Pharmacogenomics Network for Drug Safety (CPNDS). 2020. Available at: http://cpnds.ubc.ca/. Accessed March 5, 2020.

[13] FDA. FDA Announces Collaborative Review of Scientific Evidence to Support Associations Between Genetic Information and Specific Medications | FDA. 2020. Available at: https://www.fda.gov/news-events/press-announcements/fda-announces-collaborative-review-scientific-evidence-support-associations-between-genetic. Accessed February 28, 2020.

[14] PharmGKB. PharmGKB. Available at: https://www.pharmgkb.org/. Accessed March 14, 2020.

[15] Relling MV, Klein TE. CPIC-Guidelines 2009. Available at: https://cpicpgx.org/guidelines/. Accessed March 11, 2020.

[16] DPWG. Pharmacogenomics guidelines (DPWG). Available at: http://upgx.eu/guidelines/. Accessed March 14, 2020.

[17] Hicks JK, Sangkuhl K, Swen JJ, et al. Clinical pharmacogenetics implementation consortium guideline (CPIC) for CYP2D6 and CYP2C19 genotypes and dosing of tricyclic antidepressants: 2016 update. Clin Pharmacol Ther 2017;102(1):37–44.

[18] FDA. Table of Pharmacogenetic Associations. 2020. Available at: https://www.fda.gov/medical-devices/precision-medicine/table-pharmacogenetic-associations. Accessed March 11, 2020.

[19] Scott SA, Jaremko M, Lubitz SA, et al. CYP2C9*8 is prevalent among African-Americans: implications for pharmacogenetic dosing. Pharmacogenomics 2009;10(8):1243–55.

[20] Perera MA, Cavallari LH, Limdi NA, et al. Genetic variants associated with warfarin dose in African-American individuals: a genome-wide association study. Lancet 2013;382(9894):790–6.

[21] Mayzent [Package Insert]. 2019. Available at: https://www.accessdata.fda.gov/drugsatfda_docs/label/2019/209884s000lbl.pdf. Accessed November 22, 2019.

[22] Caudle KE, Sangkuhl K, Whirl-Carrillo M, et al. Standardizing CYP2D6 genotype to phenotype translation: consensus recommendations from the clinical pharmacogenetics implementation consortium and dutch pharmacogenetics working group. Clin Transl Sci 2019. https://doi.org/10.1111/cts.12692.

[23] Software T. Making sense of pharmacogenomics testing | translational software 2020. Available at: https://www.translationalsoftware.com/. Accessed March 14, 2020.

[24] Sorich MJ, Polasek TM, Wiese MD. Systematic review and meta-analysis of the association between cytochrome P450 2C19 genotype and bleeding. Thromb Haemost 2012;108(1):199–200.

[25] Vos HI, Guchelaar H-J, Gelderblom H, et al. Replication of a genetic variant in ACYP2 associated with cisplatin-induced hearing loss in patients with osteosarcoma. Pharmacogenet Genomics 2016;26(5):243–7.

[26] Drogemoller BI, Brooks B, Critchley C, et al. Further investigation of the role of ACYP2 and WFS1 pharmacogenomic variants in the development of cisplatin-induced ototoxicity in testicular cancer patients. Clin Cancer Res 2018;24(8):1866–71.

[27] Driessen CM, Ham JC, Te Loo M, et al. Genetic variants as predictive markers for ototoxicity and nephrotoxicity in patients with locally advanced head and neck cancer treated with cisplatin-containing chemoradiotherapy (the PRONE study). Cancers (Basel) 2019;11(4). https://doi.org/10.3390/cancers11040551.

[28] Bousman CA, Dunlop BW. Genotype, phenotype, and medication recommendation agreement among commercial pharmacogenetic-based decision support tools. Pharmacogenomics J 2018;18(5):613–22.

[29] Shah RR, Smith RL. Addressing phenoconversion: the Achilles' heel of personalized medicine. Br J Clin Pharmacol 2015;79(2):222–40.

[30] Borges S, Desta Z, Jin Y, et al. Composite functional genetic and comedication CYP2D6 activity score in predicting tamoxifen drug exposure among breast cancer patients. J Clin Pharmacol 2010;50(4):450–8.

[31] Gaedigk A, Simon SD, Pearce RE, et al. The CYP2D6 activity score: translating genotype information into a qualitative measure of phenotype. Clin Pharmacol Ther 2008;83(2):234–42.

[32] Nofziger C, Turner AJ, Sangkuhl K, et al. PharmVar GeneFocus: CYP2D6. Clin Pharmacol Ther 2020;107(1):154–70.

[33] Pratt VM, Cavallari LH, Del Tredici AL, et al. Recommendations for Clinical CYP2C9 genotyping allele selection: a joint recommendation of the association for molecular pathology and college of american pathologists. J Mol Diagn 2019;21(5):746–55.

[34] Pratt VM, Del Tredici AL, Hachad H, et al. Recommendations for Clinical CYP2C19 Genotyping Allele Selection: A Report of the Association for Molecular Pathology. J Mol Diagn 2018;20(3):269–76.

[35] PharmVar. PharmVar - CYP2D6. 2020. Available at: https://www.pharmvar.org/gene/CYP2D6. Accessed March 13, 2020.

[36] Gaedigk A, Turner A, Everts RE, et al. Characterization of reference materials for genetic testing of CYP2D6 Alleles: A GeT-RM Collaborative Project. J Mol Diagn 2019; 21(6):1034–52.

[37] Ujiie S, Sasaki T, Mizugaki M, et al. Functional characterization of 23 allelic variants of thiopurine S-methyltransferase gene (TPMT*2 - *24). Pharmacogenet Genomics 2008;18(10):887–93.

[38] Clinical Pharmacogenomics Implementation Consortium, PharmGKB. Annotation of CPIC Guideline for Capecitabine and DPYD. Available at: https://www.pharmgkb.org/guidelineAnnotation/PA166109594. Accessed January 14, 2020.

[39] Caudle KE, Dunnenberger HM, Freimuth RR, et al. Standardizing terms for clinical pharmacogenetic test results: consensus terms from the Clinical Pharmacogenetics Implementation Consortium (CPIC). Genet Med 2017; 19(2):215–23.

[40] Goodspeed A, Kostman N, Kriete TE, et al. Leveraging the utility of pharmacogenomics in psychiatry through clinical decision support: a focus group study. Ann Gen Psychiatry 2019;18:13.

[41] Kim W-Y, Kim H-S, Oh M, et al. Survey of physicians' views on the clinical implementation of pharmacogenomics-based personalized therapy. Transl Clin Pharmacol 2020;28(1):34–42.

[42] DeLuca J, Selig D, Poon L, et al. Toward personalized medicine implementation: survey of military medicine providers in the area of pharmacogenomics. Mil Med 2020;185(3–4):336–40.

[43] Rahawi S, Naik H, Blake KV, et al. Knowledge and attitudes on pharmacogenetics among pediatricians. J Hum Genet 2020. https://doi.org/10.1038/s10038-020-0723-0.

[44] Walden LM, Brandl EJ, Changasi A, et al. Physicians' opinions following pharmacogenetic testing for psychotropic medication. Psychiatry Res 2015;229(3):913–8.

[45] Lemke AA, Hutten Selkirk CG, Glaser NS, et al. Primary care physician experiences with integrated pharmacogenomic testing in a community health system. Per Med 2017;14(5):389–400.

[46] Bain KT, Schwartz EJ, Knowlton OV, et al. Implementation of a pharmacist-led pharmacogenomics service for the Program of All-Inclusive Care for the Elderly (PHARM-GENOME-PACE). J Am Pharm Assoc 2018; 58(3):281–9.e1.

[47] Blagec K, Koopmann R, Crommentuijn-van Rhenen M, et al. Implementing pharmacogenomics decision support across seven European countries: The Ubiquitous Pharmacogenomics (U-PGx) project. J Am Med Inform Assoc 2018;25(7):893–8.

[48] Bell GC, Crews KR, Wilkinson MR, et al. Development and use of active clinical decision support for preemptive pharmacogenomics. J Am Med Inform Assoc 2014; 21(e1):e93–9.

[49] Petry N, Baye J, Aifaoui A, et al. Implementation of wide-scale pharmacogenetic testing in primary care. Pharmacogenomics 2019;20(12):903–13.

[50] Finkelstein J, Friedman C, Hripcsak G, et al. Potential utility of precision medicine for older adults with polypharmacy: a case series study. Pharmgenomics Pers Med 2016;9:31–45.

[51] Brockmoller J, Stingl JC. Multimorbidity, polypharmacy and pharmacogenomics in old age. Pharmacogenomics 2017;18(6):515–7.

[52] Ramsey LB, Prows CA, Zhang K, et al. Implementation of pharmacogenetics at cincinnati children's hospital medical center: lessons learned over 14 years of personalizing medicine. Clin Pharmacol Ther 2019;105(1):49–52.

[53] Smith DM, Peshkin BN, Springfield TB, et al. Pharmacogenetics in practice: estimating the clinical actionability of pharmacogenetic testing in perioperative and ambulatory settings. Clin Transl Sci 2020. https://doi.org/10.1111/cts.12748.

[54] Hicks JK, Dunnenberger HM, Gumpper KF, et al. Integrating pharmacogenomics into electronic health records with clinical decision support. Am J Health Syst Pharm 2016;73(23):1967–76.

[55] Dunnenberger HM, Crews KR, Hoffman JM, et al. Preemptive clinical pharmacogenetics implementation: current programs in five US medical centers. Annu Rev Pharmacol Toxicol 2015;55:89–106.

[56] Empey PE, Stevenson JM, Tuteja S, et al. Multisite Investigation of Strategies for the Implementation of CYP2C19 Genotype-Guided Antiplatelet Therapy. Clin Pharmacol Ther 2018;104(4):664–74.

[57] Hicks JK, Shealy A, Schreiber A, et al. Patient decisions to receive secondary pharmacogenomic findings and development of a multidisciplinary practice model to integrate results into patient care. Clin Transl Sci 2018; 11(1):71–6.

[58] Rx Clinic Pharmacy. Rx Clinic Pharmacy. 2018. Available at: https://rxclinicpharmacy.com/. Accessed March 11, 2020.

[59] van der Wouden CH, Bank PCD, Ozokcu K, et al. Pharmacist-initiated pre-emptive pharmacogenetic panel testing with clinical decision support in primary care: record of pgx results and real-world impact. Genes (Basel) 2019;10(6). https://doi.org/10.3390/genes10060416.

Advances in Molecular Pathology 3 (2020) 131–142

ADVANCES IN MOLECULAR PATHOLOGY

Precision Medicine Using Pharmacogenomic Panel-Testing

Current Status and Future Perspectives

Cathelijne H. van der Wouden, PharmD[a,b], Henk-Jan Guchelaar, PharmD, PhD[a,b],
Jesse J. Swen, PharmD, PhD[a,b,*]

[a]Department of Clinical Pharmacy & Toxicology, Leiden University Medical Center, Albinusdreef 2, Leiden 2333ZA, The Netherlands; [b]Leiden Network for Personalised Therapeutics, Leiden, The Netherlands

---

KEYWORDS
• Pharmacogenomics • Panel-testing • Implementation • Adverse drug reactions

KEY POINTS

- Logistics and cost-effectiveness of pharmacogenomics (PGx)-guided prescribing may be optimized when delivered in a preemptive panel approach.
- Barriers impeding implementation of a preemptive PGx-panel approach include the lack of evidence of (cost-)effectiveness, the undetermined optimal target population and timing for delivering PGx, and the lack of tools supporting implementation.
- Developments in sequencing and artificial intelligence will further improve the predictive utility of genetic variation to predict drug response.

INTRODUCTION

Although drug treatment is often successful, adverse drug reactions (ADRs) and lack of efficacy present a significant burden for individual patients and society as a whole. ADRs are an important cause of emergency department visits and hospital admissions. A study in 2 large UK hospitals showed that 6.5% of hospital admissions were attributable to ADRs [1]. In the United States, ADR-related morbidity and mortality have been estimated at $30 billion to $136 billion annually [2]. In parallel, lack of efficacy also results in a significant burden. Its magnitude can be estimated by inspecting the number needed to treat of commonly used drugs [3], which are commonly more than 10. As a result, most patients will not benefit from drug treatment and, in contrast, may experience harm from unsuccessfully treated disease. It has been estimated that $100 billion a year is wasted on ineffective drug treatment [4].

Precision medicine aims to individualize or stratify application of pharmacotherapy, as opposed to the current population-based application, in an effort to optimize the benefit/risk ratio [5,6]. By enabling identification of individuals who are at higher risk for ADRs or lack of efficacy, before drug initiation and potential harm, an individualized dose and drug selection may be applied to reduce this risk. An individual's germline genetic variation is a particularly promising

---

Funding: The research leading to these results has received funding from the European Community's Horizon 2020 Program under grant agreement no. 668353 (U-PGx).

*Corresponding author. Albinusdreef 2, Postzone L0-P, Leiden 2333ZA, The Netherlands. *E-mail address:* j.j.swen@lumc.nl

https://doi.org/10.1016/j.yamp.2020.07.012

predictive factor that can enable drug response prediction. This notion is supported by its pharmacologic plausibility and has been demonstrated in various studies [7–10]. Drug-gene interactions (DGIs) can be categorized into 3 groups (Fig. 1A–C): pharmacokinetic-dependent ADRs (see Fig. 1A), pharmacodynamic-dependent ADRs (see Fig. 1B), and idiosyncratic ADRs (see Fig. 1C).

Pharmacogenomics (PGx) uses an individual's germline genetic profile to identify those who are at higher risk for ADRs or lack of efficacy (see Fig. 1D) [11–13]. This information can be used by health care professionals (HCPs) to guide dose and drug selection before drug initiation in an effort to optimize drug therapy [14]. Within germline PGx, the focus lies on inherited variation in genes, which play a role in drug absorption, distribution, metabolism, and elimination (ADME). To date, several randomized controlled trials (RCT) support the clinical utility of individual DGIs

to either optimize dosing [15–18] or drug selection [19,20]. Following the completion of the Human Genome Project, the Royal Dutch Pharmacists Association anticipated a proximate future where patients would present themselves in the pharmacy with their genetic information. In anticipation, the Dutch Pharmacogenetics Working Group (DPWG) was established in 2005 with the objective to develop clear guidelines for HCPs on how to interpret and apply PGx test results [21,22]. In parallel, the Clinical Pharmacogenetics Implementation Consortium was initiated in 2008 and devises similar guidelines [23].

Significant debate persists regarding the optimal timing and methodology of testing for delivering PGx testing in clinical care [24]. Some support a pretherapeutic single gene–drug approach, in which a PGx test of a single relevant gene is ordered once a target drug is prescribed, while others advocate for a preemptive

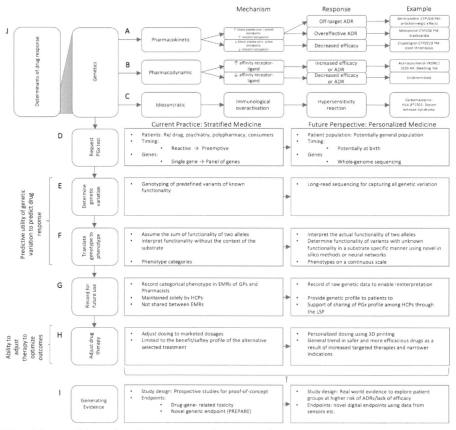

FIG. 1 Precision medicine using pharmacogenomic panel testing: current status and future perspectives. conc., concentration; PM, poor metabolizers; Rx, prescription.

panel-based strategy, in which multiple genes are tested simultaneously and saved for later use in preparation of future prescriptions throughout a patient's lifetime [25]. When combined with a clinical decision support system (CDSS), the corresponding PGx guideline can be deployed by the CDSS at the point of care, thereby providing clinicians with the necessary information to optimize drug prescribing, when a target drug is prescribed. A CDSS is deemed useful because patients will receive multiple drug prescriptions with potential DGIs within their lifetime [24,26]. It has been estimated that half of the patients older than 65 years will use at least one of the drugs for which PGx guidelines are available during a 4-year period, and one-fourth to one-third will use 2 or more of these drugs [27]. Logistics and cost-effectiveness are therefore optimized when delivered in a preemptive panel-based approach; pharmacotherapy does not have to be delayed, in awaiting single-gene testing results, and costs for genotyping are minimized, because marginal acquisition costs of testing and interpreting additional pharmacogenes is near zero [28]. When PGx is adopted in such a model, it has been estimated that 23.6% of all indecent prescriptions will have a relevant DGI [29]. To date, a small number of individual genes are tested pretherapeutically to guide pharmacotherapy of high-risk drugs. For example, *DPYD*-guided initial drug and dose selection of fluoropyridines to reduce risk of severe toxicity has been widely implemented in the Netherlands [30]. Despite the progress in application of PGx in single-gene scenarios, a preemptive PGx-panel approach is still not routinely applied. As such, several barriers preventing the implementation of preemptive panel testing have been identified [31–33]. Remaining barriers include the lack of evidence of (cost-)effectiveness supporting a PGx-panel approach, the undetermined optimal target population, and timing for delivering a PGx panel and the lack of tools supporting implementation. These remaining barriers and steps to overcome them are discussed in this review. Furthermore, the authors discuss future perspectives of these domains.

THE LACK OF EVIDENCE OF (COST-) EFFECTIVENESS SUPPORTING A PHARMACOGENOMICS-PANEL APPROACH

Several of the reported hurdles obstructing the implementation of PGx-panel testing are currently being addressed by various initiatives, in both the United States and the European Union. Overviews of these initiatives have previously been published [24,34]. Despite these initiatives, a major hurdle preventing

implementation is the absence of evidence presenting the collective clinical utility of a panel of PGx markers for preemptive PGx testing. Although several RCT support the clinical utility of individual gene-drug pairs, delivered in a single-gene reactive approach [15–20], evidence supporting clinical utility of the remaining DGIs for which recommendations are available when delivered in a preemptive panel approach is lacking. Significant debate persists regarding both the nature and the strength of evidence required for the clinical application of these remaining DGIs. Some argue an RCT is required for each individual DGI before clinical implementation is substantiated [35]. Others argue that a mandatory requirement for prospective evidence to support the clinical validity for each PGx interaction is incongruous and excessive [36–39]. Generating gold-standard evidence for each individual DGI for which PGx guidelines are available separately would require unrealistically large amounts of funds. On the other hand, extrapolating efficacy of all of these DGIs based on the conclusions of the previously mentioned RCTs, supporting clinical utility for a subset of individual DGIs, is also not substantiated.

Regardless of the inconvenience, there is still a demand for evidence substantiating patient benefit and cost-effectiveness, to enable stakeholders to practice evidence-based medicine. The Ubiquitous Pharmacogenomics Consortium (U-PGx), a European Consortium funded by the Horizon 2020 program, aims to generate such evidence [34]. The U-PGx consortium set out to quantify the collective clinical utility of a panel of PGx markers (50 variants in 13 pharmacogenes) within a single trial (the PREPARE study, ClinicalTrials.gov: NCT03093818) as a proof-of-concept across multiple potentially clinically relevant DGIs [34,40]. It is a block RCT aiming to enroll 8100 patients across 7 European countries. Additional outcomes include cost-effectiveness, process indicators for implementation, and provider adoption of PGx.

In the meantime, several smaller randomized and observational studies indicate the cost-effectiveness of PGx panel–based testing in psychiatry and polypharmacy patients [41–44]. Observed cost savings ranged from $218 [42] to $2778 [45] per patient. Others have modeled the cost-effectiveness of one-time genetic testing to minimize a lifetime of ADRs and concluded an incremental cost-effectiveness ratio (ICER) of $43,165 per additional life-year and $53,680 per additional quality-adjusted life-year, therefore considered cost-effective [46]. However, cost-effectiveness may vary across ethnic populations, as a result of differences in allele frequencies, differences in prescription patterns, and differences in health care costs and ICER cost-effectiveness thresholds. The study designed by the U-PGx consortium (the PREPARE Study) will enable the quantification of the cost-effectiveness over a 12-week time horizon.

Clinical trials and prospective cohorts typically measure short-term benefits of PGx testing, whereas the time horizon for the benefits and risks of PGx testing is over a lifetime and therefore unable to be captured within regular trials. As such, the life-long cost-effectiveness of one-time preemptive panel-based testing to prevent ADRs is yet undetermined. Other methodologies, such as Markov models, can be deployed to simulate effectiveness over longer time horizons. The results of such models will be of interest to reimbursement policymakers, who require evidence that panel-based testing will yield downstream improved health outcomes at acceptable costs. Therefore, once the effectiveness of PGx-panel testing has been established, future research should model the cost-effectiveness of preemptive PGx testing to prevent a lifetime of ADRs. Optimally, such an analysis could be run on a longitudinal cohort of patients for which both prescription data and PGx results are available. Furthermore, such a data set could be used to explore the optimal timing and subgroup application of testing to optimize cost-effectiveness.

FINDING THE OPTIMAL TARGET POPULATION AND TIMING FOR DELIVERING PHARMACOGENOMICS

The optimal target population and time at which panel-based testing should be performed remain to be determined. In the most progressive application of PGx panel-testing could be performed when no drug initiation is indicated, in anticipation of future drug prescriptions. However, if no drug is initiated in the near future, PGx testing would be a waste of resources. Alternatively, in a more efficient scenario, panel testing could be performed once a patient plans to initiate a drug for which PGx testing may be useful and reuse these results when future DGIs are encountered. Such a model was deployed in a pilot study [47], whereby pharmacists requested a PGx-panel test when patients planned to initiate one of 10 drugs for which PGx guidelines are available. Here, 97% of patients (re)used PGx-panel results for at least one, and 33% for up to 4 newly initiated prescriptions with possible DGIs within a 2.5-year follow-up. In this case, 24% were actionable DGIs, requiring pharmacotherapy adjustment. This high rate of reuse indicates that such a model may be promising for delivering PGx panel-based testing. As an alternative

model, another initiative at Vanderbilt University Medical Center has used a prediction model to select patients who may benefit from PGx testing in the near future algorithmically and using prescription data [48,49].

In addition to undetermined timing and methodology, the most optimal target group for testing is also yet undetermined. Current studies have identified potential patient subgroups for which preemptive PGx-panel testing may be most useful. Some initiatives have selected patients with particular indications in psychiatry [43,44,50,51]. Others have selected patients with particular characteristics, such as polypharmacy and elderly patients [41,42].

Alternatively, consumers who have an interest in their PGx profile may also obtain their PGx test results outside the realm of health care and without the intervention of an HCP. In 2018, direct-to-consumer (DTC) PGx testing for specific DGIs was approved by the Food and Drug Administration (FDA). However, in contrast to DTC tests provided before 2013, the FDA has approved only a limited scope of 33 variants in 8 genes, and providers have mandated the need to retest. Concerns of DTC PGx testing have been reported to relate to patient actions (eg, to stop taking a prescribed medication or adjusting the regimen based on genotype without consultation with a health provider) [52]. However, a longitudinal study of DTC consumers showed that only 5.6% of consumers reported changing a medication they were taking or starting a new medication because of their PGx results. Of these, 45 (83.3%) reported consulting with an HCP regarding the change [53]. Nonetheless, the involvement of HCPs will optimize the use of PGx results when delivered in a DTC setting. In the same longitudinal study, the authors found that 63% of consumers planned to share their results with a primary care provider. However, at 6-month follow-up, only 27% reported having done so, and 8% reported sharing with another HCP. Among participants who discussed results with their PCP, 35% were very satisfied with the encounter, and 18% were not at all satisfied. These results indicate that PGx testing in a DTC model may be a safe model for obtaining PGx testing.

THE LACK OF TOOLS SUPPORTING IMPLEMENTATION OF PHARMACOGENOMICS-PANEL TESTING
Development of a Pharmacogenomics Panel to Facilitate Implementation

Another important challenge hampering adoption of preemptive panel testing is the lack of standardization regarding variants included in such panels. Standardization would enable clinicians to understand PGx test results without extensive scrutiny of the alleles included in the panel. Despite the identification of standardization as a potential accelerator for PGx adoption, exchange, and continuity [54], there are currently no standards defining which variants should be tested [55,56]. Although some initiatives have developed standardized panels of relevant variants within individual genes [57], and other initiatives across multiple genes [58], a panel covering widely accepted genetic variants reflecting an entire set of guidelines is not yet available. Thus, in order to facilitate the clinical implementation of PGx testing, the U-PGx consortium set out to develop a pan-European panel based on actionable DPWG guidelines, called the "PGx-Passport" [59]. Here, germline variant alleles were systematically selected using predefined criteria regarding allele population frequencies, effect on protein functionality, and association with drug response. A "PGx-Passport" of 58 germline variant alleles, located within 14 genes (CYP2B6, CYP2C9, CYP2C19, CYP2D6, CYP3A5, DPYD, F5, HLA-A, HLA-B, NUDT15, SLCO1B1, TPMT, UGT1A1 and VKORC1), was composed. This "PGx-Passport" can be used in combination with the DPWG guidelines to optimize drug prescribing for 49 commonly prescribed drugs. An advantage of the approach is that the number of clinically interpretable results within their "PGx-Passport" is maximized, while costs remain reasonable.

Importantly, the presented panel will not be able to fully identify those at risk for unwanted drug response. The overall ability of a panel to predict drug response is dependent on, first, the predictive utility of genetic variation to predict drug response and, second, the ability to adjust pharmacotherapy to reduce the risk of unwanted effects among high-risk individuals. In the following sections, the current limitations of both domains are further elaborated.

Current predictive utility of genetic variation to predict drug response

Even though multiple genetic variants have been discovered, the authors currently restrict testing to a subset of these variants. However, restricting testing to individual variants disregards untested or undiscovered variants that may also influence the functionality of the gene product. Therefore, the functionality of the gene product cannot be fully predicted (see Fig. 1E). Reasons for restriction of testing are twofold. First, technical limitations regarding the sequencing of complex loci prevent complete determination of both the gene of interest and other areas in the genome, which may have an effect on the gene product. Determining genetic variation is specifically difficult in highly polymorphic genes, such as the HLA genes, or genes located near pseudogenes, such as CYP2D6. Although sequencing of these loci is technically possible, it are costly and time-consuming. Second, even if one were to determine all genetic variation, the downstream effect on protein functionality may be unknown and therefore impossible to interpret clinically [60].

However, progress in the interpretation of functional consequences of such uncharacterized variations may support future interpretation in silico [61], in vitro, or in vivo [62]. Importantly, a study has shown that 92.9% of genetic variation in ADME genes is rare, and an estimated 30% to 40% of functional variability in pharmacogenes can be attributed to these variants [63]. In addition to the downstream functionality, the penetrance (ie, the potential of a variant to accurately predict the genetic component of drug response) is also unknown. The penetrance is a function of both the variant's effect on protein functionality and the extent to which the protein functionality is associated with clinical outcome. Significant debate persists regarding both the nature and the strength of evidence required for the clinical application of variant alleles of unknown functionality. Because the strength of these functions differs across genes and DGIs, the authors do not foresee a one-size-fits-all consensus regarding and evidence threshold across all DGIs, but rather a different evidence threshold per individual DGI based on the genetics and pharmacology of the interaction. For example, in the case of the TPMT-thiopurine interaction, the effect of TPMT variation on protein functionality has been firmly established because it exhibits behavior similar to monogenetic codominant traits [64]. Therefore, identified variants in TPMT (*3A/*3B/*3C) are considered to have sufficient evidence to be applied in the clinic. The clinical interpretation has been clinically validated in a study specifically investigating clinical effects in patients carrying these variants [18]. On the other hand, clinically relevant variant alleles in CYP2D6 are based on the pharmacology of the interaction. For example, the flecainide-CYP2D6 interaction is based on the associations between decreasing CYP2D6 activity leading to increasing flecainide plasma levels, which in turn leads to increased risk for flecainide intoxication. Therefore, all identified variants in CYP2D6, shown to have a significant effect on CYP2D6 enzyme activity, are considered clinically applicable. As such, both the functional effects and the penetrance of many rare variants are yet unknown. As an additional complication, these may also differ across substrates and drug responses. Even more fundamentally, variants may impact each other's functionality, and therefore, individual variants may have different functionalities depending on the absence or presence of other variants.

Another significant limitation, which is applicable to PGx testing and interpretation as it is performed today, is that predicted phenotypes are interpreted as categories rather than continuous scores, and it is assumed the sum of both alleles equals total metabolic capacity (see Fig. 1F). For example, for CYP2D6, patients are categorized into normal metabolizers, intermediate metabolizers, poor metabolizers, or ultrarapid metabolizers. However, the actual CYP2D6 phenotype is likely normally distributed [65,66]. Imposing categorization, as opposed to the interpretation of the actual diplotype, therefore sacrifices information in order to simplify clinical interpretation. In the process, the functionality of each allele is interpreted individually, and it is assumed that the sum of these activity scores equals the total activity of the diplotype. Furthermore, these categorizations are currently substrate independent, even though the effects on metabolic capacity are known to differ between substrates [67].

Current ability to adjust pharmacotherapy to optimize outcomes

In addition to the ability of genetic variation to predict drug response, the second component determining the utility of PGx-guided pharmacotherapy is the ability to adjust pharmacotherapy to the specific genetic variants. Currently, there are 2 options to reduce the risk of ADRs and lack of efficacy: (1) selecting another drug and (2) adjusting the dose (see Fig. 1H).

A successful example of choosing an alternative therapy to avoid an ADR is preemptive testing for HLA-B*57:01 to guide drug selection for abacavir or another antiretroviral. Here, 0% of the prospectively screened group versus 2.7% of the control group experienced immunologically confirmed hypersensitivity [19]. In this example, the PGx intervention and subsequent adjustment completely eliminated the risk of hypersensitivity.

An example of adjusting the dose to reduce the risk of ADRs is preemptive testing for TPMT to guide dose selection of thiopurines to reduce the risk of severe hematologic ADRs [18]. In contrast to the previously described abacavir/HLA-B*57:01 example, this intervention has a smaller effect size. Here, severe hematologic ADRs still occurred in 2.6% of TPMT variant carriers who received an adjusted dose, compared

with 22.9% of TPMT variant carriers treated with a normal dose. Although dose adjustment prevented ∼89% of severe hematologic ADRs, the remaining ∼11% could not be prevented by this intervention. Indeed, this could partially be a result of the sensitivity of TPMT testing not reaching 100%, but could also be due to the fact that dose reduction was not sufficient for avoiding this ADR. Furthermore, the incidence of severe hematological ADRs among noncarriers of TPMT variants was 7.3%, indicating that other (genetic) factors, such as NUDT15, may play a role in the risk of severe hematological ADRs.

Enable Recording of Pharmacogenomics-Panel Results for Future Use

To enable preemptive PGx testing, it is imperative that the PGx test results are recorded in the electronic medical records (EMRs) for future use (see Fig. 1G). Within a pilot study, the authors found that both pharmacists and general practitioners (GPs) are able to record PGx results in their EMRs as contraindications (96% and 33% of pharmacists and GPs, respectively), enabling the deployment of relevant guidelines by the CDSS when a DGI is encountered at both prescribing and dispensing [47]. In contrast, a recent study showed that genotyping results were sparsely communicated and recorded correctly; only 3.1% and 5.9% of reported genotyping results were recorded by GPs and pharmacists, respectively, within a similar follow-up time of 2.36 years [68].

FUTURE PERSPECTIVES

Generating Evidence for Effectiveness of Precision Medicine Approaches

In an era where digitalization is driving data accumulation and a concomitant increase in stratification of patient groups and a more precise diagnosis, we are moving toward the utilization of real-world data to support precision medicine (see Fig. 1I). Several investigators have pointed out that precision medicine, and genomic medicine, in particular, would benefit from a convergence of implementation science and a learning health system to measure outcomes and generate evidence across a large population [69,70]. However, this requires standardization of outcomes in EMRs to enable aggregation of phenotype data across large populations for both discovery and outcomes assessment within a genomic medicine implementation [71]. Many nationwide, large-scale initiatives are generating prospective   longitudinal   evidence   supporting precision medicine approaches [72–74]. For example, a landmark project specifically generating evidence for PGx is the All of Us project [75]. Alternatively, pragmatic clinical trials offer researchers a means to study precision medicine interventions in real-world settings [76,77]. In contrast to traditional clinical trials that are performed in ideal conditions, these pragmatic trials are conducted in the context of usual care [77]. Pragmatic clinical trials easily transition into existing health care infrastructures and therefore make them particularly appealing to comparative effectiveness research and the evidence-based mission of learning health care systems [78,79]. An example of such a pragmatic trial for generating evidence for preemptive PGx testing is the I-PICC study [80].

In parallel, evolving digital health technologies are driving data accumulation. Data collected by sensors (in smartphones, wearables, and ingestibles), mobile apps, and social media can be processed by machine learning to support medical decision making [81]. Raw sensor data can also be processed into digital biomarkers and endpoints [82]. This development may be particularly useful for endpoint definition in disease areas where biological endpoints are lacking, such as in psychiatry and neurology, to enable quantification of disease progression and drug response. For example, novel digital endpoints are being developed to stratify mental health conditions and predict remission using passively collected smartphone data [83]. Another example is the development of a digital biomarker for Parkinson disease using motor active tests and passive monitoring through a smartphone [84]. For precision medicine, in particular, we may also be more able to stratify patient groups into responders and nonresponders with improved endpoint development in these disease areas. Increased stratification of patient groups on the basis of genetic, (digital) biomarker, phenotypic, of psychosocial characteristics will drive more precise diagnoses and pharmacotherapy optimization [85,86]. This trend will drive demand for innovations for more efficient study designs because of increasing numbers of indications, whereas resources to fund these trials remain constant [87].

Determining Optimal Timing and Target Group for Pharmacogenomics-Panel Testing

Consensus regarding who should be tested, and when it is most cost-effective to perform preemptive panel-testing, remains undetermined [28]. Moreover, the most cost-effective technique to determine the PGx profile is also undetermined. As novel DGIs are discovered, it may be more efficient to sequence whole genomes, to

avoid testing of additional variants through genotyping over time. Clinically relevant PGx variants can successfully be extracted from sequencing data using bioinformatics pipelines [88,89]. As the cost of sequencing techniques decrease, genotype-based testing will become obsolete. In this case, it may be more cost-effective to perform population-wide sequencing at birth, to ensure the maximization of instances in which a PGx result is available when a DGI is encountered. However, whole-exome sequencing and whole-genome sequencing are increasingly applied for other medical indications and objectives [90,91]. As this development expands, determining the cost-effectiveness of implementing PGx testing may become redundant, because the information on PGx variants becomes secondary findings, free of additional costs.

Improving Predictive Utility of Genetic Variation to Predict Drug Response

Recent advances have been made to improve the ability to determine an individual's genetic variation. Technical limitations regarding the sequencing of complex loci may be overcome by advances in long-read sequencing technologies and synthetic long-read assembly [92]. As a result, an increasing number of variants with unknown functionality will need to be interpreted. Because of the vast increasing number of rare variants, it is impossible to determine functionality in traditional expression systems. To overcome this challenge, advances have been made in the development of in silico methods to predict functionality. However, these methods are based on genes that are evolutionarily highly conserved. Because many ADME genes are only poorly conserved, steps have been taken to calibrate in silico models on data sets. For example, recently investigators developed a novel computational functionality prediction model optimized for pharmacogenetic assessments, which substantially outperformed standard algorithms [62].

Nonetheless, these models still do not enable prediction of the functionality of synonymous mutations, intronic variants, or variants in noncoding regions of the genome. Recent initiatives have provided an alternative method for the interpretation of variants with unknown functionality using machine learning [65,93], one using an existing data set for model training and the other using a mock data set. In the first, the investigators trained a neural network model on the long-read sequencing profiles of CYP2D6 of 561 patients and used the metabolic ratio between tamoxifen and endoxifen as an outcome measure. The model explains 79% of the interindividual variability in CYP2D6 activity compared with 55% with the conventional categorization approach. In addition, this model is capable of assigning accurate enzyme activity to alleles containing previously uncharacterized combinations of variants. The suggested model has provided a method to determine predicted phenotype on a continuous scale. Indeed, enzyme activity may be expected to be normally distributed within a population and therefore better described by such a scale. A future is envisioned where phenotypes can be predicted more precisely by using all of an individual's genetic variation, as opposed to limiting the view only to those variants included in a tested panel.

Following a further understanding of the effects of individual variants to inform phenotype prediction on a continuous scale, one can imagine that this phenotype prediction will ultimately become substrate specific on top of gene specific. More fundamentally, in PGx, the view is currently limited to a single DGI, whereas multiple genes may be involved in the metabolism of drugs and their metabolites. If one were to expand their view to multiple genes involved to predict drug response, the predictive utility will further improve. To incorporate genetic variations of multiple genes, polygenic risk scores may prove useful [94].

Although genetics is considered the causal anchor of biological processes [95], the biological mechanism underlying drug response may be downstream of a genetic variant. In these cases, genetics will have no predictive utility for drug response (see Fig. 1J, top left). Therefore, incorporating processes downstream of the genome, such as the epigenome [96], transcriptome, microbiome [97], and metabolome [98], may further optimize the ability to predict drug response to enable more accurate stratification of patient populations. Combining these profiles in a systems medicine approach may have a synergistic effect.

Improving Ability to Adjust Pharmacotherapy to Optimize Outcomes

In the future, pharmacotherapy adjustment may be further improved by imminent technologies, such as 3-dimensional (3D) printing to enable personalized dosing and delivery [99]. Currently, the DPWG calculates specific dose adjustments based on pharmacokinetic studies and rounds the recommended dose to the nearest corresponding marketed dose for clinical feasibility. The utilization of 3D-printing technologies may enable rapid compounding of tablets with a specific dose based on an individual's genetic profile. In any case, adjustment of the pharmacotherapy will always be limited by the safety profile of available drugs.

Opportunely, over the last decades, newly developed drugs have been shifting from unspecific small molecules to more targeted drugs in the form of humanized monoclonal antibodies [100], cell therapies [101], and gene therapies [102] with fewer off-target ADRs.

Recording Pharmacogenomics-Panel Results for Future Use

Future initiatives should focus on the development of automated sharing of PGx results across EMRs. In the Netherlands, such an initiative has been launched but requires patient consent before it can be used. The National Exchange Point ("Landelijk Schakel Punt" [LSP]) is a nationwide secured EMR infrastructure to which nearly all HCPs can access [103]. Only when a patient has provided written consent for the LSP can a professional summary of the local pharmacy or GP EMR, including PGx results, be downloaded by another treating HCP in the same region, unless the patient chose to shield this information. Alternatively, providing the PGx results directly to patients may resolve the issue in terms of communicating and recording PGx results; for example, using the MSC safety-code card as used in the PREPARE study [104,105].

SUMMARY

In conclusion, developments in evidence generation and in genetic sequencing and interpretation will revolutionize current stratified medicine to enable true precision medicine, whereby multiple -omics profiles of an individual are combined to predict drug response and optimize pharmacotherapy accordingly.

DISCLOSURE

The authors have nothing to disclose.

REFERENCES

[1] Pirmohamed M, James S, Meakin S, et al. Adverse drug reactions as cause of admission to hospital: prospective analysis of 18 820 patients. BMJ 2004;329(7456):15–9.

[2] Johnson JA, Bootman JL. Drug-related morbidity and mortality. A cost-of-illness model. Arch Intern Med 1995;155(18):1949–56.

[3] Therapy (NNT) Reviews. Available at: https://www.thennt.com/home-nnt/#nntblack. Accessed November 11, 2019.

[4] Harper AR, Topol EJ. Pharmacogenomics in clinical practice and drug development. Nat Biotechnol 2012; 30(11):1117–24.

[5] Jameson JL, Longo DL. Precision medicine–personalized, problematic, and promising. N Engl J Med 2015; 372(23):2229–34.

[6] Peck RW. Precision medicine is not just genomics: the right dose for every patient. Annu Rev Pharmacol Toxicol 2018;58:105–22.

[7] Matthaei J, Brockmoller J, Tzvetkov MV, et al. Heritability of metoprolol and torsemide pharmacokinetics. Clin Pharmacol Ther 2015;98(6):611–21.

[8] Alexanderson B, Evans DA, Sjoqvist F. Steady-state plasma levels of nortriptyline in twins: influence of genetic factors and drug therapy. Br Med J 1969;4(5686): 764–8.

[9] Vesell ES, Page JG. Genetic control of drug levels in man: phenylbutazone. Science 1968;159(3822): 1479–80.

[10] Stage TB, Damkier P, Pedersen RS, et al. A twin study of the trough plasma steady-state concentration of metformin. Pharmacogenet Genomics 2015;25(5): 259–62.

[11] Relling MV, Evans WE. Pharmacogenomics in the clinic. Nature 2015;526(7573):343–50.

[12] Weinshilboum R, Wang L. Pharmacogenomics: bench to bedside. Nat Rev Drug Discov 2004;3(9):739–48.

[13] Roden DM, McLeod HL, Relling MV, et al. Pharmacogenomics. Lancet 2019;394(10197):521–32.

[14] Pirmohamed M. Personalized pharmacogenomics: predicting efficacy and adverse drug reactions. Annu Rev Genomics Hum Genet 2014;15:349–70.

[15] Pirmohamed M, Burnside G, Eriksson N, et al. A randomized trial of genotype-guided dosing of warfarin. N Engl J Med 2013;369(24):2294–303.

[16] Wu AH. Pharmacogenomic testing and response to warfarin. Lancet 2015;385(9984):2231–2.

[17] Verhoef TI, Ragia G, de Boer A, et al. A randomized trial of genotype-guided dosing of acenocoumarol and phenprocoumon. New Engl J Med 2013;369(24): 2304–12.

[18] Coenen MJ, de Jong DJ, van Marrewijk CJ, et al. Identification of patients with variants in TPMT and dose reduction reduces hematologic events during thiopurine treatment of inflammatory bowel disease. Gastroenterology 2015;149(4):907–17.e7.

[19] Mallal S, Phillips E, Carosi G, et al. HLA-B*5701 screening for hypersensitivity to abacavir. N Engl J Med 2008;358(6):568–79.

[20] Claassens DMF, Vos GJA, Bergmeijer TO, et al. A genotype-guided strategy for oral P2Y12 inhibitors in primary PCI. N Engl J Med 2019;381(17):1621–31.

[21] Swen JJ, Nijenhuis M, de Boer A, et al. Pharmacogenetics: from bench to byte–an update of guidelines. Clin Pharmacol Ther 2011;89(5):662–73.

[22] Swen JJ, Wilting I, de Goede AL, et al. Pharmacogenetics: from bench to byte. Clin Pharmacol Ther 2008;83(5):781–7.

[23] Relling MV, Klein TE. CPIC: clinical pharmacogenetics implementation consortium of the pharmacogenomics research network. Clin Pharmacol Ther 2011;89(3): 464–7.

[24] Dunnenberger HM, Crews KR, Hoffman JM, et al. Preemptive clinical pharmacogenetics implementation: current programs in five US medical centers. Annu Rev Pharmacol Toxicol 2015;55:89–106.

[25] Weitzel KW, Cavallari LH, Lesko LJ. Preemptive panel-based pharmacogenetic testing: the time is now. Pharm Res 2017;34(8):1551–5.

[26] Driest VSL, Shi Y, Bowton EA, et al. Clinically actionable genotypes among 10,000 patients with preemptive pharmacogenomic testing. Clin Pharmacol Ther 2014; 95(4):423–31.

[27] Samwald M, Xu H, Blagec K, et al. Incidence of exposure of patients in the United States to multiple drugs for which pharmacogenomic guidelines are available. PLoS One 2016;11(10):e0164972.

[28] Roden DM, Van Driest SL, Mosley JD, et al. Benefit of preemptive pharmacogenetic information on clinical outcome. Clin Pharmacol Ther 2018;103(5):787–94.

[29] Bank PCD, Swen JJ, Guchelaar HJ. Estimated nationwide impact of implementing a preemptive pharmacogenetic panel approach to guide drug prescribing in primary care in The Netherlands. BMC Med 2019; 17(1):110.

[30] Lunenburg CA, van Staveren MC, Gelderblom H, et al. Evaluation of clinical implementation of prospective DPYD genotyping in 5-fluorouracil- or capecitabine-treated patients. Pharmacogenomics 2016;17(7):721–9.

[31] Abbasi J. Getting pharmacogenomics into the clinic. JAMA 2016;316(15):1533–5.

[32] Haga SB, Burke W. Pharmacogenetic testing: not as simple as it seems. Genet Med 2008;10(6):391–5.

[33] Swen JJ, Huizinga TW, Gelderblom H, et al. Translating pharmacogenomics: challenges on the road to the clinic. PLoS Med 2007;4(8):e209.

[34] van der Wouden CH, Cambon-Thomsen A, Cecchin E, et al. Implementing pharmacogenomics in Europe: design and implementation strategy of the Ubiquitous Pharmacogenomics consortium. Clin Pharmacol Ther 2017;101(3):341–58.

[35] Janssens AC, Deverka PA. Useless until proven effective: the clinical utility of preemptive pharmacogenetic testing. Clin Pharmacol Ther 2014;96(6):652–4.

[36] Altman RB. Pharmacogenomics: "noninferiority" is sufficient for initial implementation. Clin Pharmacol Ther 2011;89(3):348–50.

[37] van der Wouden CH, Swen JJ, Schwab M, et al. A brighter future for the implementation of pharmacogenomic testing. Eur J Hum Genet 2016;24(12): 1658–60.

[38] Pirmohamed M, Hughes DA. Pharmacogenetic tests: the need for a level playing field. Nat Rev Drug Discov 2013;12(1):3–4.

[39] Khoury MJ. Dealing with the evidence dilemma in genomics and personalized medicine. Clin Pharmacol Ther 2010;87(6):635–8.

[40] Manson LE, van der Wouden CH, Swen JJ, et al. The Ubiquitous Pharmacogenomics Consortium: making effective treatment optimization accessible to every European citizen. Pharmacogenomics 2017;18(11): 1041–5.

[41] Elliott LS, Henderson JC, Neradilek MB, et al. Clinical impact of pharmacogenetic profiling with a clinical decision support tool in polypharmacy home health patients: a prospective pilot randomized controlled trial. PLoS One 2017;12(2):e0170905.

[42] Brixner D, Biltaji E, Bress A, et al. The effect of pharmacogenetic profiling with a clinical decision support tool on healthcare resource utilization and estimated costs in the elderly exposed to polypharmacy. J Med Econ 2016;19(3):213–28.

[43] Pérez V, Salavert A, Espadaler J, et al. Efficacy of prospective pharmacogenetic testing in the treatment of major depressive disorder: results of a randomized, double-blind clinical trial. BMC Psychiatry 2017; 17(1):250.

[44] Espadaler J, Tuson M, Lopez-Ibor JM, et al. Pharmacogenetic testing for the guidance of psychiatric treatment: a multicenter retrospective analysis. CNS Spectr 2017; 22(4):315–24.

[45] Winner JG, Carhart JM, Altar CA, et al. Combinatorial pharmacogenomic guidance for psychiatric medications reduces overall pharmacy costs in a 1 year prospective evaluation. Curr Med Res Opin 2015;31(9): 1633–43.

[46] Alagoz O, Durham D, Kasirajan K. Cost-effectiveness of one-time genetic testing to minimize lifetime adverse drug reactions. Pharmacogenomics J 2015;16(2): 129–36.

[47] van der Wouden CH, Bank PCD, Ozokcu K, et al. Pharmacist-initiated pre-emptive pharmacogenetic panel testing with clinical decision support in primary care: record of PGx results and real-world impact. Genes (Basel) 2019;10(6):416.

[48] Pulley JM, Denny JC, Peterson JF, et al. Operational implementation of prospective genotyping for personalized medicine: the design of the Vanderbilt PREDICT project. Clin Pharmacol Ther 2012;92(1):87–95.

[49] Grice GR, Seaton TL, Woodland AM, et al. Defining the opportunity for pharmacogenetic intervention in primary care. Pharmacogenomics 2006;7(1):61–5.

[50] Bradley P, Shiekh M, Mehra V, et al. Improved efficacy with targeted pharmacogenetic-guided treatment of patients with depression and anxiety: a randomized clinical trial demonstrating clinical utility. J Psychiatr Res 2018;96:100–7.

[51] Walden LM, Brandl EJ, Tiwari AK, et al. Genetic testing for CYP2D6 and CYP2C19 suggests improved outcome for antidepressant and antipsychotic medication. Psychiatry Res 2018;279:111–5.

[52] Haga SB. Managing increased accessibility to pharmacogenomic data. Clin Pharmacol Ther 2019;106(5): 922–4.

[53] Carere DA, VanderWeele TJ, Vassy JL, et al. Prescription medication changes following direct-to-consumer personal genomic testing: findings from the Impact of Personal Genomics (PGen) Study. Genet Med 2017;19(5):537–45.

[54] Caudle KE, Keeling NJ, Klein TE, et al. Standardization can accelerate the adoption of pharmacogenomics: current status and the path forward. Pharmacogenomics 2018;19(10):847–60.

[55] Pratt VM, Everts RE, Aggarwal P, et al. Characterization of 137 genomic DNA reference materials for 28 pharmacogenetic genes: a GeT-RM collaborative project. J Mol Diagn 2016;18(1):109–23.

[56] Pratt VM, Zehnbauer B, Wilson J, et al. Characterization of 107 genomic DNA reference materials for CYP2D6, CYP2C19, CYP2C9, VKORC1, and UGT1A1: a GeT-RM and Association for Molecular Pathology collaborative project. J Mol Diagn 2010;12(6): 835–46.

[57] Pratt VM, Del Tredici AL, Hachad H, et al. Recommendations for clinical CYP2C19 genotyping allele selection: a report of the association for molecular pathology. J Mol Diagn 2018;20(3):269–76.

[58] Bush WS, Crosslin DR, Owusu-Obeng A, et al. Genetic variation among 82 pharmacogenes: the PGRNseq data from the eMERGE network. Clin Pharmacol Ther 2016;100(2):160–9.

[59] Van der Wouden CH, Van Rhenen MH, Jama W, et al. Development of the PGx-passport: a panel of actionable germline genetic variants for pre-emptive pharmacogenetic testing. Clin Pharmacol Ther 2019;106(4): 866–73.

[60] Drogemoller BI, Wright GE, Warnich L. Considerations for rare variants in drug metabolism genes and the clinical implications. Expert Opin Drug Metab Toxicol 2014;10(6):873–84.

[61] Li B, Seligman C, Thusberg J, et al. In silico comparative characterization of pharmacogenomic missense variants. BMC Genomics 2014;15(Suppl 4):S4.

[62] Zhou Y, Mkrtchian S, Kumondai M, et al. An optimized prediction framework to assess the functional impact of pharmacogenetic variants. Pharmacogenomics J 2019; 19(2):115–26.

[63] Kozyra M, Ingelman-Sundberg M, Lauschke VM. Rare genetic variants in cellular transporters, metabolic enzymes, and nuclear receptors can be important determinants of interindividual differences in drug response. Genet Med 2016;19(1):20–9.

[64] Weinshilboum RM, Sladek SL. Mercaptopurine pharmacogenetics: monogenic inheritance of erythrocyte thiopurine methyltransferase activity. Am J Hum Genet 1980;32(5):651–62.

[65] van der Lee M, Allard WG, Vossen RHAM, et al. A unifying model to predict variable drug response for personalised medicine. Biorxiv. 2020: 2020.2003.2002.967554.

[66] Hertz DL, Rae J. Pharmacogenetics of cancer drugs. Annu Rev Med 2015;66:65–81.

[67] Hicks JK, Swen JJ, Gaedigk A. Challenges in CYP2D6 phenotype assignment from genotype data: a critical assessment and call for standardization. Curr Drug Metab 2014;15(2):218–32.

[68] Simoons M, Mulder H, Schoevers RA, et al. Availability of CYP2D6 genotyping results in general practitioner and community pharmacy medical records. Pharmacogenomics 2017;18(9):843–51.

[69] Chambers DA, Feero WG, Khoury MJ. Convergence of implementation science, precision medicine, and the learning health care system: a new model for biomedical research. JAMA 2016;315(18):1941–2.

[70] Lu CY, Williams MS, Ginsburg GS, et al. A proposed approach to accelerate evidence generation for genomic-based technologies in the context of a learning health system. Genet Med 2018;20(4):390–6.

[71] Peterson JF, Roden DM, Orlando LA, et al. Building evidence and measuring clinical outcomes for genomic medicine. Lancet 2019;394(10198):604–10.

[72] Turnbull C, Scott RH, Thomas E, et al. The 100 000 Genomes Project: bringing whole genome sequencing to the NHS. BMJ 2018;361:k1687.

[73] Gottesman O, Scott SA, Ellis SB, et al. The CLIPMERGE PGx Program: clinical implementation of personalized medicine through electronic health records and genomics-pharmacogenomics. Clin Pharmacol Ther 2013; 94(2):214–7.

[74] Leitsalu L, Haller T, Esko T, et al. Cohort profile: estonian biobank of the Estonian Genome Center, University of Tartu. Int J Epidemiol 2015;44(4):1137–47.

[75] Collins FS, Varmus H. A new initiative on precision medicine. N Engl J Med 2015;372(9):793–5.

[76] Khoury MJ, Rich EC, Randhawa G, et al. Comparative effectiveness research and genomic medicine: an evolving partnership for 21st century medicine. Genet Med 2009;11(10):707–11.

[77] Ford I, Norrie J. Pragmatic trials. N Engl J Med 2016; 375(5):454–63.

[78] Fiore LD, Lavori PW. Integrating randomized comparative effectiveness research with patient care. N Engl J Med 2016;374(22):2152–8.

[79] Weinfurt KP, Hernandez AF, Coronado GD, et al. Pragmatic clinical trials embedded in healthcare systems: generalizable lessons from the NIH Collaboratory. BMC Med Res Methodol 2017;17(1):144.

[80] Brunette CA, Miller SJ, Majahalme N, et al. Pragmatic trials in genomic medicine: the Integrating Pharmacogenetics in Clinical Care (I-PICC) study. Clin Transl Sci 2019. https://doi.org/10.1111/cts.12723.

[81] Sim I. Mobile devices and health. N Engl J Med 2019; 381(10):956–68.

[82] Coravos A, Khozin S, Mandl KD. Developing and adopting safe and effective digital biomarkers to improve patient outcomes. NPJ Digit Med 2019; 2(1):14.

[83] Mindstrong health and Takeda partner to explore development of digital biomarkers for mental health conditions. Available at: https://www.prnewswire.com/news-releases/mindstrong-health-and-takeda-partner-to-explore-development-of-digital-biomarkers-for-mental-health-conditions-300604553.html. Accessed December 10, 2020.

[84] Lipsmeier F, Taylor KI, Kilchenmann T, et al. Evaluation of smartphone-based testing to generate exploratory outcome measures in a phase 1 Parkinson's disease clinical trial. Mov Disord 2018;33(8):1287–97.

[85] Clay I. Impact of digital technologies on novel endpoint capture in clinical trials. Clin Pharmacol Ther 2017;102(6):912–3.

[86] Haendel MA, Chute CG, Robinson PN. Classification, ontology, and precision medicine. N Engl J Med 2018;379(15):1452–62.

[87] Miksad RA, Samant MK, Sarkar S, et al. Small but mighty: the use of real-world evidence to inform precision medicine. Clin Pharmacol Ther 2019;106(1): 87–90.

[88] Yang W, Wu G, Broeckel U, et al. Comparison of genome sequencing and clinical genotyping for pharmacogenes. Clin Pharmacol Ther 2016;100(4): 380–8.

[89] van der Lee M, Allard WG, Bollen S, et al. Repurposing of diagnostic whole exome sequencing data of 1,583 individuals for clinical pharmacogenetics. Clin Pharmacol Ther 2019. https://doi.org/10.1002/cpt.1665.

[90] Holm IA, Agrawal PB, Ceyhan-Birsoy O, et al. The BabySeq project: implementing genomic sequencing in newborns. BMC Pediatr 2018;18(1):225.

[91] Kalia SS, Adelman K, Bale SJ, et al. Recommendations for reporting of secondary findings in clinical exome and genome sequencing, 2016 update (ACMG SF v2.0): a policy statement of the American College of Medical Genetics and Genomics. Genet Med 2017; 19(2):249–55.

[92] Lauschke VM, Ingelman-Sundberg M. How to consider rare genetic variants in personalized drug therapy. Clin Pharmacol Ther 2018;103(5):745–8.

[93] McInnes G, Dalton R, Sangkuhl K, et al. Transfer learning enables prediction of CYP2D6 haplotype function. Biorxiv 2020:684357.

[94] Gibson G. On the utilization of polygenic risk scores for therapeutic targeting. PLoS Genet 2019;15(4): e1008060.

[95] Watson JD, Crick FH. Genetical implications of the structure of deoxyribonucleic acid. Nature 1953; 171(4361):964–7.

[96] Lauschke VM, Zhou Y, Ingelman-Sundberg M. Novel genetic an epigenetic factors of importance for interindividual differences in drug disposition, response and toxicity. Pharmacol Ther 2019;197:122–52.

[97] Sun L, Xie C, Wang G, et al. Gut microbiota and intestinal FXR mediate the clinical benefits of metformin. Nat Med 2018;24(12):1919–29.

[98] Kaddurah-Daouk R, Weinshilboum R. Metabolomic signatures for drug response phenotypes:

pharmacometabolomics enables precision medicine. Clin Pharmacol Ther 2015;98(1):71–5.

[99] Afsana, Jain V, Haider N, et al. 3D printing in personalized drug delivery. Curr Pharm Des 2018;24(42): 5062–71.

[100] Hansel TT, Kropshofer H, Singer T, et al. The safety and side effects of monoclonal antibodies. Nat Rev Drug Discov 2010;9(4):325–38.

[101] Jackson HJ, Rafiq S, Brentjens RJ. Driving CAR T-cells forward. Nat Rev Clin Oncol 2016;13(6):370–83.

[102] Naldini L. Gene therapy returns to centre stage. Nature 2015;526(7573):351–60.

[103] Track your own healthcare with 'Volgjezorg. Available at: https://www.volgjezorg.nl/en. Accessed January 18, 2019.

[104] Samwald M, Minarro-Giménez JAA, Blagec K, et al. Towards a global IT system for personalized medicine: the Medicine Safety Code initiative. Stud Health Technol Inform 2014;205:261–5.

[105] Blagec K, Koopmann R, Crommentuijn-van Rhenen M, et al. Implementing pharmacogenomics decision support across seven European countries: the Ubiquitous Pharmacogenomics (U-PGx) project. J Am Med Inform Assoc 2018;25(7):893–8.

Informatics

Advances in Molecular Pathology 3 (2020) 143–155

ADVANCES IN MOLECULAR PATHOLOGY

Artificial Intelligence in the Genetic Diagnosis of Rare Disease

Check for updates

Kiely N. James, PhD[a,1], Sujal Phadke, PhD[a,1], Terence C. Wong, PhD[a,1], Shimul Chowdhury, PhD[b,1,*]

[a]Genomics, Rady Children's Institute for Genomic Medicine, 7910 Frost Street, MC5129, San Diego, CA 92123, USA; [b]Rady Children's Institute for Genomic Medicine, 7910 Frost Street, MC5129, San Diego, CA 92123, USA

KEYWORDS

- Genomics • Precision medicine • Natural language processing • Artificial intelligence

KEY POINTS

- The use of artificial intelligence can streamline the lengthy process currently required to clinically interpret a genome.
- Natural language processing can eliminate much of the human variability and bias that is involved in translating information from the medical record.
- Deep learning approaches can expedite the prioritization of genetic variants during interpretation of genomic data.
- The promise of genomic medicine will be fully realized only if the time and cost of analyzing genomic data continue to decrease.

INTRODUCTION

More than 7000 rare diseases have been described, with prevalence ranging from fewer than 1 in a million (eg, metachromatic leukodystrophy) to greater than 1 in 10,000 (eg, sickle cell anemia), and of these, approximately 70% are largely genetic in origin [1]. In total, an estimated 263 to 446 million individuals are thought to be afflicted by rare diseases worldwide [1]. The identification of causal genetic variants in these individuals enables patient-specific clinical management, referred to as genomic or precision medicine, which has the potential to improve patient survival and quality of life, and reduce health care costs [2,3].

Genetic diagnosis is achieved through testing of specific genes or by more comprehensive interrogation via whole exome sequencing (WES) or whole genome sequencing (WGS; Box 1). The typical workflow for diagnostic genomic sequencing in affected individuals involves sample collection and processing, phenotypic evaluation, genetic variant detection, genetic variant interpretation, and reporting (Fig. 1). In cases in which the pretest differential diagnosis is narrow and pathognomonic features are present, a single gene or gene panel test is likely to be ordered. However, the use of clinical WES and WGS is growing more widespread as costs and turn-around-times drop. In both methods, primary phenotypes are used during genomic analysis to inform gene review and variant prioritization based on the overlap of canonical disease descriptions with the patient's phenotype, a necessary step, as WES and WGS can produce approximately 25,000 genetic variants and upward of 4 to 5 million variants, respectively [4].

Artificial intelligence (AI) has the potential to transform many aspects of the practice of medicine, including rare disease diagnosis. Defined as the ability of a computer or machine to perform tasks that are normally associated with human intelligence, AI can be divided into subfields, such as natural language processing, machine

---

[1] All authors contributed equally to this work.

*Corresponding author, E-mail address: schowdhury@rchsd.org

BOX 1
Glossary of Key Terms

Bayesian Probability Model: probability expressed as a degree of belief in an event based on prior knowledge about the event, such as the results of previous experiments [40].

Computer Vision: a subfield of artificial intelligence concerned with understanding, analyzing, and interpreting visual images

Deep Learning: a branch of machine learning that combines large multilayered neural networks with large computing power to learn and recognize patterns

Electronic Health Record: a digital version of a patient's medical chart over time, including medical history, diagnoses, medications, treatment plans, immunizations, radiology images, and laboratory and genetic test results

Machine Learning: a subfield of artificial intelligence concerned with developing computer algorithms to learn from data, identify patterns, and build models without predefined assumptions

Natural Language Processing: a subfield of artificial intelligence concerned with understanding, analyzing, and interpreting human language

Neural Network: a statistical model used in machine learning based on neurons in the human brain to process data through multiple layers, with adaptive weights tuned to optimize results.

Ontology: a representation of entities and the relationships between them, often visualized as nodes connected by labeled paths. Example: in the Human Phenotype Ontology, the node/term "Short stature" is connected to its parent node/term "Abnormality of height" by the path "is a"

Random Forest: a machine learning algorithm that outputs the mode or median of multiple decision trees for classification. This aggregation protects against overfitting to training datasets

Random Walk: a machine learning algorithm that involves random sampling from large amounts of data to iteratively pinpoint which sources to use for classification

Whole Exome Sequencing: the process of determining the sequence of the coding regions of the genome. This is approximately 1% to 2% of the entire genome.

Whole Genome Sequencing: the process of determining the complete DNA sequence of an individual

---

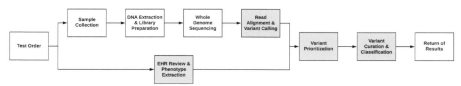

FIG. 1 Typical genome sequencing workflow to diagnose genetic diseases. A test order is placed for genomic sequencing and a biological sample is collected. For rare genetic disease, blood is often the preferred sample type. DNA is extracted from blood and sequencing libraries are prepared. Genomic sequencing is performed and the resulting sequencing reads are aligned to the reference human genome and variants are called. In parallel, phenotypic features are extracted from a patient's EHR and translated into phenotypic terms. Annotated variants and phenotypic terms are integrated to identify genetic variants that are the likely cause of disease. These variants are curated, classified according to standard guidelines, and reported to the clinical team. Phenotype extraction and variant prioritization (highlighted in *orange*) can potentially be automated with the use of computational or artificial intelligence methods. Note that read alignment and variant calling (highlighted in *blue*) typically incorporates AI methods to achieve an increased sensitivity and specificity [39]. Variant curation and classification (highlighted in *blue*) is another area in which AI may prove helpful.

learning (including neural networks and deep learning), computer vision (including image recognition), and cognitive computing (see Box 1). Since its initial development in the 1950s, AI has achieved more widespread use in recent decades due to decreased data storage costs, advances in computer algorithms, and gains in computing power. Through its ability to analyze increasingly large amounts of data in an unbiased manner, AI has been applied to improve patient outcomes through more accurate diagnoses and more comprehensive monitoring [5].

In the field of rare and ultra-rare disease, the use of AI may help overcome the limits of human experience-based reasoning and reduce the time needed to reach a diagnosis. Because there are many rare genetic disorders, clinicians may have never seen a particular genetic disorder before encountering it in their patient. Here, we review the current landscape of AI platforms for phenotype extraction and phenotype-driven variant prioritization in WGS for the diagnosis of rare disease. Currently, automatic phenotypic extraction from the electronic health record (EHR) is quite rare, whereas the use of phenotype-aware automated variant prioritization tools is fairly common. We survey the available tools for both processes, highlight strengths and weaknesses, and provide examples of their application in the clinical setting. Finally, we end with a discussion of the limitations and challenges of AI-assisted diagnosis of rare disease and considerations of confidentiality and security related to genomic data.

SIGNIFICANCE
Artificial Intelligence in Phenotype Extraction
Linking phenotypes to known genetic disease descriptions is essential for diagnosis. The primary source of clinical phenotypic information is the EHR, which collects granular, individual-level clinical information. EHRs have been widely implemented in most major hospital systems to meet regulatory and billing requirements. EHRs present a comprehensive, quantitative portrait of the patient's observed symptoms and signs as well as additional information including ongoing or resolved prior diagnoses, medical and surgical history, family history, birth history, medications, interventions and responses, laboratory tests, and diagnostic investigations. The medical data contained in EHRs takes the form of time-stamped unstructured data or "free text," as well as structured data. The abundance of unstructured textual data and the remarkable diversity of synonyms, abbreviations, and qualifiers used by clinicians make manual EHR

curation error-prone, time-consuming, and inaccessible to nonexperts.

Clinical Natural Language Processing (NLP) tools can mitigate these burdens by automatically extracting phenotypic information from EHRs, but several challenges have slowed their adoption. In addition to privacy concerns regarding storage or use of EHR data (see *Limitations and Challenges*), the matching of both structured and unstructured EHR data to potential diagnoses or genes requires translation across vocabularies or ontologies that were not expressly designed to be linked. Two forms of structured data commonly present in EHRs are International Classification of Diseases (ICD) codes, which represent diagnoses and are used mainly for billing purposes, and Systematized Nomenclature of Medicine (SNOMED) terms, which represent clinical findings and were developed to allow for precise, controlled information sharing among clinicians caring for a patient (Table 1). Unstructured EHR data must be extracted into some structured format, such as Unified Medical Language System (UMLS) concepts, Human Phenotype Ontology (HPO), and SNOMED Clinical Terms (SNOMED CT), or Current Procedural Terminology (CPT) and ICD codes, often sorted by frequency or probability (Fig. 2, Table 2). In addition, tools such as the Monarch Initiative can be used to map between different ontologies. Variant prioritization tools accept phenotypic data in specific formats, most commonly HPO (Table 3). Some tools for automated phenotype extraction include a mapping step to translate phenotype terms from other ontologies or vocabularies into HPO terms, but robust tools for this translation step are still needed. In this context, the Monarch Initiative promises to fill an important unmet need to leverage semantic relationships between biological concepts by developing key ontological resources to harmonize phenotype ontologies in the Unified Phenotype Ontology [6]. The Monarch Initiative uses uPheno (http://obofoundry.org/ontology/upheno) to find candidate genes and potential animal models for human diseases. Allowing for inexact matching during intervocabulary translation while retaining accuracy and high information content remains an important challenge [7].

Multiple clinical NLP solutions are available for extraction of phenotypic information. A representative sample is reviewed in Table 2.

Unified Medical Language System–based clinical Natural Language Processing tools
UMLS, which is a collection of several controlled vocabularies in biomedical sciences, provides a base mapping structure for 2 popular clinical NLP tools: MetaMap and

TABLE 1
Ontologies Used in Natural Language Processing/Artificial Intelligence Tools for Genetic Diagnosis

Abbreviation	Ontology	Description	References
DO	Disease Ontology	Hierarchy of disease descriptions, with embedded information about inheritance patterns and OMIM phenotype terms.	Schriml et al [41], 2019
GO	Gene Ontology	Loosely hierarchical computational model of biological systems, which includes 3 sub-ontologies: GO-BP (biological process), GO-CC (cellular component), GO-MF (molecular function).	Ashburner et al [22], 2000
HPO	Human Phenotype Ontology	Collaboratively developed hierarchical ontology, originally based on OMIM disease descriptions. Terms are connected by "is-a" (ie, subset) relationships.	Köhler et al [42], 2019
ICD	International Classification of Diseases	Set of alphanumeric codes representing diagnoses, with some characters optional for specifying body regions, etiology or severity. Used for medical billing and research; maintained by the World Health Organization.	World Health Organization [43], 2004
OMIM	Online Mendelian Inheritance in Man	Catalog of human diseases and their genetic causes.	McKusick-Nathans Institute of Genetic Medicine [44]
SNOMED	Systematized Nomenclature of Medicine	Large collaboratively developed medical vocabulary used for precise recording and sharing of clinical information. Merger of 2 ontologies, developed by the College of American Pathologists and the UK's National Health Service (NHS).	Cornet & de Keizer [45], 2008
UMLS	Unified Medical Language System	A set of tools for translating between clinical and biomedical vocabularies including SNOMED and ICD. Maintained by the US National Library of Medicine.	Bodenreider [38], 2004
uPheno	The Unified Phenotype Ontology	A key resource to map and harmonize between various ontologies and facilitate discovery of candidate genes and potential animal models for human diseases. Developed and maintained by The Monarch Initiative.	Mungall et al [46], 2017

Clinical Text Analysis and Knowledge Extraction System (cTAKES) [8].

• *MetaMap:* MetaMap (https://metamap.nlm.nih.gov/) is a public resource developed by the National Library of Medicine to extract and standardize biomedical text to medical concepts in UMLS [9]. It integrates knowledge-intensive approach and computational linguistic techniques. MetaMap uses a nonstandard input text that is frequently found in the form of MEDLINE/PubMed citations. For

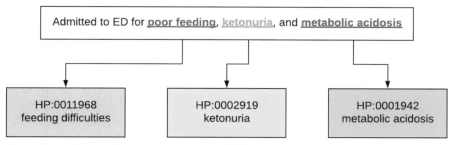

FIG. 2 Extraction and translation of phenotypes from EHRs to ontology terms. Automated NLP methods can be used to extract a patient's phenotypes from the EHR and translate them into a standardized vocabulary in an ontology, such as HPO.

each phrase in input text, MetaMap produces default output as a human-readable list of candidate Meta-thesaurus concepts matching or part of the phrase.

- *cTAKES*: cTAKES combines the UMLS framework with the OpenNLP natural language processing toolkit to offer an open-source NLP system that extracts clinical information from unstructured data in clinical notes [10]. cTAKES accepts either plain text or clinical document architecture—compliant XML documents as input. cTAKES is a modular system of pipelined components combining rule-based and machine learning algorithms. cTAKES is available at http://www.ohnlp.org/.

Human Phenotype Ontology–based clinical Natural Language Processing tools

The HPO is an atlas of standardized vocabulary of phenotypic abnormalities reported in human disease with the aim of facilitating phenotype-driven differential diagnostics, genomic diagnostics, and translational research. NLP tools such as ClinPhen, use HPO as a phenotype mapping structure for clinical phenotypes. In addition, tools such as Phenolyzer or Phenomizer (not discussed) can take HPO terms and create patient-specific gene lists to help guide genomic analysis [11,12].

- *ClinPhen*: ClinPhen (http://bejerano.stanford.edu/clinphen/) is a fast, easy-to-use, high-precision, and high-sensitivity tool that scans through free-text notes in a patient's clinical notes and returns a prioritized list of patient phenotypes using HPO terms [13]. These phenotypes can be input to gene ranking tools that rank the causative gene for Mendelian diseases. ClinPhen uses hash tables created from sentences, subsentences, and words in clinical notes. It was benchmarked as performing 20 times faster than cTAKES and MetaMap [14].

Semi-supervised clustering-based clinical Natural Language Processing tools

Semi-supervised approaches to phenotypic extraction integrate prior knowledge with cluster analyses to generate a priority or rank list of phenotypes to aid clinical diagnostics.

- *DAPS*: Denoising Autoencoders for Phenotype Stratification (DAPS; https://github.com/greenelab/DAPS) is a machine learning algorithm that uses semi-supervised technique for exploring phenotypes in the EHR. The algorithm is trained using clustering via principal components analysis and t-distributed stochastic neighbor embedding [15]. A typical output includes a list of cosegregating phenotypes describing distinct disease conditions.
- *PheCap*: PheCAP uses a semi-supervised approach to automated extraction of phenotypes from clinical notes [16]. PheCap accepts high-throughput structured and unstructured data from the EHR and produces a phenotype algorithm, the probability of the phenotype for all patients, and a binary (yes or no) phenotype classification. PheCAP suffers in being substantially slower in performance than other tools such as ClinPhen and CLiX ENRICH [16].

Systematized Nomenclature of Medicine Clinical Terms–based clinical Natural Language Processing tools

SNOMED CT is a comprehensive and multilingual health terminology standard developed to assist electronic exchange of clinical health information. It is also a required standard in interoperability specifications of the US Healthcare Information Technology Standards Panel. SNOMED CT can be mapped to other coding systems including ICD-9 and ICD-10 to facilitate semantic interoperability. CliniThink is a leading

TABLE 2
Clinical Natural Language Processing Tools for Phenotypic Extraction

Tool	Artificial Intelligence	Input	Output	References
MetaMap	Unsupervised approaches for automatic indexing to map medical text to Metathesaurus concepts, unsupervised approaches to automatic disambiguation of Metathesaurus concepts (also called as Word Sense Disambiguation)	Unstructured and structured data from electronic health record (EHR)	Human-readable and machine-readable list of candidate Metathesaurus concepts in MetaMap machine output (MMO), XML and colorized MetaMap formats	Aronson & Lang [9], 2010
cTAKES (2010)	Rule-based and machine learning algorithms used to generate outputs	Unstructured and structured data from EHR	Machine-readable XMI CAS file including annotations for anatomic sites, signs and symptoms, medical procedures, diseases/disorders and medications, normalized Unified Medical Language System concept unique identifiers, uncertainty score and patient specific	Savova et al [10], 2010
ClinPhen	Rule-based sentence analysis process	Unstructured and structured data from EHR	Machine-readable hash tables created from sentences, subsentences, and words, human-readable sorted list of all Human Phenotype Ontology (HPO) phenotypes found, with the most frequent- and earliest-appearing phenotypes at the top	Deisseroth et al [13], 2019
DAPS	Machine learning used for training	Unstructured and structured data from EHR	Human and machine-readable list of cosegregating phenotypes describing distinct disease conditions	Beaulieu-Jones & Greene [15], 2016, https://github.com/greenelab/DAPS

PheCap	Semi-supervised approach used in phenotype extraction	Unstructured and structured data from EHR	Human-readable and machine-readable probability of the phenotype for a patient, a binary phenotype classification (yes or no)	Zhang et al [16], 2019
CliniThink	Proprietary artificial intelligence technology to parse EHR Data into Systemized Nomenclature of Medicine (SNOMED) terms	Unstructured and structured data from EHR	List of SNOMED terms; optional step to map SNOMED to HPO terms	Clark et al [17], 2019

TABLE 3
Phenotype-Driven Variant Prioritization Tools

Tool (Year)	Artificial Intelligence	Input	Output	References
eXtasy (2013)	Machine learning training (random forests)	VCF + HPO terms	Annotated variant list including phenotype-derived gene-level rank	Aerts et al [19], 2006 & Sifrim et al [20], 2013
Phevor (2014)	Ontological propagation algorithm used to assess likelihood of gene involvement in disease (including for novel genes)	Ranked variant list (eg, VAAST format) + HPO/DO/GO/OMIM terms	Re-ranked variant list	Singleton et al [21], 2014
Phen-Gen (2014)	Machine learning (Random walk with restart algorithm) used for phenotype (ie, disease) risk estimation. Bayesian framework integrates patient genetic and phenotypic risk estimates.	VCF + HPO terms + pedigree (PED) file	Ranked gene list (for genes present on input VCF) and separate file of annotated variants from those genes	Javed et al [24], 2014
Exomiser (2015)	Machine learning (random walk algorithm) used for novel disease gene discovery mode (ExomeWalker)	VCF + HPO/OMIM/ DECIPHER/ORDO terms	VCF: ranked variant list HTML: ranked gene list with associated diseases and variants in the gene embedded, in HTML format	Smedley et al [26], 2015
Xrare (2019)	Machine learning (gradient boosting decision tree algorithm) used to generate gene-phenotype scores and to train the Xrare variant classifier	VCF + HPO terms	Ranked variant list	Li et al [18], 2019
DeepPVP (2019)	Deep neural network used for training and variant classification	VCF + HPO terms	Ranked variant list	Boudellioua et al [27], 2019
eDiva (2019)	Machine learning (random forest model) used for variant pathogenicity prediction (eDiva-Score) eDiva-Prioritize: incorporates HPO term similarity scoring underlying the Phenomizer tool (see Kohler et al)	VCF + HPO terms	Ranked variant list	Bosio et al [28], 2019 Kohler et al [25], 2009
Moon (2019)	Bayesian framework combines gene-phenotype similarity score and variant pathogenicity scores	VCF + HPO terms	Ranked variant list	Clark et al [17], 2019

Abbreviations: DECIPHER, DatabasE of genomiC variation and Phenotype in Humans using Ensembl Resources; DO, Disease Ontology; GO, Gene Ontology; HPO, Human Phenotype Ontology; OMIM, Online Inheritance in Man; VAAST, ORDO, Orphanet Rare Disease Ontology; Variant Annotation, Analysis and Search Tool; VCF, variant call format.

phenotype extraction platform that primarily uses SNOMED CT ontologies.

- *CliniThink*: The CliniThink platform CLiX ENRICH uses SNOMED CT for phenotypic extraction. The proprietary CLiX (Corporate Learning and Information Exchange) system encodes clinical free text (pre-coordinated) to enrich for SNOMED dictionary terms and select contextually correct SNOMED concepts (post-coordinated). The standard output from CLiX ENRICH is in the form of SNOMED CT that includes diagnosis, medication, sign/symptoms, and contextual concepts, such as historical reference and negation [17].

Artificial Intelligence in Phenotype-Driven Variant Prioritization

As WES began to become more widely available as a clinical test approximately 2012 to 2015, numerous groups developed tools to aid in the evaluation of the large number of genomic variants generated per case. Many recent variant prioritization tools have incorporated AI methods into their training and implementation, and a subset uses patient phenotype information input to rank variants in a phenotype-driven manner. Several AI methods have emerged as of particular importance for these tools:

- Machine learning during tool training with positive and negative control variant datasets to optimize sensitivity and specificity
- Incorporation of multiple gene interactomes and similarity metrics to enable disease prediction for novel genes
- Calculation of a similarity score between the patient phenotype and gene or disease phenotypes, often relying on one or more phenotypic ontology

The exact format of the phenotypic input required has varied among variant prioritization tools as the clinical genomics field has co-opted multiple biological and clinical ontologies such as Gene Ontology (GO), ICD, HPO, Disease Ontology (DO), and Online Mendelian Inheritance in Man (OMIM), with recent convergence on HPO as a consensus input vocabulary (see Tables 1 and 3). Most variant prioritization tools developed to date were designed and tested with manual input of phenotypic terms. To scale with the ongoing increase in demand for clinical next-generation sequencing (NGS), variant prioritization tools will need to be optimized to accept phenotypic terms that are automatically extracted from medical records [18].

First-Generation Phenotype-Based Variant Prioritization Tools

A first generation of phenotype-based variant prioritization tools for NGS was published in 2013 to 2014. All accepted HPO terms as input, but some also accepted phenotypic terms in other formats, reflecting the lack of early consensus on a phenotypic ontology.

- *EXtasy*: One of the first published phenotype-driven variant prioritization tools, EXtasy was trained on positive and negative control variant datasets using a random forest algorithm, a form of machine learning. EXtasy incorporates patient phenotype data input as HPO terms to derive a gene-level metric, which is integrated with metrics of variant pathogenicity to rank variants in a phenotype-driven manner [19,20]. The gene-level metric integrates information about disease phenotypes and gene function, similarity and interaction from multiple sources including biomedical literature, GO functional annotation (see Table 1), gene expression datasets, and protein interactomes. This tool's reliance on machine learning for training and integration of multiple data sources for gene-disease modeling was prescient of approaches that have become widely adopted.

- *Phevor*: In Phevor, patient phenotypic terms are input together with annotated variants, to a propagation algorithm, which transmits weighted values across and within several biomedical ontologies containing information about relationships between phenotypic features (HPO, DO, Mammalian Phenotype Ontology) or about gene function and interaction (GO) [21]. Earlier work linking HPO terms to genes and genes to GO terms allows for propagation between phenotypic and gene ontologies [22,23]. Ultimately the output of Phevor's propagation algorithm is a re-scoring of candidate variants, ranked by a combination of relevance to patient phenotype and predicted pathogenicity. Phevor's algorithm was shown to detect (ie, highly rank) variants in novel disease genes, an important marker of the algorithm's utility for gene discovery [21].

- *Phen-Gen*: Phen-Gen uses a Bayesian framework (see Box 1) to generate gene-level estimations of disease involvement based on patient phenotype and variant data, using an implementation of Phenomizer [24]. Phenomizer is a tool that calculates similarity scores between HPO input queries and genetic diseases that have been annotated with HPO terms [25].

- *Exomiser*: Exomiser can be run in several modes, depending on whether the goal is to search for variants in known or novel disease genes [26]. One mode, ExomeWalker, uses a random walk algorithm within a protein interactome, seeded by genes input by the user, to search for novel disease genes. Another mode, PhenIX, uses a similar phenotype ranking approach to that used by PhenoDB: known disease genes are scored for likelihood of disease involvement based on similarity of the input patient phenotype terms to those in OMIM disease entries; then the gene-level score is combined with variant pathogenicity scoring to generate an overall variant ranking.

Second-Generation Phenotype-Based Variant Prioritization Tools

Several new phenotype-based variant prioritization tools were published in 2019, including Xrare, DeepPVP, eDiva, and Moon. These tools showcase the increasing integration of machine learning, including use of neural networks (DeepPVP). All of these tools accept HPO terms as input, perhaps reflecting growing consensus in the field for adoption of that ontology.

- *Xrare*: The development of Xrare incorporated a gradient-boosting decision tree (GBDT) algorithm, a form of machine learning that can robustly handle redundant, highly correlated inputs, for training [18]. The GBDT approach was also used to generate the model's gene-phenotype scores, seeded by genes with known phenotypes. The gene-phenotype scores are static scores determined for each gene-phenotype pair, calculated using 10 gene interactomes, among them the 3 GO sub-ontologies (see Table 1), BLAST for sequence similarity, and Reactome for shared pathways [18]. This gene-phenotype score is combined with variant-level features such as allele frequency, gene constraint and in silico variant pathogenicity predictions, to rank input variants. Xrare also includes a phenotype similarity measure developed to handle noisy, imprecise patient phenotypic data and compare it to phenotype sets associated with disease or genes within its model. Xrare is notable for its consideration of input data imprecision and redundancy, which will likely prove important in the development of tools designed to accept phenotypic data automatically generated from EMRs.

- *DeepPVP*: DeepPVP uses a deep neural network to classify variants (see Box 1) [27]. Similar to Xrare and Exomiser-PhenIX, DeepPVP scores genes for

similarity between their associated phenotypes (drawn from multiple databases spanning animal model results, gene expression data, and GO) (see Table 1) and the input patient phenotype, both of which are instantiated by sets of HPO terms [27]. This similarity score is one of the features input to the neural network–based variant classifier.

- *eDiva*: The training of eDiva's variant pathogenicity classifier, eDiva-Score, used a random forest machine learning approach [28]. A downstream module, eDiva-Prioritize, relies on an HPO similarity scoring metric built on the Phenomizer tool (as does Phen-Gen's phenotype-driven risk estimate; see Table 3) to compute similarity between patient phenotype and the disease association of genes.

- *Moon*: Moon computes a similarity score between the patient's phenotype term set and many disease-specific phenotype term sets to rank diseases by likelihood [17]. An interesting innovation by Moon is that the disease-specific phenotype term sets are generated using NLP of the medical literature, as opposed to, for example, OMIM-derived phenotype term lists used by other prioritization tools. A Bayesian model combines this disease likelihood ranking with variant pathogenicity scores derived from numerous sources.

DISCUSSION/SUMMARY
Limitations and Challenges

The promise of AI and the potential benefits it could provide to a health care system [29] have led to a large number of research studies demonstrating AI's applications in various fields of medicine [30], including its application in genomics and precision medicine [17,31,32]. However, the vast majority of these studies have been performed retrospectively, testing against already performed expert interpretation [30]. In addition, robust randomized control trials are limited in assessing AI-based approaches compared with current clinical practice. Thus, the true impact and implementation of AI in genomic interpretation has not yet been realized.

Recent review articles have framed the current challenges of AI in medicine [33] as well as the challenges associated with the clinical interpretation of genomic data more broadly [34]. The current bottlenecks of time-intensive clinical variant interpretation, and the lack of qualified experts to clinically interpret genomic data continue to hinder the widespread adoption of AI implementation in genomic analysis.

Current Challenges and Barriers to Address

- *Privacy*: Privacy issues related to genomic analysis remain regardless of the incorporation of AI-based approaches [35]. Genomic testing is highly sensitive (https://www.genome.gov/about-genomics/policy-issues/Privacy) in part because: (1) it can be interpreted as "identifiable information," (2) the potential for genomic analysis to reveal findings not related to the patient's current phenotype (incidental findings), and (3) potential impact to family members if pathogenic variants are inherited. The use of AI and the introduction of new applications into the genomic data analysis process requires careful consideration to ensure the tools and processes respect and protect patient privacy.

- *Human Resistance*: The field of genetics and genomics has traditionally been shepherded by clinical genetics and laboratory genetics professionals. However, as genomics becomes applied to all areas of medicine, the ability to allow other subspecialties and individuals with different backgrounds and training will be essential to scale genomic sequencing to all the patients that may benefit from this testing. Currently, there are approximately 5000 genetic counselors and 1500 clinical geneticists in the United States, numbers well below what would be required to deploy broader genomic sequencing (https://www.nsgc.org/). Thus, technology-based solutions will be required to serve the patient base for genomic sequencing that may benefit from this technology.

- *Lack of Regulation and Quality Control*: The vast majority of genetic tests fall under the category of laboratory developed tests that are governed and regulated by accreditation bodies such as the Clinical Laboratory Improvement Amendment and the College of American Pathologists. However, there are no current guidance for the validation and implementation of AI in the diagnosis of genetic disease, and the question of what is the right regulatory framework for AI remains unresolved [36]. The regulatory considerations for these novel approaches and technologies must be addressed before AI can be widely adopted across laboratories. There is a lack of published studies on AI implementation within genetic diagnostic pipelines. A collaborative, cross-laboratory effort to establish best practices for AI implementation in genetic testing would be valuable.

- *Lack of Gold Standard Truth Sets*: Genomic sequencing has benefited from the establishment of gold standard truth sets to assess the validity of genomic data generated via NGS [37]. Standards to assess the interpretation and clinical reporting of genomic data lag behind these sequencing validation truth sets, and will be required to allow laboratories to benchmark AI-based approaches.

- *Phenotypic Complexity*: Many diseases manifest as multiple phenotypes with variable severity, necessitating modeling of the phenotypic spectrum through NLP to facilitate (1) identification of core symptoms of the disease, (2) delineation of disease subtypes, (3) refinement of differential diagnoses, and (4) discovery of new genetic and pathophysiological mechanisms through hypothesis-driven research.

One Laboratory's Experience with Artificial Intelligence and Genetic Disease

In Clark and colleagues [17], the Rady Children's Institute for Genomic Medicine conducted a pilot study in which automated clinical NLP phenotype extraction from the EHR was performed, and that phenotypic information was then automatically incorporated into the rapid WGS analysis. Various steps in this process

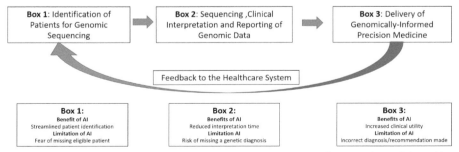

FIG. 3 Described are 3 major areas in which AI could advance and benefit genomic medicine with a continuous feedback loop as part of a learning health care system. One potential benefit and 1 potential limitation is described for each box.

required thorough testing and development. Challenges included (1) thorough testing and validation on real patient data with genetic diagnoses at each step in the process; (2) the mappings of SNOMED CT and HPO were incomplete; (3) the accuracy of the NLP approach had to be thoroughly assessed; (4) the large phenotypic output (20 times greater than manual curation) had to be incorporated into the genomic analysis pipeline to prioritize a genetic diagnosis. The pilot pipeline achieved very strong concordance with expert manual interpretation (97% recall and 99% precision in 95 children with 97 genetic diseases) in retrospective cases. The investigators showed a proof of concept of how NLP and AI could aid in the rapid genetic diagnosis of children in the intensive care unit.

Final Thoughts

AI holds the potential to not just aid in the analysis of genomic data, but potentially in other areas of genomic medicine, including patient selection criteria and delivery of treatment guidance to maximize the utility of genomic sequencing (Fig. 3). To maximize the potential that genomic medicine has promised, the ability to deliver genetic diagnoses in a timeframe conducive to impacting clinical management is essential. Currently, many individuals with rare disease, who stand to benefit from genomic testing, lack access to it. Meanwhile, sequencing technologies continue to develop and drop in cost. Thus, the ability to comprehensively and efficiently analyze genomic data must maintain pace with sequencing improvements to ensure laboratories can meet the demand for genomic testing. The use of AI to aid genomic diagnosis presents a unique opportunity to address many of the current challenges and barriers that exist today, including the dearth of laboratory geneticists and trained workforce, and the cost and effort required to analyze genomic data. AI can help foster collaboration between academia and industry to ensure rapid developments in this evolving field. Realizing the potential of AI to aid genomic diagnosis will require a collaborative effort from the entire genomics community to ensure that these technologies can be deployed in a robust and responsible manner.

DISCLOSURE

This study was supported by grant U19HD077693, U01TR002271, UL1TR002550 from NICHD and NHGRI and NCATS.

REFERENCES

[1] Nguengang Wakap S, Lambert DM, Olry A, et al. Estimating cumulative point prevalence of rare diseases: analysis of the Orphanet database. Eur J Hum Genet 2020;28(2):165–73.

[2] Farnaes L, Hildreth A, Sweeney NM, et al. Rapid whole-genome sequencing decreases infant morbidity and cost of hospitalization. NPJ Genom Med 2018; 3(1):10.

[3] Melbourne Genomics Health Alliance, Stark Z, Lunke S, et al. Meeting the challenges of implementing rapid genomic testing in acute pediatric care. Genet Med 2018;20(12):1554–63.

[4] Kingsmore SF, Cakici JA, Clark MM, et al. A randomized, controlled trial of the analytic and diagnostic performance of singleton and trio, rapid genome and exome sequencing in ill infants. Am J Hum Genet 2019; 105(4):719–33.

[5] Brasil S, Pascoal C, Francisco R, et al. Artificial Intelligence (AI) in rare diseases: is the future brighter? Genes 2019;10(12):978.

[6] Shefchek KA, Harris NL, Gargano M, et al. The Monarch Initiative in 2019: an integrative data and analytic platform connecting phenotypes to genotypes across species. Nucleic Acids Res 2020;48(D1):D704–15.

[7] Dhombres F, Bodenreider O. Interoperability between phenotypes in research and healthcare terminologies—Investigating partial mappings between HPO and SNOMED CT. J Biomed Semantics 2016;7(1):3.

[8] Reátegui R, Ratté S. Comparison of MetaMap and cTAKES for entity extraction in clinical notes. BMC Med Inform Decis Mak 2018 14;18(Suppl 3):74.

[9] Aronson AR, Lang F-M. An overview of MetaMap: historical perspective and recent advances. J Am Med Inform Assoc 2010;17(3):229–36.

[10] Savova GK, Masanz JJ, Ogren PV, et al. Mayo clinical Text Analysis and Knowledge Extraction System (cTAKES): architecture, component evaluation and applications. J Am Med Inform Assoc 2010;17(5):507–13.

[11] Yang H, Robinson PN, Wang K. Phenolyzer: phenotype-based prioritization of candidate genes for human diseases. Nat Methods 2015;12(9):841–3.

[12] Ullah MZ, Aono M, Seddiqui MH. Estimating a ranked list of human hereditary diseases for clinical phenotypes by using weighted bipartite network. Conf Proc IEEE Eng Med Biol Soc 2013;2013:3475–8.

[13] Deisseroth CA, Birgmeier J, Bodle EE, et al. ClinPhen extracts and prioritizes patient phenotypes directly from medical records to expedite genetic disease diagnosis. Genet Med 2019;21(7):1585–93.

[14] Liu C, Ta CN, Rogers JR, et al. Ensembles of natural language processing systems for portable phenotyping solutions. J Biomed Inform 2019;100:103318.

[15] Beaulieu-Jones BK, Greene CS. Semi-supervised learning of the electronic health record for phenotype stratification. J Biomed Inform 2016;64:168–78.

[16] Zhang Y, Cai T, Yu S, et al. High-throughput phenotyping with electronic medical record data using a common semi-supervised approach (PheCAP). Nat Protoc 2019; 14(12):3426–44.

[17] Clark MM, Hildreth A, Batalov S, et al. Diagnosis of genetic diseases in seriously ill children by rapid whole-genome sequencing and automated phenotyping and interpretation. Sci Transl Med 2019;11(489): eaat6177.

[18] Li Q, Zhao K, Bustamante CD, et al. Xrare: a machine learning method jointly modeling phenotypes and genetic evidence for rare disease diagnosis. Genet Med 2019;21(9):2126–34.

[19] Aerts S, Lambrechts D, Maity S, et al. Gene prioritization through genomic data fusion. Nat Biotechnol 2006; 24(5):537–44.

[20] Sifrim A, Popovic D, Tranchevent L-C, et al. eXtasy: variant prioritization by genomic data fusion. Nat Methods 2013;10(11):1083–4.

[21] Singleton MV, Guthery SL, Voelkerding KV, et al. Phevor combines multiple biomedical ontologies for accurate identification of disease-causing alleles in single individuals and small nuclear families. Am J Hum Genet 2014; 94(4):599–610.

[22] Ashburner M, Ball CA, Blake JA, et al. Gene ontology: tool for the unification of biology. The Gene Ontology Consortium. Nat Genet 2000;25(1):25–9.

[23] Robinson PN, Köhler S, Bauer S, et al. The human phenotype ontology: a tool for annotating and analyzing human hereditary disease. Am J Hum Genet 2008;83(5): 610–5.

[24] Javed A, Agrawal S, Ng PC. Phen-Gen: combining phenotype and genotype to analyze rare disorders. Nat Methods 2014;11(9):935–7.

[25] Köhler S, Schulz MH, Krawitz P, et al. Clinical diagnostics in human genetics with semantic similarity searches in ontologies. Am J Hum Genet 2009;85(4): 457–64.

[26] Smedley D, Jacobsen JOB, Jäger M, et al. Next-generation diagnostics and disease-gene discovery with the Exomiser. Nat Protoc 2015;10(12):2004–15.

[27] Boudellioua I, Kulmanov M, Schofield PN, et al. DeepPVP: phenotype-based prioritization of causative variants using deep learning. BMC Bioinformatics 2019;20(1):65.

[28] Bosio M, Drechsel O, Rahman R, et al. eDiVA—Classification and prioritization of pathogenic variants for clinical diagnostics. Hum Mutat 2019;40(7):865–78.

[29] Bodenheimer T, Sinsky C. From triple to quadruple aim: care of the patient requires care of the provider. Ann Fam Med 2014;12(6):573–6.

[30] Kelly CJ, Karthikesalingam A, Suleyman M, et al. Key challenges for delivering clinical impact with artificial intelligence. BMC Med 2019;17(1):195.

[31] Xu J, Yang P, Xue S, et al. Translating cancer genomics into precision medicine with artificial intelligence: applications, challenges and future perspectives. Hum Genet 2019;138(2):109–24.

[32] Uddin M, Wang Y, Woodbury-Smith M. Artificial intelligence for precision medicine in neurodevelopmental disorders. NPJ Digit Med 2019;2(1):112.

[33] Yu K-H, Kohane IS. Framing the challenges of artificial intelligence in medicine. BMJ Qual Saf 2019;28(3): 238–41.

[34] Kim Y-E, Ki C-S, Jang M-A. Challenges and considerations in sequence variant interpretation for mendelian disorders. Ann Lab Med 2019;39(5):421.

[35] Schwab AP, Luu HS, Wang J, et al. Genomic privacy. Clin Chem 2018;64(12):1696–703.

[36] Gerke S, Babic B, Evgeniou T, et al. The need for a system view to regulate artificial intelligence/machine learning-based software as medical device. NPJ Digit Med 2020; 3(1):53.

[37] Zook JM, McDaniel J, Olson ND, et al. An open resource for accurately benchmarking small variant and reference calls. Nat Biotechnol 2019;37(5):561–6.

[38] Bodenreider O. The Unified Medical Language System (UMLS): integrating biomedical terminology. Nucleic Acids Res 2004;32(Database issue):D267–70.

[39] DePristo MA, Banks E, Poplin R, et al. A framework for variation discovery and genotyping using next-generation DNA sequencing data. Nat Genet 2011; 43(5):491–8.

[40] Gelman A, Carlin JB, Stern HS, et al. Bayesian data analysis. 3rd edition. Chapman and Hall/CRC Press Taylor and Francis Group; 2013.

[41] Schriml LM, Mitraka E, Munro J, et al. Human Disease Ontology 2018 update: classification, content and workflow expansion. Nucleic Acids Res 2019;47(D1): D955–62.

[42] Köhler S, Carmody L, Vasilevsky N, et al. Expansion of the Human Phenotype Ontology (HPO) knowledge base and resources. Nucleic Acids Res 2019;47(D1): D1018–27.

[43] World Health Organization. ICD-10: international statistical classification of diseases and related health problems/World Health Organization. 10th revision, 2nd edition. Geneva (Switzerland): World Health Organization; 2004.

[44] McKusick-Nathans Institute of Genetic Medicine. Online Mendelian Inheritance in Man, OMIM®. [Internet]. Available at: https://omim.org/. Accessed January 1, 2020.

[45] Cornet R, de Keizer N. Forty years of SNOMED: a literature review. BMC Med Inform Decis Mak 2008;8(Suppl 1):S2.

[46] Mungall CJ, McMurry JA, Köhler S, et al. The Monarch Initiative: an integrative data and analytic platform connecting phenotypes to genotypes across species. Nucleic Acids Res 2017;45(D1):D712–22.

Advances in Molecular Pathology 3 (2020) 157–167

ADVANCES IN MOLECULAR PATHOLOGY

Building Infrastructure and Workflows for Clinical Bioinformatics Pipelines

Sabah Kadri, PhD[1]

Department of Pathology, Ann and Robert H. Lurie Children's Hospital, Northwestern University Feinberg School of Medicine, Chicago, IL 60611, USA

KEYWORDS

- Clinical bioinformatics • Infrastructure • Container technology • Nextflow • Docker • Singularity
- Cloud computing • Bioinformatics pipeline

KEY POINTS

- Clinical bioinformatics pipelines require high-performance computational infrastructure and implementation practices that can support robustness and reproducibility requirements.
- This review describes the heterogeneity in computational infrastructure used by clinical laboratories to process next generation sequencing data, both on-premise and cloud service providers.
- Advanced technologies such as containerization (for example, Docker) and workflow management systems (for example, Nextflow) allow for reproducible, reliable, modular, and scalable bioinformatics pipeline implementations, although these are more common in research than clinical environments at this time.

INTRODUCTION

Next generation sequencing (NGS) assays operate on large amounts of data, making bioinformatics analyses an integral part of all NGS assays [1,2]. These assays have been evolving both in size, from small gene panels to clinical whole genome sequencing, as well as complexity of analysis, and number and types of analytes.

Clinical molecular laboratories performing NGS testing must be in compliance with accreditation checklist requirements provided by the College of American Pathologists (CAP) and regulations listed by the Clinical Laboratory Improvement Amendments. In 2018, the Association for Molecular Pathology (AMP) and CAP provided recommendations for validation of clinical bioinformatics pipelines including their design and development [3]. However, details about computational infrastructure and pipeline frameworks are few across all these guidelines.

One of the main reasons for this is that there is lack of standardization in implementation of bioinformatics pipelines for clinical NGS assays and there are multiple reasons for this. The range of assays available in each laboratory is vast, and these assays vary in technology, design, target analytes, and limits of detection. Even if the same assay is implemented at different institutions, there is a lot of variability due to major differences in hardware and bioinformatics pipeline orchestration. Computing paradigms and technology vary immensely across institutions, which makes portability and standardization very difficult. The availability of skilled bioinformatics staff also can contribute to these differences. A laboratory might not have the flexibility to design complex pipeline modules in the absence of skilled staff and might adopt less-flexible out-of-the-box vendor-supplied solutions.

This article describes the heterogeneity in computational infrastructure used across clinical laboratories

[1] Present address: 225 East Chicago Avenue, Box 82, Chicago, IL 60611, USA.
E-mail address: skadri@luriechildrens.org

https://doi.org/10.1016/j.yamp.2020.07.014
2589-4080/20/

and lays out considerations for those moving or planning to move computing and/or storage to cloud-based systems. This review also describes the various approaches to workflow orchestration used in clinical bioinformatics pipelines, and explains advances in available technology and approaches that can eventually move us toward standardization and reproducibility. The infrastructure and pipeline frameworks discussed here are not an exhaustive list, but were found to be most relevant from a clinical bioinformatics perspective.

This review does not dive into specific tools and detailed pipeline steps for specific bioinformatics workflows, for example, DNA, RNA, or metabolomics. Instead, it focuses on design and methodologies that would apply to any clinical bioinformatics pipeline, irrespective of the application or sequencing technology. Other articles have previously reviewed software tools, specific to various clinical NGS applications [2,4,5].

SIGNIFICANCE

There has been much focus in the literature on specific bioinformatics pipeline tools and guidelines to build and validate a clinical NGS bioinformatics pipeline. This article puts together the building blocks on which to design clinical bioinformatics pipelines; the underlying infrastructure and workflow frameworks to put these pipelines together. The various types of on-premise and cloud-based computational infrastructure and related considerations about privacy, security, and compliance are also visited. Some basic good software practices are listed to help with implementation and maintenance. With recent advances in modern workflow management systems and container technology, laboratories can build pipelines that are portable and eventually independent of the underlying hardware systems and dependencies, making these implementations robust and reliable.

COMPUTATIONAL INFRASTRUCTURE FOR BIOINFORMATICS

NGS data analysis requires significant computing and storage requirements due to the large amounts of data generated from each sample. There is a large variability in the computing architecture for clinical bioinformatics across different institutions and laboratories, including, but not limited to hardware, operating systems (OSs), and versions of the software and tools. Here, we review some common types of computational

infrastructure being used for clinical NGS data processing. The appropriate architecture should be determined by the expected data size and volume, coupled with the institution's cost considerations and available personnel and resources. Clinical laboratories should also invest in a development and QA environment that is separate from the production environment to test new software or changes to existing software, although it should closely emulate the production environment [3]. The typical computational infrastructure models are shown in Fig. 1 and described as follows.

ON-PREMISE COMPUTING INFRASTRUCTURE

On-premise options for computing are the conventional approaches used by institutions, typically containing infrastructure within the firewall of the institute (see Fig. 1A). These are the following:

i.   Smaller-scale, locally installed and maintained servers in the clinical laboratory. In some cases, vendors provide preconfigured bioinformatics solutions on servers accompanying sequencing instruments.

ii. Larger high-performance computing clusters (HPCs) usually maintained by the institutional information technology (IT) teams. It has also been indicated that running data through a priority queue dedicated to the clinical laboratory instead of the usual queue in an HPC cluster might ensure better privacy measures [6] (Box 1).

The local IT team might also provide virtual machines (VMs) on existing local hardware. VMs use a virtualization layer on top of the physical hardware but require the installation of a complete operating system (OS), as it runs independently of the underlying OS. Consistency of bioinformatics software installations on these on-premise systems can be challenging due to complex or conflicting dependencies. If container technology is not being used, package managers such as Conda (https://docs.conda.io/en/latest/) and Bioconda [11] can be used (Table 1), as they provide reliable software components and automatically install necessary dependencies in isolated virtual execution environments. These are still not perfect and can be influenced by the host OS based on the specifications [12].

CLOUD-BASED SERVICE PROVIDERS

At many institutions, internal IT infrastructure is unable to support the growing NGS needs, either for storage or

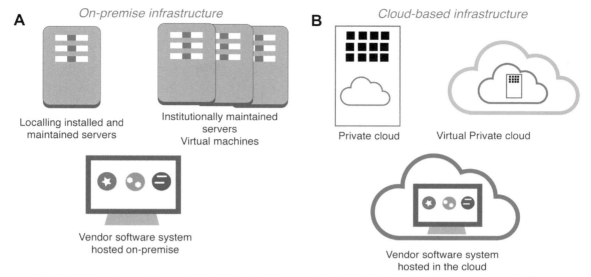

FIG. 1 Various types of computational infrastructure used by clinical laboratories (**A**) on-premise and (**B**) using cloud-based service providers.

computing or both. As a result, laboratories looking for scalable and affordable options are turning to cloud-based services due to their scalability, elasticity, and cost-efficiency in the long run. The National Institute of Standards and Technology (NIST) defines cloud infrastructure as hardware and software that enables convenient and on-demand network access to a shared pool of configurable computing resources that can be provisioned and released with minimal management [16]. Cloud services essentially provide a virtualization

---

BOX 1
Privacy and Security

An important consideration for any hardware or software solution decision in a molecular pathology laboratory is security and privacy of patient data, both related but with differences [3,7,8]. Security of the data is concerned with safeguarding the data from unauthorized access and actions, whereas privacy is concerned with policies regarding use and governance of the data (https://iapp.org/about/what-is-privacy/).

All NGS data are considered electronic Protected Health Information (ePHI) protected under Health Insurance Portability and Accountability Act (HIPAA) protocols [9]. Under HIPAA, ePHI is defined as identifiable health information generated and transmitted via electronic media. All clinical laboratories must be mindful of HIPAA compliance and safety requirements pertaining to NGS data, especially, when on-boarding third-party software systems or infrastructure. It is also the responsibility of the laboratory to be compliant with their local, state, and national laws [3].

If using on-premise servers or HPC clusters, it is the responsibility of the laboratory to ensure that the compute and storage servers/nodes have the necessary safeguards in place regarding who can access and modify the data and execute the pipelines [6].

Adoption of a cloud-based system requires a shared responsibility model such that the cloud service provider is responsible for the physical infrastructure and its security, whereas the institution is responsible for controlling access and implementation that is both secure and compliant. This latter responsibility can be split between the local IT and clinical bioinformatics teams as deemed appropriate. Many cloud services are advertised as HIPAA-eligible, which requires that the users using that service set it up with the appropriate settings to make it HIPAA-compliant.

When using cloud-based platforms for clinical data storage and/or processing, the institutions must involve appropriate legal counsel for the business associate agreements and other agreements, as well as IT personnel to ensure that the cloud-based solutions are in compliance with the institutional IT security policies [9,10]. Carter [9] provides a detailed review about genomic data privacy and security in cloud-based systems.

TABLE 1
Useful Projects with Packages and Tools for Bioinformatics for Robust Software Management

Name of Project	Programming Language or Technology	Comment
Bioconductor [13]	R	Large collection of packages useful for bioinformatics in R. A detailed review on the most useful packages and their functionality can be found [14].
Bioconda [11]	Language-agnostic	Repository within open-source package manager Conda that provides packaged scientific software focused on bioinformatics.
Biocontainers [15]	Docker and Singularity	Community-driven project with container images for packages from Conda and Bioconda.

layer on top of high-performance hardware. The most commonly used platforms for bioinformatics and informatics are Amazon's Amazon Web Services (AWS), Google's Cloud Platform (GCP), and Microsoft's Azure. The adoption of cloud computing for genomics first started in research laboratories but has gradually been expanding to clinical laboratories as well [17]. Special attention should be given to ensure that cloud systems are used in a secure and compliant manner (see Box 1).

According to the NIST [16], cloud-based systems use 3 main service models:

i. Software as a Service (SaaS): Software is hosted and runs in the cloud and the application is accessible to users through client devices.

ii. Platform as a Service (PaaS): The user deploys either a custom-developed or acquired software application onto the cloud. Examples include commercial companies such as DNANexus (https://www.dnanexus.com/), and Seven Bridges (https://www.sevenbridges.com/), Basespace (www.basespace.illumina.com/), and institute-based projects like Globus Genomics [18].

iii. Infrastructure as a Service (IaaS): The user can provision compute, storage, networks, and other resources and deploy software, OS, and applications, for example, Amazon Elastic Compute Cloud (Amazon EC2).

In each of these models, the user does not have access to the underlying cloud hardware and operating systems.

There are multiple ways to deploy a cloud-based infrastructure in a clinical laboratory [16]. The most popular method (see Fig. 1B) is

i. Private cloud, either on-premise (such as OpenStack [openstack.org] and OpenNebula [opennebula.org]) or Virtual private cloud in commercial public clouds. In such a case, the access settings for the cloud are restricted to the institution or specific laboratories at the institution.

Other ways to deploy the cloud, although not useful for clinical environments (no reports in literature) are the following:

ii. A community cloud provides limited access among multiple users across different organizations (good for data sharing), whereas

iii. A public cloud is open to the public. The latter is not a good option for a clinical environment.

iv. A fourth option is a hybrid cloud solution that allows for a combination of one or more of the preceding infrastructures, and can also contain a combination of on-premise and cloud solutions. For example, data storage in the cloud and computing on-premise.

DATA STORAGE

NGS data can be quite large, including intermediate files that are created at various points in the bioinformatics pipeline [1]. It is important for the clinical molecular laboratory to not only define data retention, compression, and archival policies for the raw and final processed files, but also for the intermediate files [3]. Similar to the computing infrastructure defined previously, storage can also be local, vendor-based, or cloud-based. It is also important to recognize the different needs of short-term storage (typically more expensive) for current test data, compared with longer-term storage systems (slower retrieval but cheaper). The appropriate features, such as redundancy and off-site backup location(s), as well as disaster recovery protocols, should be put into place. The protocols for moving specific NGS files to long-term storage should be specified in the laboratory's data retention policies [1,3].

DATA TRANSFER

One of the bottlenecks in the use of cloud services is speed of file transfer over the Internet. High-bandwidth fiberoptic based infrastructure can be adopted to allow faster speeds of up to 10 Gbps, but these are associated with higher costs [1]. However, whenever possible, investment in dedicated network resources, with appropriate security measures, will allow for uninterrupted and reliable data transfers, especially, if the laboratory plans to transfer large amounts of NGS data to the systems such as cloud storage over the Internet.

CONTAINER TECHNOLOGY

Bioinformatics software tools often have very complex and sometimes conflicting dependencies, causing issues with installations and updating software versions. A container is a lightweight, encapsulated unit of a software with all its dependencies, including the OS components required for execution. Containers are platform-agnostic, which in turn helps ensure reproducibility and providing an unprecedented level of isolation from the host system.

Docker (https://www.docker.com/) and Singularity [19] are the most popular container technologies, out of many. Adopting containers in bioinformatics pipeline development can ensure easy and reliable software deployment. Docker images require root privileges causing some security concerns for local systems and, thus, Singularity is more popular in HPC systems. This review does not discuss these technologies in detail; however, detailed reviews on these technologies can be found elsewhere [12,20]. Implementation of container-based virtualization systems require some experience and familiarity with command-line interface. Projects such as Biocontainers [15] and Dockstore [21] contain containerized bioinformatics tools and entire workflows respectively (see Box 5, Table 1). Efforts should be taken in selecting the right container images to use in one's clinical bioinformatics pipelines.

BIOINFORMATICS PIPELINE DESIGN AND IMPLEMENTATION FRAMEWORKS

A bioinformatics pipeline typically consists of primary, secondary, and tertiary analysis steps [1,2,22]. This workflow consists of several serial and parallel steps, each converting input files generated by another step into output file(s). This can be viewed as a directional acyclic graph (DAG) defining dependencies between the steps based on the order of the input and output file generation [23]. A simplified example of a generic variant calling pipeline as a DAG is shown in Fig. 2.

Depending on availability of resources and skilled personnel, institutions either use purchased software systems or implement pipelines based on best-practices [24], publications, or most often, establish customized workflows for the specific NGS test (Box 2). Table 1 shows a selected list of projects with collections of software packages with curated and good-quality software that can be used in bioinformatics pipelines (with and without containerization).

There is a variety of frameworks to choose from for any pipeline implementation, and these vary in their design philosophies [23]. The most popular frameworks have been outlined in sections that follow.

PRINCIPLES FOR ROBUST PIPELINE IMPLEMENTATION

As mentioned previously, AMP and CAP published standards and guidelines for validating clinical bioinformatics pipelines for NGS assays [3]. They made 17 best practice recommendations that guide readers through validation of bioinformatics pipelines, software tools, code as well as computing paradigms.

One of the most critical aspects of clinical bioinformatics pipeline validation is reproducibility, which essentially means that a pipeline should return the same results when run on the same data multiple times. Certain software use a random seed or have a heuristic algorithm, for example, BWA-MEM [25] and thus, a very small amount of variability in quantitative values should be permitted; however, the main results should not change. Box 3 lists some recommended good practices to improve clinical bioinformatics pipeline implementations.

NATIVE/BASIC PIPELINE FRAMEWORKS

The most basic pipeline frameworks are scripts written in Unix shell scripting languages, Perl and Python. These pipelines are the least robust due to the lack of dependency specifications (changes to an upstream task does not automatically update downstream steps) and reentrancy (restart the pipeline from the point of failure) [23]. Unless explicit logic has been implemented, a pipeline written in these native frameworks will have to be restarted from the beginning in case there is a failure at some point in the pipeline execution.

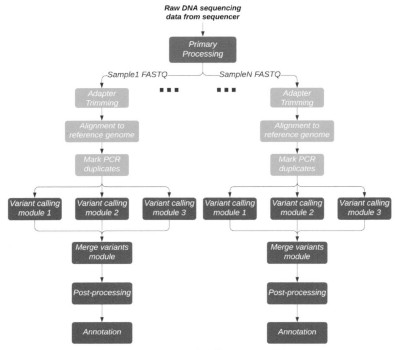

FIG. 2 A simplified example directed acyclic graph (DAG) representing a generic bioinformatics variant calling pipeline, showing parallel processing of N samples. The raw data from sequencing undergoes primary processing, converting the raw base calls and demultiplexing the read data to FASTQ files. Each Sample FASTQ file (or files in case of paired-end sequencing) undergoes processing using a modular pipeline with serial and some parallel steps.

A less popular programming language for clinical pipeline development is R, but there are options to build pipelines if needed such as systemPipeR [26], a package that provides a framework to design end-to-end analysis pipelines and reports. R is used widely for research purposes; however, the absence of certain common NGS data processing tools in R packages further requires interfaces to the OS for system calls to other tools. Thus, this language does not have the same widespread clinical use for NGS pipeline development as some other programming languages [14]. The common workflow languages (CWL) (https://www.commonwl.org/) is a shared platform in an effort to standardize workflow description languages and has

---

BOX 2
Bioinformatics Implementation Approaches

Clinical laboratories use a combination of in-house expertise, financial budgets, and functionality to determine the best option for bioinformatics implementation. Sometimes, a combination of options is integrated together to fill in for performance gaps.

1. End-to-end solution from a commercial vendor, implemented on-premise or in the cloud, often with the trade-off of limited flexibility and customization.

2. Implementation of a well-established best-practice pipeline, such as Genome Analysis Tool Kit [24].

3. Custom assembly of tools, both licensed and/or open source. The latter allows users to better understand the functions and limitations of the software, troubleshoot errors, and optimize parameters, if appropriate expertise is present.

BOX 3
Recommended Good Practices for Custom Clinical Bioinformatics Pipeline Development Based on Published Best Practices

1. *Microservice architecture:* A framework in which complex systems are divided into simplified easily managed constitutive units. This allows for optimization, easy maintenance, and testing of each unit individually, which in turn leads to higher reliability and stability [20]. Containers are a good framework to use to implement a microservice architecture.

2. *Version control:* Using version control systems, such as Github (https://github.com/), subversion (www.subversion. apache.org/), or bitbucket (www.bitbucket.org), can ensure reliable tracking of the pipeline changes. Versions also should be tracked for any resource files, for example, files representing the target regions of an NGS targeted assay or transcript versions for annotation.

3. *Unique version tags for production releases:* Assign a release version tag to each pipeline release in the version control system.

4. *Documentation:* Each pipeline and all of its releases should be accompanied with detailed documentation on changes and versions of each component software. Some guidelines for this are provided in Roy and colleagues [3]. Please note that for custom software, developer documentation should provide details on the tools design and intended use, whereas the user documentation should explain protocols for how to use the software, wherever applicable.

5. *Single pipeline command:* The pipeline should be designed such that it can be run in a single command instead of being split in multiple sub-pipelines, each invoked manually. This reduces the risk for error and also automates the process of execution.

6. *Error handling:* Wherever possible, the pipeline should be able to catch potential errors that might lead to termination of the pipeline, and/or allow for reentrancy, that is, restarting the pipeline from the failure instead of the beginning. This is not possible in all implementation frameworks, as discussed as follows.

7. *Common pipeline structure and usage:* If the laboratory runs multiple NGS tests, each with its own bioinformatics pipeline, trying to maintain a similar implementation design and usage will promote consistency between pipelines and make it easy to maintain them.

---

gained popularity in cancer genomics [21]. A package in R, called Rcwl allows users to write workflows using CWL in R.

MODERN WORKFLOW MANAGEMENT FRAMEWORKS

A major problem for building reproducible and portable clinical bioinformatics pipelines stems from the dependency of the implementation on the associated computing environment, which is most commonly on-premise servers or HPC clusters. This methodology is being challenged by recent advances in container technology and specialized workflow management systems that can be run efficiently on high-performance parallel systems [23]. Projects such as CWL (https://www.commonwl.org/), Nextflow [27], and Snakemake [28] provide portable and robust frameworks to implement complex pipelines (see later in this article).

The main principle of these systems lies in separation of the underlying physical infrastructure from the analysis workflow/pipeline. This is important because dependencies between the computing environment and software installations hinder portability. This can allow for sharing of clinical bioinformatics pipelines, standardization efforts, and portability of pipelines between test and production environments and computing infrastructure. Any changes to the pipeline or infrastructure still require appropriate validation but these technologies make it easier. *Choice of a workflow framework should be determined by its performance, scalability capabilities and design philosophy, based on the demands of the pipeline as well as the users of the pipeline.*

Box 4 lists selected popular workflow frameworks for clinical pipeline development, with a few of them discussed in detail in sections that follow. An exhaustive list of workflow frameworks can be found at https://github.com/pditommaso/awesome-pipeline.

DOMAIN SPECIFIC LANGUAGE SYSTEMS: NEXTFLOW AND SNAKEMAKE

Nextflow [27] and Snakemake [28] both infer the dependency tree of the pipeline modules using the specified input and output requirements, without any requirement to explicitly specify the task dependencies. These systems have developed independently but in parallel around the same time and are becoming

---

BOX 4
Popular Modern Workflow Frameworks for Bioinformatics Pipeline Implementation

As described in some detail [23], workflow frameworks can either

i. infer the dependencies between tasks from input and output specifications, for example, Nextflow [27] and Snakemake [28] (see later in this article), or

ii. explicitly declare dependencies between the tasks, somewhat similar to scripting such as Queue and Toil (https://github.com/bd2kgenomics/toil).

Another class of frameworks are platforms (PaaS) that are

i. open-source such as Galaxy [29] and

ii. commercial cloud-based platforms such as DNANexus and SevenBridges.

---

increasingly popular for writing bioinformatics workflows because they allow the development of reproducible and portable workflows. They provide detailed documentation along with pipeline templates and guidelines for developers. These systems have integrated support for container such as Docker and Singularity.

Nextflow is the more mature of the two because of its built-in support for package managers, such as Conda, Kubernetes, and most common HPC schedulers, as well as cloud platforms such as AWS and Google Cloud. A comparison between Nextflow and Snakemake is provided in Table 2. More details can be found in Di Tommaso and colleagues [27], with more up-to-date information on the individual system Web sites. Different bioinformatics tools have different requirements, such that some might require a higher number of processing cores and memory, whereas others might require fewer cores and more or less memory. Using a microservicelike architecture and optimizing the workflow to execute modules with similar computing and memory requirements on appropriate cloud instances can allow for a workflow with optimized resource utilization.

Two community-based projects for bioinformatics pipelines written in Nextflow (nf-core [30]) and Snakemake (https://github.com/snakemake-workflows) domain-specific language (DSL) exist (Box 5). These can be used as frameworks and templates to build on

---

TABLE 2
Comparison Between Snakemake and Nextflow

Feature	Nextflow	Snakemake
Code syntax	Less human-readable	Simpler and more human-readable
Modularization	Modular implementation is undergoing beta testing (https://www.nextflow.io/blog/2019/one-more-step-towards-modules.html)	Modularization functionality is native
Technology/Programming language of framework implementation	Groovy/Java virtual machine	Python
Built-in integration with Conda	Yes	Yes
Built-in integration with container technology	Docker and Singularity	Singularity
Execution in the cloud	Built-in support for AWS and Google Cloud	Yes, through Kubernetes

---

BOX 5
Community-Based Projects of Bioinformatics Pipelines

There are numerous example customizable pipeline implementations and templates for the user.

nf-core [30]: Community-based project of bioinformatics pipelines written in Nextflow [27]. These pipelines have a defined set of guidelines for developers to create, test, and synchronize bioinformatics pipelines.

Snakemake [28] *workflows* (https://github.com/snakemake-workflows): Github repository of community-based bioinformatics pipelines written in Snakemake.

Dockstore [21]: Platform developed by the Cancer Genome Collaboratory and used by the Global Alliance for Genomics & Health (GA4GH) (https://www.ga4gh.org) to share Docker-based tools described using CWL, WDL, or Nextflow.

Galaxy [29] (https://galaxyproject.org/): Makes tools accessible for researchers or tool testing but not appropriate for a clinical production environment.

These are not clinical pipelines but provide example frameworks on which to build pipelines.

and write clinical pipelines, although they require the same amount of thorough validation and testing as any other pipeline implementation.

One of the main advantages of using a DSL such as Nextflow is portability. Workflows written in Nextflow DSL are highly portable, and thus can be run in different computing environments such as HPC or Cloud with no changes to the main workflow. It is important to state that changing the computing environment still requires clinical validation but the workflow itself remains the same.

COMMERCIAL PLATFORMS: DNANexus AND SevenBridges

This class of frameworks is popular among clinical groups with limited software development expertise, especially in the cloud. They provide intuitive graphical interfaces to build the pipelines, typically using drag-and-drop functionality. These platforms (PaaS) use underlying cloud provider resources to execute the pipeline implementations. There is a trade-off between flexibility and ease of development versus accessibility and speed. Laboratories must consider "return on investment" while considering these options [23].

TERTIARY ANALYSIS SYSTEMS

Tertiary analysis is the process of clinical interpretation and reporting using the results from the secondary analysis of the pipeline [22]. This typically consists of variant annotation, filtration, prioritization, and interpretation. This step requires special mention because as NGS assays increase in size, many laboratories use independent systems to perform this step, either from a

commercial vendor [1] or built in-house [31] or a combination of both based on the needs of the laboratory. The main features in a such a system should include Human Genome Variation Society (HGVS; https://varnomen.hgvs.org/) nomenclature, functional effects, integration of data from variant databases such as ClinVar [32] and population databases such as gnomAD [33], and a user-friendly interface for variant filtration and prioritization [2,3,22]. But it is important to note that similar considerations as those mentioned under Infrastructure apply to these systems along with integration challenges (see the following section). Many health care institutions have adopted tertiary analysis software that runs in the cloud (SaaS), and typically accessed using a Web browser. This prevents any local installations or maintenance.

INTEROPERABILITY AND DATA INTEGRATION WITH CLINICAL INFORMATICS

As discussed previously, clinical laboratories performing testing using NGS require high-throughput computing infrastructure and advanced bioinformatics implementations. In many cases, institutions try to keep up with the pace of NGS test advancements and make short-term decisions to satisfy their infrastructure needs. Unfortunately, this can lead to a disconnect between the clinical informatics and bioinformatics infrastructures at many institutions, causing scalability and data integration issues.

An informatics system is ideally supposed to capture the flow of data in the laboratory from test order and specimen tracking to NGS results and reporting to the electronic health records (EHR) system. Detailed architectural discussion is out of scope for this review but it is important to acknowledge the increasing need to integrate bioinformatics workflows with informatics systems to avoid fragmented processes with manual components leading to potential errors.

Similar to bioinformatics solutions, there is a large variety in laboratory information management systems (LIMS). Some institutions develop in-house LIMS systems [31] and others might purchase plug-and-play commercial systems, either implemented on-premise or adopted as a cloud-based solution [1]. An important CAP checklist item also requires every clinical laboratory to maintain a variant database.

Due to the diversity in the number of software and tests provided by a molecular pathology laboratory, it is common that the laboratory might have multiple informatics systems and tools. Bioinformatics pipelines are not run in isolation and computational infrastructure requires integration with other systems. For example, a laboratory might have 1 or more of the following.

  i. Tools with graphical interfaces for interpretation, for example, copy number analysis or tertiary analysis software
 ii. Command-line Linux system for bioinformatics pipelines
iii. Laboratory information management system
 iv. EHR system
  v. Downstream research data warehouse that collates genotype and phenotype data to create biomedical resources for research, and so forth

Interoperability refers to the communication and data exchange across these various systems [1], such as health level 7 messaging between the LIMS and EHR systems. Although one might want seamless integration between these various systems, it is not always possible due to interface, network, or data format issues.

Wherever possible, it might be helpful to evaluate the interoperability capabilities of a platform, software, or system before on-boarding into an established data workflow in a clinical laboratory.

DISCUSSION

Advances in NGS assays for molecular pathology have led to the need for high-performance infrastructure, complex software installations, and orchestration to build clinical bioinformatics pipelines. Even if commercial vendor solutions are adopted, there is a need for bioinformatics validation, security and privacy considerations, and interoperability across multiple laboratory systems [3]. A wide range of on-premise and

cloud-based systems are available for laboratories; however, the latter provides significant scalability advantages. *Successful implementation and maintenance of modern clinical NGS bioinformatics pipelines depends both on appropriate and scalable computational infrastructure and clinical staff with technical bioinformatics knowledge.*

While creating custom workflows, bioinformatics developers must pay attention to unintentional effects on their pipelines during hardware and/or software updates. For example, updates made to one software package or tool might inadvertently affect another software or tool due to complex dependency chains. Special care must be taken to separate development and production environments and any updates made to even a single software must be thoroughly validated in the context of the entire pipeline.

Using a combination of advanced technologies and practices like (i) containerization and virtualization technology in a (ii) microservice-like architecture using (iii) workflow management systems that automatically orchestrate the pipeline components, will not only increase the reliability and reproducibility of bioinformatics pipelines but also provide computational robustness to clinical NGS testing. However, these are more common in research than clinical environments at this time. Adoption of good programming practices and attention to scalability, security, and privacy measures will increase the robustness of clinical bioinformatics pipelines over time, thus improving the quality of clinical service as well.

DISCLOSURE

The author has nothing to disclose.

REFERENCES

[1] Roy S, LaFramboise WA, Nikiforov YE, et al. Next-generation sequencing informatics: challenges and strategies for implementation in a clinical environment. Arch Pathol Lab Med 2016;140(9):958–75.

[2] Oliver GR, Hart SN, Klee EW. Bioinformatics for clinical next generation sequencing. Clin Chem 2015;61(1): 124–35.

[3] Roy S, Coldren C, Karunamurthy A, et al. Standards and guidelines for validating next-generation sequencing bioinformatics pipelines: a joint recommendation of the Association for Molecular Pathology and the College of American Pathologists. J Mol Diagn 2018;20(1):4–27.

[4] Pabinger S, Dander A, Fischer M, et al. A survey of tools for variant analysis of next-generation genome sequencing data. Brief Bioinformatics 2014;15(2): 256–78.

[5] SoRelle JA, Wachsmann M, Cantarel BL. Assembling and validating bioinformatic pipelines for next-generation sequencing clinical assays. Arch Pathol Lab Med 2020. https://doi.org/10.5858/arpa.2019-0476-RA.

[6] Santani A, Simen BB, Briggs M, et al. Designing and implementing NGS tests for inherited disorders: a practical framework with step-by-step guidance for clinical laboratories. J Mol Diagn 2019;21(3):369–74.

[7] Cucoranu IC, Parwani AV, West AJ, et al. Privacy and security of patient data in the pathology laboratory. J Pathol Inform 2013;4(1):4.

[8] Dove ES, Joly Y, Tassé A-M, et al. Genomic cloud computing: legal and ethical points to consider. Eur J Hum Genet 2015;23(10):1271–8.

[9] Carter AB. Considerations for genomic data privacy and security when working in the cloud. J Mol Diagn 2019; 21(4):542–52.

[10] Datta S, Bettinger K, Snyder M. Secure cloud computing for genomic data. Nat Biotechnol 2016;34(6):588–91.

[11] Grüning B, Dale R, Sjödin A, et al. Bioconda: sustainable and comprehensive software distribution for the life sciences. Nat Methods 2018;15(7):475–6.

[12] Grüning B, Chilton J, Köster J, et al. Practical computational reproducibility in the life sciences. Cell Syst 2018;6(6):631–5.

[13] Huber W, Carey VJ, Gentleman R, et al. Orchestrating high-throughput genomic analysis with Bioconductor. Nat Methods 2015;12(2):115–21.

[14] Sepulveda JL. Using R and bioconductor in clinical genomics and transcriptomics. J Mol Diagn 2020;22(1):3–20.

[15] da Veiga Leprevost F, Grüning BA, Alves Aflitos S, et al. BioContainers: an open-source and community-driven framework for software standardization. Bioinformatics 2017;33(16):2580–2.

[16] Mell P, Grance T. The NIST Definition of Cloud Computing. 7. Available at: https://csrc.nist.gov/publications/detail/sp/800-145/final.

[17] Charlebois K, Palmour N, Knoppers BM. The adoption of cloud computing in the field of genomics research: the influence of ethical and legal issues. PLoS One 2016; 11(10):e0164347.

[18] Madduri RK, Sulakhe D, Lacinski L, et al. Experiences building globus genomics: a next-generation sequencing analysis service using Galaxy, Globus, and Amazon Web services. Concurr Comput 2014;26(13):2266–79.

[19] Kurtzer GM, Sochat V, Bauer MW. Singularity: scientific containers for mobility of compute. PLoS One 2017; 12(5):e0177459.

[20] Williams CL, Sica JC, Killen RT, et al. The growing need for microservices in bioinformatics. J Pathol Inform 2016;7:45.

[21] O'Connor BD, Yuen D, Chung V, et al. The Dockstore: enabling modular, community-focused sharing of Docker-based genomics tools and workflows. F1000Res 2017;6:52.

[22] Lebo MS, Hao L, Lin C-F, et al. Bioinformatics in clinical genomic sequencing. Clin Lab Med 2018;1(1):9–26.

[23] Leipzig J. A review of bioinformatic pipeline frameworks. Brief Bioinformatics 2017;18(3):530–6.

[24] Poplin R, Ruano-Rubio V, DePristo MA, et al. Scaling accurate genetic variant discovery to tens of thousands of samples. bioRxiv 2017;14:201178.

[25] Li H, Durbin R. Fast and accurate short read alignment with Burrows-Wheeler transform. Bioinformatics 2009; 25(14):1754–60.

[26] Backman TWH, Girke T. systemPipeR: NGS workflow and report generation environment. BMC Bioinformatics 2016;17(1):388.

[27] Di Tommaso P, Chatzou M, Floden EW, et al. Nextflow enables reproducible computational workflows. Nat Biotechnol 2017;35(4):316–9.

[28] Köster J, Rahmann S. Snakemake—a scalable bioinformatics workflow engine. Bioinformatics 2012;28(19): 2520–2.

[29] Afgan E, Baker D, Batut B, et al. The Galaxy platform for accessible, reproducible and collaborative biomedical analyses: 2018 update. Nucleic Acids Res 2018;46(W1): W537–44.

[30] Ewels PA, Peltzer A, Fillinger S, et al. The nf-core framework for community-curated bioinformatics pipelines. Nat Biotechnol 2020;38(3):276–8.

[31] Kang W, Kadri S, Puranik R, et al. System for informatics in the molecular pathology laboratory: an open-source end-to-end solution for next-generation sequencing clinical data management. J Mol Diagn 2018;20(4):522–32.

[32] Landrum MJ, Lee JM, Benson M, et al. ClinVar: improving access to variant interpretations and supporting evidence. Nucleic Acids Res 2018;46(D1):D1062–7.

[33] Karczewski KJ, Francioli LC, Tiao G, et al. The mutational constraint spectrum quantified from variation in 141,456 humans. Nature 2020;581(7809):434–43.

Solid Tumors

Advances in Molecular Pathology 3 (2020) 169–188

ADVANCES IN MOLECULAR PATHOLOGY

Microsatellite Instability Testing and Therapy Implications

David B. Chapel, MD[a], Lauren L. Ritterhouse, MD, PhD[b],*

[a]Division of Women's and Perinatal Pathology, Department of Pathology, Brigham and Women's Hospital, Amory 3, 75 Francis Street, Boston, MA 02115, USA; [b]Department of Pathology, Center for Integrated Diagnostics, Harvard Medical School, Massachusetts General Hospital, Jackson Building, Suite 1015, 55 Fruit Street, Boston, MA 02114, USA

KEYWORDS
- Cancer • Immunotherapy • Immune checkpoint inhibitor • Microsatellite instability • Mismatch repair
- Lynch syndrome • Familial cancer syndromes • Next-generation sequencing

KEY POINTS
- Frameshift mutations in coding microsatellites are under strong selective pressure in both treatment-naive and treated tumors.
- Immunohistochemistry and polymerase chain reaction–based assays remain the tests of choice for Lynch syndrome screening.
- Next-generation sequencing can be used to detect, quantify, and profile tumor microsatellite instability.

INTRODUCTION

Microsatellite instability (MSI) is found in 1.5% to 3.5% of all human cancers, and it plays a central role in tumor biology and clinical management. Some tumors with MSI are secondary to Lynch syndrome. Immunohistochemistry (IHC) and the polymerase chain reaction (PCR)–based sizing assays have been the standard methods for detecting MSI for more than 2 decades. However, a variety of robust next-generation sequencing (NGS)–based methods for detecting, quantifying, and profiling tumor MSI are now available. The precise role for each of these assays is evolving, because detection of MSI continues to play a central role in LS screening, as well as having a new and growing role in predicting tumor responsiveness to immunotherapy.

This article begins with a brief review of mismatch repair (MMR) biology, followed by a detailed comparison of methods for detecting MSI, emphasizing novel NGS-based techniques. The article concludes with a discussion of the clinical applications of these tests, as well as a brief discussion of areas of continued uncertainty and ongoing investigation.

CLINICAL BIOLOGY OF DNA MISMATCH REPAIR DEFICIENCY AND MICROSATELLITE INSTABILITY

The human genome contains more than 19 million microsatellites; short tandem repeats of motifs of 1 to 6 nucleotides, typically spanning 10 to 60 nucleotides in total length [1]. Slippage of DNA polymerase can alter microsatellite length, but DNA MMR mechanisms normally correct these errors, and microsatellites generally show low somatic mutation rates within individuals. In contrast, accumulated replication errors over a generational timescale yield considerable population-level variability in microsatellite length. As a result,

---

*Corresponding author, *E-mail address:* LRitterhouse@partners.org

https://doi.org/10.1016/j.yamp.2020.07.019
2589-4080/20/

certain polymorphic microsatellites can serve as an individual's molecular barcode, which can be used in forensic identification, paternity testing, and diagnostic classification of products of conception.

DNA MMR proteins form active heterodimers to repair single nucleotide variants and short insertions and deletions (indels), including indels that alter microsatellite length [2–4]. The main MMR dimers, comprising the 4 main MMR proteins, are MLH1-PMS2 and MSH2-MSH6. In approximately 1.5% to 3.5% of all human cancers, deleterious germline or somatic alterations in MMR genes lead to functional loss of 1 or more MMR proteins, termed MMR deficiency (dMMR) [1,5–9]. dMMR, in turn, produces MSI, a molecular phenotype characterized by increased genome-wide variation in microsatellite length. It should be emphasized that dMMR and MSI are intimately linked but distinct concepts: dMMR refers to functional loss of 1 or more MMR proteins, whereas MSI develops over time through accumulation of unrepaired DNA replication errors [6,10,11]. dMMR and MSI are most frequently seen in endometrial, colorectal, small bowel, and gastric adenocarcinomas but is also detected at low frequency in many other tumor types [1,5,6,9,12,13] (Fig. 1).

TESTING FOR MISMATCH REPAIR DEFICIENCY AND MICROSATELLITE INSTABILITY

IHC for MMR proteins is the most practical test for dMMR, whereas PCR-based amplification of small microsatellite panels is the most widely available method for detecting MSI directly. In recent years, NGS-based algorithms for direct detection and quantification of MSI have been developed and increasingly refined. These methods, including their advantages, shortcomings, and clinical applications, are discussed in this article.

Polymerase Chain Reaction-Based Microsatellite Instability Testing

In 1997, Dietmaier and colleagues [14] profiled 31 microsatellite loci, creating the first standardized PCR-based MSI panel using 5 microsatellites that accurately segregated 200 colorectal carcinomas with and without MSI [15]. The following year, a National Cancer Institute working group adopted a modified microsatellite panel (termed the Bethesda panel), which included 2 poly-A homopolymers (BAT-25, BAT-26) and 3 dinucleotide repeats (D5S346, D2S123, D17S250) [16]. Microsatellite panels composed only of mononucleotide

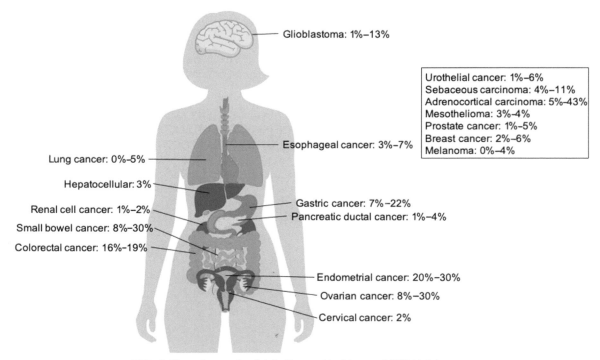

Glioblastoma: 1%–13%

Urothelial cancer: 1%–6%
Sebaceous carcinoma: 4%–11%
Adrenocortical carcinoma: 5%–43%
Mesothelioma: 3%–4%
Prostate cancer: 1%–5%
Breast cancer: 2%–6%
Melanoma: 0%–4%

Esophageal cancer: 3%–7%

Lung cancer: 0%–5%

Hepatocellular: 3%

Renal cell cancer: 1%–2%

Small bowel cancer: 8%–30%

Colorectal cancer: 16%–19%

Gastric cancer: 7%–22%
Pancreatic ductal cancer: 1%–4%

Endometrial cancer: 20%–30%

Ovarian cancer: 8%–30%

Cervical cancer: 2%

FIG. 1 The primary site distribution and incidence of MSI-high tumors.

loci (eg, poly-A homopolymers BAT-25, BAT-26, NR-21, NR-24, NR-27/MONO-27) are now preferred, because mononucleotides offer greater sensitivity than dinucleotides for detecting MSI-high (MSI-H) tumors [1,17]. One commercially available 7-locus panel from Promega (Madison, WI) includes 5 mononucleotides for MSI testing and 2 pentanucleotides for patient identification (ie, to prevent sample swap errors), and is currently seeking companion diagnostic status for pembrolizumab [18].

Classification of microsatellite instability

In PCR-based MSI testing, the targeted microsatellites are amplified from both tumor and matched normal tissue (ie, from the patient). The tumor and matched normal amplicons from each locus are then separated by capillary electrophoresis and assessed for fragment size via electropherograms, and a locus is considered unstable if the length and distribution of the tumor microsatellite differs (on qualitative analysis) from the

normal tissue (Fig. 2). After each microsatellite locus is assessed individually, the tumor is assigned an MSI status, using the following schema:

1. MSI-H: greater than or equal to 40% of loci unstable
2. MSI-low (MSI-L): greater than 0 but less than 40% of loci unstable
3. Microsatellite stable (MSS): 0 loci unstable

Test performance. PCR-based MSI testing shows good concordance (96%–99%) with other molecular-based tests, including NGS-based MSI testing [5,8,9,13,19]. PCR-based testing has been reported as 66.7% to 100% sensitive for detecting MSI-H status in LS-associated colorectal carcinoma [20–22], with higher sensitivity for MSI-H LS-associated tumors with *MLH1* or *MSH2* mutation (91%) than with *MSH6* or *PMS2* mutation (77%), because of smaller microsatellite shifts in *MSH6* or *PMS2* mutation [6]. Variable sensitivity across studies is likely also

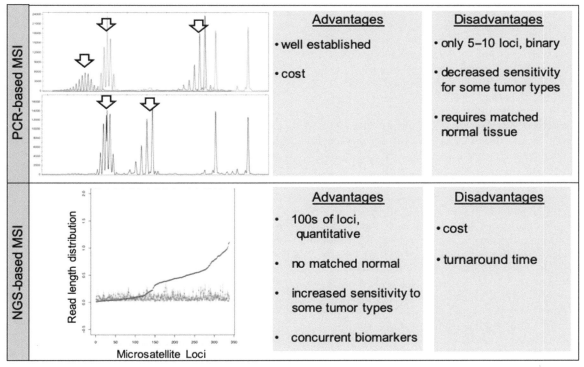

FIG. 2 PCR-based and NGS-based MSI calling. PCR-based (*top*) fragment size analysis via electropherograms with arrows highlighting the 5 microsatellite loci that are assessed for length and distribution. NGS-based (*bottom*) analysis evaluating read length distribution across hundreds of microsatellite loci.

attributable, at least in part, to variability in diagnostic methods [20].

Because microsatellite panels for PCR-based MSI testing were designed for screening in colorectal carcinoma, they can give false-negative results in other tumor types, with 1 study showing approximately 82% and 75% sensitivity for MSI-H status in prostatic and endometrial carcinoma, respectively [14,23]. PCR-based assays have decreased sensitivity in MSH6-deficient tumors (including a substantial proportion of endometrial carcinomas) because of subtle peak shifts, which are more difficult to spot on electropherogram analysis (see Fig. 2) [24–26].

These false-negative errors stem from tumor type–specific differences in genome-wide MSI profiles, which could be overcome by using more comprehensive microsatellite panels. Whole-exome and whole-genome studies have shown that certain microsatellites are highly informative with significant discriminatory capacity between MSS and MSI-H tumors, whereas some 57% of microsatellites seem virtually impervious to alterations, even in dMMR tumors [13]. Some highly informative microsatellites are specific to a particular tumor type [13,27], whereas others are highly informative across all tumor types (ie, pan-cancer loci) [1]. These highly informative microsatellites (which can be intronic or intergenic) could provide the basis for more accurate tumor type–specific or pan-cancer microsatellite panels, which could be designed for either PCR-based or NGS-based MSI testing.

Caveats. A 3-tier scoring system for PCR-based MSI testing was introduced in early studies to account for clinical abnormalities that seemed to be specific to the MSI-L group [14]. However, this system was based on few cases with technical constraints on the number of tested loci, and quantitative whole-genome sequencing–based analysis of thousands of microsatellites in many tumor types has shown that MSI is a continuously distributed variable, rather than 3 discrete molecular phenotypes [1,11,13,27,28]. Moreover, 1 large study showed no difference in the number of unstable microsatellites between tumors called MSI-L versus MSS by PCR-based testing [13]. At present, a 2-tier system (ie, MSI-H vs MSS) seems most clinically applicable, and recent recommendations are to group MSI-L with MSS tumors when using PCR-based MSI testing [12,17]. However, some studies have shown that at least a subset of MSI-L tumors (and even some MSS tumors) represent capture of recently acquired dMMR, which would presumably progress to MSI-H over time [10,11,13].

As detailed later, NGS-based panels generally capture hundreds to thousands of microsatellites. In consequence, compared with a 5-locus PCR-based panel, NGS-based MSI algorithms have higher resolution for quantifying tumor MSI, and could be used to further subdivide MSI-H tumors. Recent data indicate that, among tumors called MSI-H by such quantitative NGS-based methods, tumors with quantitatively greater MSI show better immunotherapy response than tumors with less MSI [11], suggesting that modifications in our system of tumor MSI classification may ultimately be clinically useful.

Immunohistochemistry for mismatch repair proteins

Strong correlation between dMMR status as determined by IHC and MSI as determined by molecular testing was well known by the time of the first standardized panels for PCR-based MSI testing [14,29,30]. MMR IHC is a widely available and cost-effective test for underlying MSI [31], and MMR gene alterations yield reproducible MMR IHC patterns (Fig. 3). Namely, because PMS2 and MSH6 dimerize only with MLH1 and MSH2, respectively, loss of MLH1 or MSH2 also leads to PMS2 or MSH6 loss. In contrast, MLH1 and MSH2 can also pair with other minor MMR proteins (eg, MSH3, MLH3, PMS1), so loss of PMS2 or MSH6 does not result in MLH1 or MSH2 loss [32].

Test performance

MMR IHC shows 88.5% to 99% sensitivity and 95.2% to 99.6% specificity for detecting MSI-H status (using PCR as a reference standard) [6,33–38] and approximately 80% to 91% sensitivity for detecting dMMR status in LS-associated colorectal and endometrial cancers [22,34,35]. Sensitivity and specificity seem equal in biopsy and resection material [12,39,40].

False-negative MMR IHC can result from missense mutations that impair function without altering protein localization or antigenicity, from mutations in minor MMR proteins (eg, MLH3, MSH3, PMS1), and from heterogeneous MMR IHC patterns resulting from subclonal mutations and epimutations [41,42]. Tellingly, tumors with false-negative MMR IHC results (ie, MSI-H by PCR but MMR proficient by IHC) do not show a quantitative difference in unstable microsatellites compared with true-positive tumors (ie, MSI-H, dMMR) [36].

False-positive MMR IHC can result from aberrant immunostaining patterns, including punctate or stippled nuclear staining and paranuclear staining, which should be regarded as dMMR [12]. Diagnostic misinterpretation more generally also leads to false-positive

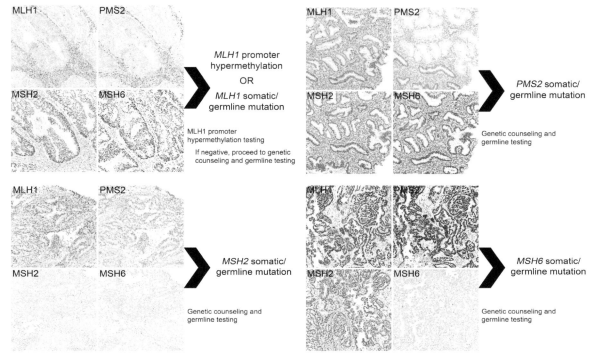

FIG. 3 MMR IHC patterns. Loss of both MLH1 and PMS2 (*top left*) indicates *MLH1* promoter hypermethylation or an *MLH1* somatic/germline mutation. Loss of both MSH2 and MSH6 (*bottom left*) indicates a *MSH2* somatic/germline mutation. Loss of PMS2 alone (*top right*) indicates a *PMS2* somatic/germline mutation. Loss of MSH6 alone (*bottom right*) indicates a *MSH6* somatic/germline mutation. Immunostains with diaminobenzidine chromogen. Original magnification, 100x.

MMR IHC, occurring in up to 10% of cases [43,44] (although 1 recent study showed excellent agreement between pathologists in MMR IHC interpretation, suggesting that MMR IHC interpretation improves with increased experience [45]). In cases with ambiguous or focal staining, confirmatory testing (ie, IHC on a second tissue block or PCR-based MSI testing) is advised, because such cases have a considerable risk of subsequent LS diagnosis [46].

Caveats. MMR heterodimer biology and some data suggest that a 2-marker PMS2 and MSH6 immunopanel offers sensitivity and specificity equal to the classic 4-marker immunopanel [47,48], although 1 recent study found that the 2-marker panel missed more than half of patients with LS with germline *MSH2* mutation [49]. The 4-marker immunopanel is currently preferred, where feasible [12].

Comparisons with polymerase chain reaction–based microsatellite instability testing. MMR IHC and PCR-based MSI testing both detect cases of

dMMR that the other assay would miss [42]. For instance, MMR IHC may detect MSH6-deficient tumors with low-level allelic shifts potentially missed by PCR-based testing. Nonetheless, at present, molecular-based MSI testing seems to have higher sensitivity and specificity than MMR IHC and is generally considered the gold standard [12,38]. However, MMR IHC is currently more widely available at a lower cost, and, unlike PCR-based testing, MMR IHC does not require matched normal patient tissue.

Some data suggest that dual MMR IHC and PCR-based MSI testing on all colorectal cancers would be a cost-effective approach [21], and 1 consensus panel recommended dual IHC and PCR-based testing on all tumors before initiation of immunotherapy, given the cost and potential side effects of such treatment (discussed later) [12].

Next-Generation Sequencing–Based Microsatellite Instability Detection

NGS is a powerful and versatile tool, scalable from small targeted panels to whole-genome sequencing, and many targeted NGS-based cancer gene panels now incorporate MSI calling [50,51]. Table 1 summarizes key details and performance characteristics for NGS-based MSI-calling methods. Table 2 details several large NGS-based studies of tumor MSI.

Unlike MMR IHC and PCR-based MSI testing, which essentially provide a binary positive or negative result, many NGS-based MSI-calling algorithms provide a quantitative tumor MSI score. This quantitative score is then converted to a clinical MSI status using thresholds obtained through cross-validation against IHC or PCR. However, because an NGS-based MSI score is a continuous variable, it could be broken into as many groups as prove clinically relevant. At present, most investigators cluster tumors into 3 groups: MSI-H, MSI-intermediate (MSI-I), and MSS. Importantly, although MSI-I occupies the same relative position as the MSI-L designation used in PCR-based testing, MSI-I is best viewed as an indeterminate or uncertain category, and there are conflicting data on its significance:

- Some data indicate that MSI-I might represent a biologically intermediate state between onset of dMMR at the level of protein function and accumulation of sufficient genomic MSI events to meet criteria for MSI-H [10,11,37].
- In contrast, 1 large study found that 97% of MSI-I tumors (by NGS) were called MSS by PCR [8], although this cohort was enriched for high-stage and recurrent tumors.
- Noncanonical (ie, neither colorectal nor endometrial) LS-associated tumors are frequently MSI-I [6], suggesting the need for tumor type–specific thresholds for assigning MSI status, more diverse tumor cohorts for method validation and threshold setting, or a combination of these 2.
- Recent data from colorectal carcinoma and melanoma cell lines with *MSH2* knockout suggest that dMMR tumors called MSI-I by NGS may show little or no response to programmed cell death protein 1 (PD-1) blockade [11].

Additional investigation of the significance of the MSI-I classification is needed.

Early next-generation sequencing–based tests for microsatellite instability

The first NGS-based test for MSI detection, Coloseq (2012), detected mutations in 6 MMR-related genes (as well as *APC*) to impute a defect in the MMR machinery, rather than sequencing microsatellites themselves [52]. In contrast, MSIseq (2012) interrogated microsatellites directly, comparing indels in 506,000 transcriptome-wide microsatellites between tumor cells and a reference genome using RNA sequencing data [28].

Read-length distribution–based algorithms

Multiple robust and versatile NGS-based MSI algorithms are based on the premise that dMMR increases the number and variance of discrete allelic lengths in tumor DNA compared with normal tissue, where functional MMR holds microsatellite lengths stable [27,53–57]. The first so-called read-length distribution–based MSI algorithms were mSINGS (2014) [53] and MSIsensor (2014) [54], which (in their original and modified forms) remain in widespread use, including in the FDA-cleared MSK-IMPACT platform [6,8]. In presenting MANTIS (2017), a third read-length distribution–based algorithm, Kautto and colleagues [55] ran mSINGS, MSIsensor, and MANTIS on the same tumor cohort and found that MANTIS provided more accurate calling MSI across a wide range of analyzed loci. Rather than separately evaluating each locus as stable or unstable (as do mSINGS and MSIsensor), MANTIS assigns a continuous instability score at each locus, which are averaged to give an aggregate tumor instability score, which more closely reflects the continuous nature of tumor MSI and improves sensitivity in tumors with low-level shifts or poor-quality reads [55]. MANTIS was also more computationally efficient than mSINGS and MSIsensor, requiring less space, memory, and run time required by mSINGS [55]. This head-to-head-to-head comparison highlights the advances in NGS-based MSI calling in the span of a few years.

Test performance. Read-length distribution–based algorithms generally show excellent (>95%) sensitivity and specificity for MSI-H detection (see Table 1), and good concordance with MMR IHC and PCR-based testing. For example, in 1 cohort, MSIsensor missed approximately 4% of MSI-H calls made by PCR and 13% of dMMR calls made by IHC [8]. However, using MMR IHC or PCR-based testing as a reference standard for performance of NGS-based assays is imperfect, because both IHC and PCR can give both false-positive and false-negative results (discussed earlier), and require more subjective interpretation than NGS. Some large NGS-based studies have more closely analyzed tumors with discordant NGS-based and PCR-based MSI calls and concluded that the NGS-based MSI status is more reliable in most cases [9,13].

Caveats. mSINGS was the first read-length distribution–based algorithm originally validated to

TABLE 1
Characteristics of Next-Generation Sequencing–Based Microsatellite Instability Calling Methods

MSI-Calling Methodology	Testing Method	Performance	Advantages	Disadvantages
MMR mutation detection	Pritchard et al [52], 2012 (Coloseq)	• Sensitivity: 99.4% • Specificity: 99.4% (for detection of targeted mutations)	—	• Provides no direct information about microsatellite instability or specific microsatellites • Limited gene panel
Microsatellite indel profiling	Lu [28], 2013 (MSIseq)	• A microsatellite insertion/deletion ratio of 0.9 accurately separated 14 MSI from 14 MSS CRC	• Compares tumor microsatellite indels with a reference transcriptome, obviating matched normal patient material	• Requires RNAseq-based transcriptome data
Read-length distribution	Salipante et al [53], 2014 (mSINGS)	• Sensitivity: 76.1% • Specificity: 98.8% • Optimal threshold for calling MSI-H: 10%	• Versatile algorithm that can be applied across NGS platforms • Performs optimally with few (~40) highly informative loci and a high threshold for MSI-H	• Developed on a CRC cohort (53% sensitivity for MSI-H endometrial cancer in 1 study) • May perform less well when using many (100s–1000s) loci
	Niu et al [54], 2014 (MSIsensor)	• Sensitivity: 96.5% • Specificity: 99.7% • Optimal threshold for calling MSI-H: 3.5%	• Versatile algorithm that can be applied across NGS platforms • Performs optimally with many (100s–1000s) highly informative loci and a low threshold for MSI-H	• May perform less well when using few (eg, <50) loci
	Kautto et al [55], 2017 (MANTIS)	• Sensitivity: 97.2% • Specificity: 99.7% • Optimal threshold for calling MSI-H: 0.4	• Versatile algorithm that can be applied across NGS platforms • Accurate MSI calling in panels with variable numbers of microsatellite loci • Energy-efficient and time-efficient computational algorithm	—
Read-length distribution + analysis of 1 highly informative microsatellite	Hause et al [13], 2016 (MOSAIC)	• Sensitivity: 95.8% • Specificity: 97.6%	• Accurate whole-exome–based algorithm validated across a wide variety of tumor types	• DEFB105A/B locus may not be captured in all NGS panels

(continued on next page)

TABLE 1
(continued)

MSI-Calling Methodology	Testing Method	Performance	Advantages	Disadvantages
Read-length distribution + mutational hotspot analysis	Hempelmann et al [56], 2015 (MSIplus)	• Sensitivity: 97.1% • Specificity: ~100%	• Amplicon-based sequencing approach with high-confidence calls at targeted loci	• Application effectively limited to CRC • Designed and validated on a single small cohort
	Zhu et al [57], 2018 (ColonCore)	• Sensitivity: 97.9% • Specificity: ~100% • Concordance with PCR: 93.4% • Concordance with IHC: 92.3%	• Validated for testing against a pooled normal comparator population, obviating need for matched normal DNA from patient	
Tumor mutational burden analysis	Nowak et al [61], 2016	• Sensitivity: 91% • Specificity: 98%	• Computationally simple test • Versatile algorithm that can be applied across NGS platforms	• May perform more poorly in non-CRC
	Stadler et al [60], 2016	• Sensitivity: 100% • Specificity: 90% • Concordance with PCR: 99%	• *POLE* exonuclease-mutated false-positives can be easily detected by *POLE* sequencing and/or mutational signature analysis	
Machine learning	Wang & Liang [62], 2018 (MSIpred)	• Sensitivity: 93.6% • Specificity: 99.6%	• Accurate MSI calling in most common MSI-H tumor types (endometrial, colonic, rectal, and gastric carcinomas) • Computationally efficient (uses MAF rather than BAM files)	• Provides no information about specific microsatellites • Validated on whole-exome sequences; applicability to other NGS platforms unclear
Vector-based prediction	Cortes-Ciriano et al [1], 2017	• Sensitivity: 92% • Specificity: 99%	• Model validated on a large and diverse cohort	• Computationally complex • Validated on whole-exome sequences; applicability to other NGS platforms unclear
Single-molecule molecular inversion probes	Waalkes et al [23], 2018	• Sensitivity: 98.5% • Specificity: 100%	• Inexpensive (~$80/sample) • Designed for application to a variety of tumor types • Can detect tumor MSI in low tumor purity samples	• Novel approach, awaiting further investigation

Abbreviations: CRC, colorectal carcinoma; RNAseq, RNA sequencing.

TABLE 2
Summary of Large Next-Generation Sequencing–Based Microsatellite Instability Studies

Study	Cohort	MSI-Calling Method	Principal Findings
Cortes-Ciriano et al [1], 2017	• 7919 whole-exome sequences and 803 whole-genome sequences • 23 tumor types • Downloaded from TCGA	Alignment and direct comparison of tumor and matched normal DNA using a Kolmogorov-Smirnov statistic and comparison with TCGA PCR-based MSI annotations	• MSI is a continuous variable, with genome-wide number of unstable microsatellites spanning 5 orders of magnitude between tumors • Identified a list of diagnostically informative microsatellites
Bonneville et al [5], 2017	• 11,139 whole-exome sequences, focused on 2539 microsatellites • 39 tumor types • Downloaded principally from TCGA	MANTIS algorithm	• Identified 22 loci that are highly predictive of MSI-H status across at least 5 tumor types, suggesting that these microsatellites could serve as a pan-cancer MSI detection panel
Latham et al [6], 2019	• 15,045 tumors, sequenced on 468-gene MSK-IMPACT NGS platform • >50 tumor types • Matched germline DNA for all patients	MSIsensor algorithm (MSI-H $\geq$10; MSI-I <10 but $\geq$3; MSS <3)	• 50% of patients with LS present with noncolorectal/nonendometrial tumors • In LS, noncolorectal/nonendometrial tumors are more likely to be MSI-I than MSI-H, but all patients with LS with MSI-I tumors were dMMR by IHC • Investigators recommend MMRP IHC for MSI-I tumors
Bailey et al [7], 2018	• 9423 tumors • >50 tumor types • Matched germline DNA for all patients	MSIsensor algorithm Gel assay validation of a subset of MSI-H tumors	• 22% of MSI-H tumors were nonendometrial/noncolorectal/nongastric • MSI-H tumors showed higher expression levels of PD-L1 and CD8, compared with MSS tumors
Hause et al [13], 2016	• 5930 whole-exome sequences, covering 223,082 microsatellites • 18 cancer types • Downloaded from TCGA	MOSAIC algorithm	• 14 of 18 tumor types had at least 1 MSI-H tumor example • 57.4% of loci were not unstable in any sequenced tumor • MSI-L and MSS tumors (as determined by PCR) showed no difference in unstable microsatellite numbers by NGS-based analysis

(continued on next page)

TABLE 2 (continued)			
Study	**Cohort**	**MSI-Calling Method**	**Principal Findings**
Middha et al [8] 2017	• 13,901 tumors, sequenced on 341–468-gene MSK-IMPACT platform • 66 tumor types	MSIsensor algorithm (MSI-H ≥10; MSI-I <10 but ≥3; MSS <3)	• Using a pooled normal comparator population, sensitivity was 96.1% and specificity 98.5%, compared with sensitivity of 96.6%–100% and specificity of 99.3%–100% for comparison with matched normal DNA • Among patients with intermediate MSIsensor score (MSI-I), 97% were MSS by PCR-based testing • MSIsensor was more sensitive than PCR-based testing for detecting MSH6-deficient patients
Vanderwalde et al [19], 2018	• 11,348 tumors, covering 7.317 microsatellites across 592 genes • 26 cancer types	Read-length distribution–based algorithm • MSI-H tumor: >45 unstable microsatellites • NGS-based called validated by PCR in 2189 cases	• 23 of 26 tumor types had at least 1 MSI-H tumor example • Sensitivity 95.8% and specificity 99.4% for MSI-H status by PCR • Sensitivity 87.1% and specificity 99.6% for dMMR status by IHC

Abbreviations: MMRP, MMR protein; TCGA, The Cancer Genome Atlas.

compare tumor microsatellites with a pooled normal comparator population, rather than with matched normal (patient) DNA [53]. With careful construction and validation, a pooled normal comparator population can, in theory, be used for any read-length distribution–based analysis. This practical approach obviates sequence-matched material from every patient but may modestly decrease sensitivity and specificity (to 96.1% and 98.5%, respectively, in 1 large study [7]). These decreases may be mitigated by enriching the evaluated microsatellites for highly informative pan-cancer or tumor type–specific loci [1,13,27,55], and a recent analysis comparing tumor samples with a reference genome using principal components analysis achieved at least 95% sensitivity and 98% specificity for detecting MSI-H (compared with a PCR-based reference standard) [9].

Adequate sequencing depth and tumor purity are important factors in NGS-based MSI calling. In general, read depth of at least 20x to 30x has been considered necessary for NGS-based MSI analysis [5,13,53], although 1 large analysis detected significantly fewer MSI events at 20x to 30x compared with 55x [1], and some studies have used minimum read depths of 200x, 250x, or 500x to ensure robust instability detection [8,9,19].

Tumor purity (percentage of tumor cells in the sequenced sample) is also important in NGS-based MSI calling. Detection of MSI events decreases in proportion to decreasing tumor purity [9], with tumor purity greater than 25% generally required for sensitive detection of MSI events [8,53]. Accurate distinction of MSI-H from MSS tumors is substantially impaired at less than 10% to 20% tumor purity [1,8,9].

In addition to MSI calling, NGS data can be used to compute a tumor mutational signature, which may provide further evidence for (or against) underlying dMMR. The dMMR mutational signature was seen in 88% of MSI-H/I tumors but just 11% of MSS tumors in 1 study [6], and was highly concordant with vector-based MSI modeling in another [1]. These findings suggest that mutational signature analysis could help clarify the significance of certain NGS results (eg, MSI-I designation, or the cause of high mutational burden in other hypermutated tumor types, including *POLE*-mutated, ultraviolet-related, or smoking-related tumors).

Read-count distribution–based assays targeting highly informative loci

Robust read-length distribution–based algorithms and NGS-based whole-exome and whole-genome MSI profiles permit development of NGS panels targeting clinically relevant tumor-related genes and highly informative microsatellites. MSIplus (2015) targets hotspot mutations in *KRAS*, *NRAS*, and *BRAF* while using an mSINGS-based algorithm on 16 highly informative microsatellites (including HSPH1), which predicts response to anticancer therapy [56,58]. Similarly, ColonCore targets somatic mutations in 36 colon cancer-related genes (including *KRAS*, *NRAS*, and *BRAF*) and evaluates 22 highly informative microsatellites using a read-length distribution–based algorithm [57]. In validation, the targeted microsatellite panel in ColonCore provided greater discrimination between MSS and MSI-H tumors than the original mSINGS and MSIsensor algorithms [57]. Although MSIplus and ColonCore are specifically designed for colorectal cancer, these assays are proof of principal for accurate MSI detection using few, highly informative microsatellites in a larger NGS panel. Further building on this concept, Waalkes and colleagues [23] (2018) used single-molecule molecular inversion probes (smMIPs) to capture and sequence 111 highly informative pancancer microsatellites, followed by mSINGS analysis. Like MSIplus and ColonCore, this smMIP technique can be adapted to simultaneously detect mutations in other genes of interest. These more targeted platforms await further independent investigation.

Non–read length distribution–based methods

Tumor mutational burden. Some NGS-based MSI-calling algorithms rely on tumor mutational burden (TMB) rather than read-length distribution comparison. TMB (discussed later) is a nonstandardized metric of all somatic tumor mutations [59]. Because dMMR inherently results in increased tumor mutations, TMB can be used as a surrogate identifying dMMR tumors (although we emphasize that TMB-high and MSI-H tumors are not synonymous [19]). In 1 study (2016), dMMR and MMR-proficient tumors were accurately separated by TMB [60], and a similar study (2017) showed that a combined metric of TMB and homopolymer indels could accurately separate dMMR from MMR-proficient tumors [61]. Advantageously, these TMB-based methods do not require matched normal DNA for comparison. Of note, TMB-based MSI calling inherently misclassifies tumors with

POLE exonuclease mutations as MSI-H, but these false-positive results can be detected by mutational signature profiling or direct *POLE* sequencing in the same NGS platform [9,60,61]. Furthermore, as in other assays, tumor type–specific validation improves the accuracy of TMB-based MSI calling, given differences in number and distribution of MSI events between tumor types [37].

Machine learning. MSIpred (2018) is a machine learning MSI-calling tool that evaluates a tumor somatic mutation profile based on 22 whole-exome sequencing–derived parameters [62]. MSIpred incorporates 9 of 10 whole-exome sequencing–derived parameters used in an earlier machine learning MSI assay, MSIseq(ML)[a] (2015) [63]. These machine learning tools show robust performance across the 4 most common MSI-H tumor types, and they analyze mutation annotated files (MAFs), [b] which require substantially less processing power than the BAM file analyses performed by read-length distribution–based algorithms. However, these machine learning algorithms do not directly quantitate MSI or provide information about specific microsatellites, which may individually have clinical relevance [58].

In a large analysis of whole-exome and wholegenome MSI distribution, Cortes-Ciriano and colleagues [1] developed a vector-based machine learning model for predicting tumor MSI status (2017). Although this approach was validated against a wide spectrum of tumor types, it is computationally complex and its applicability to smaller microsatellite panels (such as those obtained from most targeted clinical NGS panels) is unclear.

Novel Non–Next-Generation Sequencing–Based Microsatellite Instability–Calling Methods
Idylla rapid microsatellite instability–calling platform

In 2019, Samaison and colleagues [64] reported use of the Idylla sequencing platform to detect alterations at 7 microsatellite loci in 12 tumors with discordant

---

[a]Note that there are 2 NGS-based MSI-calling tools named MSIseq. The machine learning tool published by Huang and colleagues[63] in 2015 is referred to as MSIseq(ML) in this article, to distinguish it from the indel analysis method published by Lu and colleagues[28] in 2013.

[b]MIRMMR (2017) is another MSI-calling tool that analyzes MAF files, though it also requires methylation data (Foltz, and colleagues) adding an additional layer of input complexity.

MMR IHC and PCR-based MSI calling. This small study showed 100% concordance between Idylla and PCR-based MSI status. The examined microsatellites (*ACVR2A*, *BTBD7*, *DIDO1*, *MRE11*, *RYR3*, *SEC31A*, and *SULF2*) are not included in standard PCR-based panels, but 2 (*ACVR2A* and *SEC31A*) were among the most highly informative microsatellites identified in exome-wide analyses [1,13]. The tabletop Idylla platform extracts DNA from formalin-fixed paraffin-embedded tissue, amplifies target sequences, performs bioinformatic analysis, and generates a report in 150 minutes [64]. More definitive determination of performance awaits further investigation of this application.

Morphometric analysis

Kather and colleagues (2019) [65] trained convoluted neural networks to discriminate MSI-H from MSS tumors using morphologic features on hematoxylin-eosin–stained tissue. A neural network trained on 378 formalin-fixed colorectal carcinomas (with known MSI status) predicted MSI status in a validation cohort of 360 formalin-fixed colorectal carcinomas with considerable accuracy (area under the curve [AUC], 0.84). However, a neural network trained on endometrial carcinomas applied to a validation cohort of endometrial carcinomas did not perform as well (AUC, 0.75), and models trained on frozen tumor, gastric cancer, or tumors from an Asian population performed poorly on formalin-fixed tissue, colorectal carcinoma, and predominantly non-Asian populations, respectively. These data suggest that these morphometric approaches are inflexible and underperform compared with NGS-based methods.

Table 3 provides a comparative summary of available assays for detecting MSI.

Using Next-Generation Sequencing to Understand the Pathogenetic Role of Microsatellite Instability in Cancer

NGS-based whole-exome and whole-genome studies of large and diverse cohorts of dMMR tumors have provided insight into the complex role of MSI in tumorigenesis. dMMR results in both single nucleotide variants and indels, and indels in coding microsatellites can be in-frame indels or, more often, frameshifts.

Accumulated evidence shows that MSI events are predominantly under negative selection. Fewer indels are found in coding than in noncoding DNA, and coding indels are, on average, shorter and more often in-frame than noncoding indels, suggesting that coding frameshifts are evolutionarily disadvantageous [13,27]. However, certain frameshifts at coding microsatellites in cancer-related genes are highly recurrent [27,28], indicating that these loss-of-function events provide selective advantage. Some of these recurrent frameshifts are tumor type specific, such as a recurrent *JAK1* frameshift in endometrial carcinoma, associated with downregulation of multiple JAK-STAT pathway constituents [1,13]. Indels are under greater selective pressure than single nucleotide variants in both coding and noncoding DNA [1,27] and following therapeutic PD-1 blockade [11], suggesting that indels play the more significant role in tumor biology and in the immune response to tumor neoantigens.

MSI events also have a multifactorial effect on gene transcription and translation. Frameshifts in coding or splice-site microsatellites can decrease gene transcription or produce nonfunctioning transcripts [13]. Microsatellite indels in enhancers or other noncoding regulatory regions can also affect gene expression [1,66], and microsatellite indels in 3′ untranslated regions

TABLE 3
Summary of Techniques

	MMRP IHC	PCR-Based MSI Calling	NGS-Based MSI Calling
Cost	Low	Intermediate	High
Versatility	Broadly applicable across tumor types	Current panels optimized for colorectal carcinoma; show acceptable performance in endometrial carcinoma but suboptimal or unverified performance in other tumor types	• Read-length distribution–based, vector-based, and tumor mutational burden algorithms broadly applicable across tumor types • Machine learning models most applicable to tumor types on which they were trained
Availability	Broad	Intermediate	Low

(identified in 84% of MSI-H tumors vs 3% of MSS tumors) are linked to gene underexpression or overexpression and to reduced transcript stability [1,27].

PRESENT RELEVANCE AND FUTURE AVENUES OF INVESTIGATION
Lynch Syndrome
LS was first recognized in 1966 as a syndrome of familial colorectal cancer distinct from adenomatous polyposis coli [67]. LS (also termed hereditary nonpolyposis colon cancer) affects approximately 1 in 280 people [6,68] and most classically includes colorectal carcinoma and endometrial carcinoma, although patients with LS are also at increased risk of carcinomas of the small bowel, stomach, urinary tract, pancreas, adrenal cortex, and sebaceous glands, as well as glioblastoma, among other tumor types [6,67].

Seminal work in 1993 to 1994 linked LS to MSI, and ultimately to germline mutations in *MLH1*, *MSH2*, *MSH6*, and *PMS2*, with rare cases tied to *EPCAM* deletions, *MSH2* inversions, biallelic *MUTYH* mutations, and constitutional *MLH1* promoter hypermethylation [32,69–73]. Patients develop dMMR tumors following inactivation of the second wild-type allele through somatic mutation, loss of heterozygosity, or epigenetic silencing [6].

Because MLH1, MSH2, MSH6, and PMS2 each play a slightly different role in DNA MMR [32], germline mutation in each of the corresponding genes produces a slightly different clinical syndrome (Table 4) [74–78].

Rare individuals harbor biallelic deleterious germline MMR mutations, termed constitutional dMMR syndrome and associated with hematologic and central nervous system cancers in childhood, and with other LS-associated tumors in young adulthood [79].

Sporadic Microsatellite Instability
Most MSI-H tumors harbor sporadic (nongermline) dMMR, an observation dating to the original description of MSI-H LS-associated tumors [69,80]. Sporadic MSI most commonly results from epigenetic silencing of *MLH1* via promoter hypermethylation, detected in approximately 80% and 85% to 95% of MLH1-deficient colorectal and endometrial cancers, respectively [80–84]. Accordingly, promoter hypermethylation testing is critical to cost-effective use of genetic counseling and germline testing for LS.

BRAF V600E mutation is found in 46% to 70% of colorectal carcinomas with *MLH1* promoter hypermethylation, but almost never in nonmethylated colorectal carcinoma [85,86]. As a result, IHC for the *BRAF* V600E protein is a specific and cost-effective test for *MLH1*

TABLE 4 Clinical Associations with Germline Mutations				
Germline Mutation	Clinical Presentation	Lifetime Risk (%)		Population Prevalence
		Colorectal Carcinoma	Endometrial Carcinoma	
MLH1	Colorectal carcinoma at a young age	34–54	18–60	1:1946
MSH2	Colorectal carcinoma at a young age, as well as increased risk for extracolonic tumors	37–47	21–60	1:2841
MSH6	Higher relative risk of endometrial carcinoma, with a greater likelihood of minimal microsatellite shifts and lesser response to immune therapy	12	16–26	1:758
PMS2	May present later in life with endometrial or colorectal cancer; no appreciably increased risk of noncanonical LS tumors	13	13–15	1:714

promoter hypermethylation in colorectal carcinoma [87]. Importantly, the same association is not true in endometrial carcinoma, where molecular testing for *MLH1* promoter hypermethylation is indicated in tumors showing MLH1 loss.

Biallelic somatic MMR mutations also account for a substantial subset of sporadic MSI, ranging from 20% to 70% of sporadic, nonhypermethylated MSI-H tumors [6,88–90].

The proportions of sporadic and LS-associated tumors vary by tumor type. For instance, 19% of MSI-H colorectal cancers are LS associated, as are 12% to 15% of MSI-H small bowel and gastric adenocarcinomas, but just 6% of MSI-H endometrial carcinomas, despite the high percentage of MSI-H endometrial cancers overall [6]. It is more challenging to determine the precise prevalence of LS in other tumor types, because the generally small numbers of LS-associated cases makes precise estimation statistically difficult [6].

Lynch Syndrome Screening

An LS diagnosis has important clinical implications for patients and their blood relatives, making LS detection a clinical priority. Early LS screening algorithms based on personal and family cancer history show suboptimal sensitivity [67,91–95]. Furthermore, existing clinical algorithms consider only canonical LS-associated tumors (principally colorectal and endometrial), whereas large population-based studies have shown that up to half of patients with LS present with other tumor types (small bowel, gastric, urothelial, prostatic, pancreatic, and adrenocortical cancers, among others) [6,7].

Recognizing the shortcomings of clinical screening algorithms, universal LS screening is now recommended for colorectal carcinoma [96–98] and increasingly practiced for endometrial carcinoma [35,99–101]. Both MMR IHC and PCR-based MSI testing are widely used for LS screening, with repeat screening by a second method if there is high clinical concern but a negative initial screening result [12].

Robust data on the effectiveness of universal LS screening are now becoming available. Of 6649 endometrial carcinomas in 1 meta-analysis on universal screening, 206 (3.1%) were diagnosed with LS (including 32 *MLH1*, 82 *MSH2*, 75 *MSH6*, and 17 *PMS2* mutations), 44% of which would have been missed by clinical screening algorithms [80]. However, follow-through on screening results is imperfect: of 1011 screen-positive patients with endometrial carcinoma, 118 (11%) did not receive appropriate genetic counseling or germline testing, most commonly because of poor health care access and medical anxiety [75,102]. By comparison, a cohort study of 10,206 newly diagnosed colorectal carcinomas found a more modest increase in sensitivity for LS detection using universal screening compared with clinical screening criteria (100% vs 88%) [95]. Despite its improved effectiveness compared with clinical screening, current universal screening practice still omits noncanonical LS-associated tumors [6].

Prognostic and Predictive Significance of Microsatellite Instability

MSI-H colorectal carcinomas carry a favorable prognosis, irrespective of tumor stage, with a lower probability of high stage at presentation and increased sensitivity to irinotecan-based combination therapy [103–106]. dMMR endometrial cancers are also disproportionately low stage at diagnosis, and dMMR tumors carried an intermediate prognosis in a recent molecular classification of endometrial carcinoma [107,108]. One study of 1024 endometrial carcinomas found no difference in survival between dMMR tumors and MMR-proficient tumors, despite higher tumor grade and more frequent lymphovascular invasion in dMMR tumors and higher tumor stage in tumors with *MLH1* promoter hypermethylation, suggesting a complex role for MMR in endometrial cancer biology and behavior [109].

MSI-H tumors show greater response to PD-1 inhibitors across multiple tumor types [110,111]. In 1 study of 86 patients with MSI-H tumors spanning 11 tumor types and progressing through at least 1 therapy, 53% showed a durable objective response to the PD-1 inhibitor pembrolizumab [110]. In 5 subsequent clinical trials, including 149 patients with MSI-H tumors spanning 15 tumor types, 40% showed an objective response to pembrolizumab, with 78% of responses lasting at least 6 months [112]. PD-1 blockade is linked to the expansion of T cells specific for tumor neoantigens, to the number of genome-wide MSI events, and to the number of MSI-related tumor neoantigens, pointing to a robust antitumor immune response following release of PD-1–mediated suppression [11,110].

As a result of these findings, on May 23, 2017, the United States Food and Drug Administration (FDA) approved pembrolizumab "for the treatment of adult or pediatric patients with unresectable or metastatic solid tumors [that are] microsatellite instability-high or mismatch repair deficient ... that have progressed following prior treatment and who have no satisfactory alternative treatment options" [113]; this was the FDA's first tumor-agnostic drug approval [114].

A subset of tumors harbor subclonal MMR mutations or epimutations, yielding a heterogeneous dMMR pattern. Although such heterogeneous patterns are considered incompatible with underlying LS, they are relevant to immunotherapy considerations and should be documented [115]. True heterogeneous patterns should be distinguished from improper tissue fixation or technical artifacts, and recognition of a positive internal control is paramount.

Importantly, the dMMR molecular signature accounts for only half of hypermutated tumors, with the remainder composed predominantly of ultraviolet, smoking, POLE, and APOBEC (apolipoprotein B messenger RNA editing enzyme, catalytic polypeptide-like) signatures [7]. These other classes of hypermutated tumors (eg, melanoma) may show excellent response to PD-1 blockade, highlighting that MSI status is not the only arbiter of immunotherapy susceptibility.

In addition to MSI status, tumor programmed death-ligand 1 (PD-L1) expression also predicts response to immune checkpoint inhibitors [116]. TMB is an emerging biomarker that may also have clinical utility for identifying patients that are likely respond to immunotherapy; however, significant uncertainty still remains as to the true clinical utility of the biomarker, with conflicting data from multiple studies [117–119]. In addition to this, the technical component of determining TMB has yet to be standardized, although there are ongoing multi-institutional efforts to create laboratory standards for both testing and reporting TMB [59]. Because MSI tumors inherently have increased numbers of somatic mutations, tumor MSI and TMB statuses show substantial overlap, but approximately one-quarter of MSI-H tumors are TMB low, and 6% of MSS tumors were TMB high in 1 study [9,12,19].

Tumor PD-L1 expression is generally considered positive if greater than 1% of tumor cells show strong membranous expression by IHC, although optimal metrics for assessing the PD-L1–PD-1 axis are tumor type specific and remain in flux. At present, although MSI, TMB, and PD-L1 show some degree of correlation, some data suggest that they constitute independent predictive factors in tumor response to PD-1 blockade, and their precise interplay remains under investigation [11]. However, it remains possible that all 3 of these biomarkers may play complementary roles to one another in identifying patients who may respond to immune checkpoint inhibition.

In addition, MSI-H tumors are enriched in mutations in the phosphatidylinositol 3-kinase, WNT, NOTCH, JAK, and Hedgehog pathways [9], suggesting that additional targeted therapies and synthetic lethality may be effective in a subset of MSI-H tumors.

Future Directions

Despite a veritable explosion in clinical NGS applications in recent years, the precise role of NGS-based MSI calling remains unclear. Because of cost, availability, and logistical hurdles, only a minority of tumors is tested by NGS-based panels, and NGS is more often used clinically in high-stage or recurrent tumors [8,9]. High-stage and recurrent MSI-H tumors are prime candidates for immunotherapy, and, given its versatility in identifying additional therapeutic targets across hundreds of genes and pathways, NGS may offer a cost-effective means to detect MSI-H tumors, particularly for tumor types where MSI-H tumors are rare.

In contrast, NGS-based MSI calling is unlikely to become the assay of choice for LS screening, given that a high proportion of LS screening is performed on newly diagnosed, low-stage tumors with less to gain, clinically, from comprehensive NGS profiling. Furthermore, MMR IHC and PCR-based testing have proved to be excellent tools for LS screening in colorectal and endometrial cancer, and are likely to remain the tools of choice for the foreseeable future. A few institutions have expanded LS screening to small bowel, gastric, and ovarian carcinoma, but detecting LS in patients with noncanonical tumor types remains a challenge. Careful clinical attention to family history remains critical to LS detection in the absence of a practicable, cost-effective, pan-cancer LS screening assay.

At present, tumor MSI status (by IHC, PCR, or NGS) and PD-L1 expression (by IHC) should both be assessed, if possible, before initiating immunotherapy. In contrast with the varied methods available to assess tumor MSI status, PD-L1 expression is, at present, only practicably assessed by IHC. An NGS-based metric of PD-L1 and/or PD-1 expression could ultimately be feasible, allowing a single comprehensive NGS platform to assess MSI and PD-L1, as well as TMB and other relevant genetic alterations, further augmenting the clinical value of NGS in guiding treatment. Specific microsatellite alterations (such as HSPH1 in colorectal cancer [58]) could also prove to have intrinsic predictive value, warranting deliberate inclusion in targeted NGS panels. The additional value of TMB in guiding patient management remains less clear, with investigation and standardization ongoing [59,118,119].

The precise clinical significance of heterogeneous (subclonal) MMR loss remains unclear. Heterogeneous MMR IHC is seen in a minority of tumors and can be associated with either dMMR or MMR-proficient metastases [115]. Therefore, heterogeneous MMR IHC in the primary tumor should prompt repeat MMR testing before initiating immune therapy for recurrent or metastatic disease. At present, PCR-based and NGS-based assays are less suited for detecting heterogeneous MMR expression.

In less than a decade, tremendous gains in NGS-based MSI detection have improved the understanding of the role of MSI in tumorigenesis, and provided a valuable new clinical assay for MSI classification and quantification. The authors anticipate that increased awareness of NGS-based MSI calling by practicing surgical and molecular pathologists will lead to greater interest in this application, fueling broader clinical investigations and wider clinical uptake.

DISCLOSURE

The authors have nothing to disclose.

REFERENCES

[1] Cortes-Ciriano I, Lee S, Park WY, et al. A molecular portrait of microsatellite instability across multiple cancers. Nat Commun 2017;8:15180.

[2] de Wind N, Dekker M, Berns A, et al. Inactivation of the mouse Msh2 gene results in mismatch repair deficiency, methylation tolerance, hyperrecombination, and predisposition to cancer. Cell 1995;82(2):321–30.

[3] Parsons R, Li GM, Longley MJ, et al. Hypermutability and mismatch repair deficiency in RER+ tumor cells. Cell 1993;75(6):1227–36.

[4] Oki E, Oda S, Maehara Y, et al. Mutated gene-specific phenotypes of dinucleotide repeat instability in human colorectal carcinoma cell lines deficient in DNA mismatch repair. Oncogene 1999;18(12):2143–7.

[5] Bonneville R, Krook MA, Kautto EA, et al. Landscape of Microsatellite Instability Across 39 Cancer Types. JCO Precis Oncol 2017;2017.

[6] Latham A, Srinivasan P, Kemel Y, et al. Microsatellite Instability Is Associated With the Presence of Lynch Syndrome Pan-Cancer. J Clin Oncol 2019;37(4):286–95.

[7] Bailey MH, Tokheim C, Porta-Pardo E, et al. Comprehensive Characterization of Cancer Driver Genes and Mutations. Cell 2018;173(2):371–85.e18.

[8] Middha S, Zhang L, Nafa K, et al. Reliable Pan-Cancer Microsatellite Instability Assessment by Using Targeted Next-Generation Sequencing Data. JCO Precis Oncol

2017;2017. https://doi.org/10.1200/PO.17.00084. Epub 2017 Oct 3.

[9] Trabucco SE, Gowen K, Maund SL, et al. A Novel Next-Generation Sequencing Approach to Detecting Microsatellite Instability and Pan-Tumor Characterization of 1000 Microsatellite Instability-High Cases in 67,000 Patient Samples. J Mol Diagn 2019;21(6):1053–66.

[10] Chapel DB, Patil SA, Plagov A, et al. Quantitative next-generation sequencing-based analysis indicates progressive accumulation of microsatellite instability between atypical hyperplasia/endometrial intraepithelial neoplasia and paired endometrioid endometrial carcinoma. Mod Pathol 2019;32(10):1508–20.

[11] Mandal R, Samstein RM, Lee KW, et al. Genetic diversity of tumors with mismatch repair deficiency influences anti-PD-1 immunotherapy response. Science 2019;364(6439):485–91.

[12] Luchini C, Bibeau F, Ligtenberg MJL, et al. ESMO recommendations on microsatellite instability testing for immunotherapy in cancer, and its relationship with PD-1/PD-L1 expression and tumour mutational burden: a systematic review-based approach. Ann Oncol 2019;30(8):1232–43.

[13] Hause RJ, Pritchard CC, Shendure J, et al. Classification and characterization of microsatellite instability across 18 cancer types. Nat Med 2016;22(11):1342–50.

[14] Dietmaier W, Wallinger S, Bocker T, et al. Diagnostic microsatellite instability: definition and correlation with mismatch repair protein expression. Cancer Res 1997;57(21):4749–56.

[15] Bocker T, Diermann J, Friedl W, et al. Microsatellite instability analysis: a multicenter study for reliability and quality control. Cancer Res 1997;57(21):4739–43.

[16] Boland CR, Thibodeau SN, Hamilton SR, et al. A National Cancer Institute Workshop on Microsatellite Instability for cancer detection and familial predisposition: development of international criteria for the determination of microsatellite instability in colorectal cancer. Cancer Res 1998;58(22):5248–57.

[17] Umar A, Boland CR, Terdiman JP, et al. Revised Bethesda Guidelines for hereditary nonpolyposis colorectal cancer (Lynch syndrome) and microsatellite instability. J Natl Cancer Inst 2004;96(4):261–8.

[18] Promega Enters Global Collaboration with Merck to Develop Microsatellite Instability (MSI) Companion Diagnostic for Use with KEYTRUDA. 2019. Available at: https://www.promega.com/aboutus/press-releases/2019/54997940-msicompanion-dxmerckpress-release-for-partnership-agreement. Accessed March 18, 2020.

[19] Vanderwalde A, Spetzler D, Xiao N, et al. Microsatellite instability status determined by next-generation sequencing and compared with PD-L1 and tumor mutational burden in 11,348 patients. Cancer Med 2018;7(3):746–56.

[20] Coelho H, Jones-Hughes T, Snowsill T, et al. A systematic review of test accuracy studies evaluating molecular micro-satellite instability testing for the

detection of individuals with lynch syndrome. BMC Cancer 2017;17(1):836.

[21] Gould-Suarez M, El-Serag HB, Musher B, et al. Cost-effectiveness and diagnostic effectiveness analyses of multiple algorithms for the diagnosis of Lynch syndrome. Dig Dis Sci 2014;59(12):2913–26.

[22] Hampel H, Pearlman R, Beightol M, et al. Assessment of Tumor Sequencing as a Replacement for Lynch Syndrome Screening and Current Molecular Tests for Patients With Colorectal Cancer. JAMA Oncol 2018;4(6): 806–13.

[23] Waalkes A, Smith N, Penewit K, et al. Accurate Pan-Cancer Molecular Diagnosis of Microsatellite Instability by Single-Molecule Molecular Inversion Probe Capture and High-Throughput Sequencing. Clin Chem 2018; 64(6):950–8.

[24] Wu X, Snir O, Rottmann D, et al. Minimal microsatellite shift in microsatellite instability high endometrial cancer: a significant pitfall in diagnostic interpretation. Mod Pathol 2019;32(5):650–8.

[25] Edelmann W, Yang K, Umar A, et al. Mutation in the mismatch repair gene Msh6 causes cancer susceptibility. Cell 1997;91(4):467–77.

[26] Wang Y, Shi C, Eisenberg R, et al. Differences in Microsatellite Instability Profiles between Endometrioid and Colorectal Cancers: A Potential Cause for False-Negative Results? J Mol Diagn 2017;19(1):57–64.

[27] Kim TM, Laird PW, Park PJ. The landscape of microsatellite instability in colorectal and endometrial cancer genomes. Cell 2013;155(4):858–68.

[28] Lu Y, Soong TD, Elemento O. A novel approach for characterizing microsatellite instability in cancer cells. PLoS One 2013;8(5):e63056.

[29] Leach FS, Polyak K, Burrell M, et al. Expression of the human mismatch repair gene hMSH2 in normal and neoplastic tissues. Cancer Res 1996;56(2):235–40.

[30] Stone JG, Robertson D, Houlston RS. Immunohistochemistry for MSH2 and MHL1: a method for identifying mismatch repair deficient colorectal cancer. J Clin Pathol 2001;54(6):484–7.

[31] Erten MZ, Fernandez LP, Ng HK, et al. Universal Versus Targeted Screening for Lynch Syndrome: Comparing Ascertainment and Costs Based on Clinical Experience. Dig Dis Sci 2016;61(10):2887–95.

[32] Tamura K, Kaneda M, Futagawa M, et al. Genetic and genomic basis of the mismatch repair system involved in Lynch syndrome. Int J Clin Oncol 2019;24(9): 999–1011.

[33] McConechy MK, Talhouk A, Li-Chang HH, et al. Detection of DNA mismatch repair (MMR) deficiencies by immunohistochemistry can effectively diagnose the microsatellite instability (MSI) phenotype in endometrial carcinomas. Gynecol Oncol 2015; 137(2):306–10.

[34] Hampel H, Frankel WL, Martin E, et al. Screening for the Lynch syndrome (hereditary nonpolyposis colorectal cancer). N Engl J Med 2005;352(18):1851–60.

[35] Hampel H, Frankel W, Panescu J, et al. Screening for Lynch syndrome (hereditary nonpolyposis colorectal cancer) among endometrial cancer patients. Cancer Res 2006;66(15):7810–7.

[36] Hechtman JF, Rana S, Middha S, et al. Retained mismatch repair protein expression occurs in approximately 6% of microsatellite instability-high cancers and is associated with missense mutations in mismatch repair genes. Mod Pathol 2019;33(5):871–9.

[37] Dong F, Costigan DC, Howitt BE. Targeted next-generation sequencing in the detection of mismatch repair deficiency in endometrial cancers. Mod Pathol 2019;32(2):252–7.

[38] Lindor NM, Burgart LJ, Leontovich O, et al. Immunohistochemistry versus microsatellite instability testing in phenotyping colorectal tumors. J Clin Oncol 2002; 20(4):1043–8.

[39] Chapel DB, Yamada SD, Cowan M, et al. Immunohistochemistry for mismatch repair protein deficiency in endometrioid endometrial carcinoma yields equivalent results when performed on endometrial biopsy/curettage or hysterectomy specimens. Gynecol Oncol 2018; 149(3):570–4.

[40] O'Brien O, Ryan E, Creavin B, et al. Correlation of immunohistochemical mismatch repair protein status between colorectal carcinoma endoscopic biopsy and resection specimens. J Clin Pathol 2018;71(7):631–6.

[41] Chapel DB, Lengyel E, Ritterhouse LL, et al. Interpretation of Mismatch Repair Protein Immunohistochemistry in Endometrial Carcinoma Should Consider Both Lynch Syndrome Screening and Immunotherapy Susceptibility: An Illustrative Case Report. Int J Gynecol Pathol 2019;39(3):233–7.

[42] Shia J. Immunohistochemistry versus microsatellite instability testing for screening colorectal cancer patients at risk for hereditary nonpolyposis colorectal cancer syndrome. Part I. The utility of immunohistochemistry. J Mol Diagn 2008;10(4): 293–300.

[43] Chen W, Swanson BJ, Frankel WL. Molecular genetics of microsatellite-unstable colorectal cancer for pathologists. Diagn Pathol 2017;12(1):24.

[44] Cohen R, Hain E, Buhard O, et al. Association of Primary Resistance to Immune Checkpoint Inhibitors in Metastatic Colorectal Cancer With Misdiagnosis of Microsatellite Instability or Mismatch Repair Deficiency Status. JAMA Oncol 2019;5(4):551–5.

[45] Sari A, Pollett A, Eiriksson LR, et al. Interobserver Agreement for Mismatch Repair Protein Immunohistochemistry in Endometrial and Nonserous, Nonmucinous Ovarian Carcinomas. Am J Surg Pathol 2019;43(5): 591–600.

[46] Sarode VR, Robinson L. Screening for Lynch Syndrome by Immunohistochemistry of Mismatch Repair Proteins: Significance of Indeterminate Result and Correlation With Mutational Studies. Arch Pathol Lab Med 2019;143(10):1225–33.

[47] Shia J, Tang LH, Vakiani E, et al. Immunohistochemistry as first-line screening for detecting colorectal cancer patients at risk for hereditary nonpolyposis colorectal cancer syndrome: a 2-antibody panel may be as predictive as a 4-antibody panel. Am J Surg Pathol 2009;33(11):1639–45.

[48] Hall G, Clarkson A, Shi A, et al. Immunohistochemistry for PMS2 and MSH6 alone can replace a four antibody panel for mismatch repair deficiency screening in colorectal adenocarcinoma. Pathology 2010;42(5):409–13.

[49] Pearlman R, Markow M, Knight D, et al. Two-stain immunohistochemical screening for Lynch syndrome in colorectal cancer may fail to detect mismatch repair deficiency. Mod Pathol 2018;31(12): 1891–900.

[50] U.S. Food and Drug Administration. Summary of safety and effectiveness data (SSED): FoundationOne CDx. United States Food and Drug Administration; 2017. Available at. https://www.accessdata.fda.gov/cdrh_docs/pdf17/P170019S006B.pdf. Accessed December 3, 2019.

[51] US Food and Drug Administration. Evaluation of automatic class III designation for MSK-IMPACT (Integrated mutation profiling of actionable cancer targets). United States Food and Drug Administration; 2017. Available at. https://www.accessdata.fda.gov/cdrh_docs/reviews/den170058.pdf. Accessed September 4, 2020.

[52] Pritchard CC, Smith C, Salipante SJ, et al. ColoSeq provides comprehensive lynch and polyposis syndrome mutational analysis using massively parallel sequencing. J Mol Diagn 2012;14(4):357–66.

[53] Salipante SJ, Scroggins SM, Hampel HL, et al. Microsatellite instability detection by next generation sequencing. Clin Chem 2014;60(9):1192–9.

[54] Niu B, Ye K, Zhang Q, et al. MSIsensor: microsatellite instability detection using paired tumor-normal sequence data. Bioinformatics 2014;30(7):1015–6.

[55] Kautto EA, Bonneville R, Miya J, et al. Performance evaluation for rapid detection of pan-cancer microsatellite instability with MANTIS. Oncotarget 2017;8(5): 7452–63.

[56] Hempelmann JA, Scroggins SM, Pritchard CC, et al. MSIplus for Integrated Colorectal Cancer Molecular Testing by Next-Generation Sequencing. J Mol Diagn 2015;17(6):705–14.

[57] Zhu L, Huang Y, Fang X, et al. A Novel and Reliable Method to Detect Microsatellite Instability in Colorectal Cancer by Next-Generation Sequencing. J Mol Diagn 2018;20(2):225–31.

[58] Dorard C, de Thonel A, Collura A, et al. Expression of a mutant HSP110 sensitizes colorectal cancer cells to chemotherapy and improves disease prognosis. Nat Med 2011;17(10):1283–9.

[59] Stenzinger A, Allen JD, Maas J, et al. Tumor mutational burden standardization initiatives: Recommendations for consistent tumor mutational burden assessment in clinical samples to guide immunotherapy treatment decisions. Genes Chromosomes Cancer 2019;58(8): 578–88.

[60] Stadler ZK, Battaglin F, Middha S, et al. Reliable Detection of Mismatch Repair Deficiency in Colorectal Cancers Using Mutational Load in Next-Generation Sequencing Panels. J Clin Oncol 2016;34(18):2141–7.

[61] Nowak JA, Yurgelun MB, Bruce JL, et al. Detection of Mismatch Repair Deficiency and Microsatellite Instability in Colorectal Adenocarcinoma by Targeted Next-Generation Sequencing. J Mol Diagn 2017;19(1): 84–91.

[62] Wang C, Liang C. MSIpred: a python package for tumor microsatellite instability classification from tumor mutation annotation data using a support vector machine. Sci Rep 2018;8(1):17546.

[63] Huang MN, McPherson JR, Cutcutache I, et al. MSI-seq: Software for Assessing Microsatellite Instability from Catalogs of Somatic Mutations. Sci Rep 2015; 5:13321.

[64] Samaison L, Grall M, Staroz F, et al. Microsatellite instability diagnosis using the fully automated Idylla platform: feasibility study of an in-house rapid molecular testing ancillary to immunohistochemistry in pathology laboratories. J Clin Pathol 2019;72(12): 830–5.

[65] Kather JN, Pearson AT, Halama N, et al. Deep learning can predict microsatellite instability directly from histology in gastrointestinal cancer. Nat Med 2019;25(7): 1054–6.

[66] Katainen R, Dave K, Pitkanen E, et al. CTCF/cohesin-binding sites are frequently mutated in cancer. Nat Genet 2015;47(7):818–21.

[67] Lynch HT, Snyder CL, Shaw TG, et al. Milestones of Lynch syndrome: 1895-2015. Nat Rev Cancer 2015; 15:181–94.

[68] Win AK, Jenkins MA, Dowty JG, et al. Prevalence and Penetrance of Major Genes and Polygenes for Colorectal Cancer. Cancer Epidemiol Biomarkers Prev 2017;26(3):404–12.

[69] Aaltonen LA, Peltomaki P, Leach FS, et al. Clues to the pathogenesis of familial colorectal cancer. Science 1993;260(5109):812–6.

[70] Fishel R, Lescoe MK, Rao MR, et al. The human mutator gene homolog MSH2 and its association with hereditary nonpolyposis colon cancer. Cell 1993;75(5): 1027–38.

[71] Leach FS, Nicolaides NC, Papadopoulos N, et al. Mutations of a mutS homolog in hereditary nonpolyposis colorectal cancer. Cell 1993;75(6):1215–25.

[72] Papadopoulos N, Nicolaides NC, Wei YF, et al. Mutation of a mutL homolog in hereditary colon cancer. Science 1994;263(5153):1625–9.

[73] Bronner CE, Baker SM, Morrison PT, et al. Mutation in the DNA mismatch repair gene homologue hMLH1 is

associated with hereditary non-polyposis colon cancer. Nature 1994;368(6468):258–61.

[74] Bonadona V, Bonaiti B, Olschwang S, et al. Cancer risks associated with germline mutations in MLH1, MSH2, and MSH6 genes in Lynch syndrome. JAMA 2011; 305(22):2304–10.

[75] Ten Broeke SW, van der Klift HM, Tops CMJ, et al. Cancer Risks for PMS2-Associated Lynch Syndrome. J Clin Oncol 2018;36(29):2961–8.

[76] Dowty JG, Win AK, Buchanan DD, et al. Cancer risks for MLH1 and MSH2 mutation carriers. Hum Mutat 2013; 34(3):490–7.

[77] Tetzlaff MT, Singh RR, Seviour EG, et al. Next-generation sequencing identifies high frequency of mutations in potentially clinically actionable genes in sebaceous carcinoma. J Pathol 2016;240(1):84–95.

[78] Ponti G, Losi L, Di Gregorio C, et al. Identification of Muir-Torre syndrome among patients with sebaceous tumors and keratoacanthomas: role of clinical features, microsatellite instability, and immunohistochemistry. Cancer 2005;103(5):1018–25.

[79] Wimmer K, Kratz CP, Vasen HF, et al. Diagnostic criteria for constitutional mismatch repair deficiency syndrome: suggestions of the European consortium 'care for CMMRD' (C4CMMRD). J Med Genet 2014;51(6): 355–65.

[80] Kahn RM, Gordhandas S, Maddy BP, et al. Universal endometrial cancer tumor typing: How much has immunohistochemistry, microsatellite instability, and MLH1 methylation improved the diagnosis of Lynch syndrome across the population? Cancer 2019; 125(18):3172–83.

[81] Comprehensive molecular characterization of human colon and rectal cancer. Nature 2012;487(7407):330–7.

[82] Boland CR, Goel A. Microsatellite instability in colorectal cancer. Gastroenterology 2010;138(6): 2073–87.e3.

[83] Dillon JL, Gonzalez JL, DeMars L, et al. Universal screening for Lynch syndrome in endometrial cancers: frequency of germline mutations and identification of patients with Lynch-like syndrome. Hum Pathol 2017; 70:121–8.

[84] Esteller M, Levine R, Baylin SB, et al. MLH1 promoter hypermethylation is associated with the microsatellite instability phenotype in sporadic endometrial carcinomas. Oncogene 1998;17(18):2413–7.

[85] Parsons MT, Buchanan DD, Thompson B, et al. Correlation of tumour BRAF mutations and MLH1 methylation with germline mismatch repair (MMR) gene mutation status: a literature review assessing utility of tumour features for MMR variant classification. J Med Genet 2012;49(3):151–7.

[86] Domingo E, Laiho P, Ollikainen M, et al. BRAF screening as a low-cost effective strategy for simplifying HNPCC genetic testing. J Med Genet 2004;41(9): 664–8.

[87] Jin M, Hampel H, Zhou X, et al. BRAF V600E mutation analysis simplifies the testing algorithm for Lynch syndrome. Am J Clin Pathol 2013;140(2): 177–83.

[88] Haraldsdottir S, Hampel H, Tomsic J, et al. Colon and endometrial cancers with mismatch repair deficiency can arise from somatic, rather than germline, mutations. Gastroenterology 2014;147(6):1308–16.e1.

[89] Geurts-Giele WR, Leenen CH, Dubbink HJ, et al. Somatic aberrations of mismatch repair genes as a cause of microsatellite-unstable cancers. J Pathol 2014; 234(4):548–59.

[90] Mensenkamp AR, Vogelaar IP, van Zelst-Stams WA, et al. Somatic mutations in MLH1 and MSH2 are a frequent cause of mismatch-repair deficiency in Lynch syndrome-like tumors. Gastroenterology 2014;146(3):643–6.e8.

[91] Najdawi F, Crook A, Maidens J, et al. Lessons learnt from implementation of a Lynch syndrome screening program for patients with gynaecological malignancy. Pathology 2017;49(5):457–64.

[92] Musulen E, Sanz C, Munoz-Marmol AM, et al. Mismatch repair protein immunohistochemistry: a useful population screening strategy for Lynch syndrome. Hum Pathol 2014;45(7):1388–96.

[93] Perez-Carbonell L, Ruiz-Ponte C, Guarinos C, et al. Comparison between universal molecular screening for Lynch syndrome and revised Bethesda guidelines in a large population-based cohort of patients with colorectal cancer. Gut 2012;61(6):865–72.

[94] Adar T, Rodgers LH, Shannon KM, et al. Universal screening of both endometrial and colon cancers increases the detection of Lynch syndrome. Cancer 2018;124(15):3145–53.

[95] Moreira L, Balaguer F, Lindor N, et al. Identification of Lynch syndrome among patients with colorectal cancer. JAMA 2012;308(15):1555–65.

[96] Giardiello FM, Allen JI, Axilbund JE, et al. Guidelines on genetic evaluation and management of Lynch syndrome: a consensus statement by the US Multi-Society Task Force on colorectal cancer. Gastroenterology 2014;147(2):502–26.

[97] Syngal S, Brand RE, Church JM, et al. ACG clinical guideline: Genetic testing and management of hereditary gastrointestinal cancer syndromes. Am J Gastroenterol 2015;110(2):223–62 [quiz: 263].

[98] Stoffel EM, Mangu PB, Gruber SB, et al. Hereditary colorectal cancer syndromes: American Society of Clinical Oncology Clinical Practice Guideline endorsement of the familial risk-colorectal cancer: European Society for Medical Oncology Clinical Practice Guidelines. J Clin Oncol 2015;33(2):209–17.

[99] Frolova AI, Babb SA, Zantow E, et al. Impact of an immunohistochemistry-based universal screening protocol for Lynch syndrome in endometrial cancer on genetic counseling and testing. Gynecol Oncol 2015; 137(1):7–13.

[100] Watkins JC, Yang EJ, Muto MG, et al. Universal Screening for Mismatch-Repair Deficiency in Endometrial Cancers to Identify Patients With Lynch Syndrome and Lynch-like Syndrome. Int J Gynecol Pathol 2017; 36(2):115–27.

[101] Mills AM, Liou S, Ford JM, et al. Lynch syndrome screening should be considered for all patients with newly diagnosed endometrial cancer. Am J Surg Pathol 2014;38(11):1501–9.

[102] Backes FJ, Mitchell E, Hampel H, et al. Endometrial cancer patients and compliance with genetic counseling: room for improvement. Gynecol Oncol 2011;123(3): 532–6.

[103] Hamilton SR. Status of Testing for High-Level Microsatellite Instability/Deficient Mismatch Repair in Colorectal Carcinoma. JAMA Oncol 2018;4(2): e173574.

[104] Bertagnolli MM, Redston M, Compton CC, et al. Microsatellite instability and loss of heterozygosity at chromosomal location 18q: prospective evaluation of biomarkers for stages II and III colon cancer–a study of CALGB 9581 and 89803. J Clin Oncol 2011; 29(23):3153–62.

[105] Germano G, Amirouchene-Angelozzi N, Rospo G, et al. The Clinical Impact of the Genomic Landscape of Mismatch Repair-Deficient Cancers. Cancer Discov 2018;8(12):1518–28.

[106] Popat S, Hubner R, Houlston RS. Systematic review of microsatellite instability and colorectal cancer prognosis. J Clin Oncol 2005;23(3):609–18.

[107] Talhouk A, McConechy MK, Leung S, et al. Confirmation of ProMisE: A simple, genomics-based clinical classifier for endometrial cancer. Cancer 2017;123(5): 802–13.

[108] Bischoff J, Ignatov A, Semczuk A, et al. hMLH1 promoter hypermethylation and MSI status in human endometrial carcinomas with and without metastases. Clin Exp Metastasis 2012;29(8):889–900.

[109] McMeekin DS, Tritchler DL, Cohn DE, et al. Clinicopathologic Significance of Mismatch Repair Defects in Endometrial Cancer: An NRG Oncology/Gynecologic Oncology Group Study. J Clin Oncol 2016;34(25): 3062–8.

[110] Le DT, Durham JN, Smith KN, et al. Mismatch repair deficiency predicts response of solid tumors to PD-1 blockade. Science 2017;357(6349):409–13.

[111] Le DT, Uram JN, Wang H, et al. PD-1 Blockade in Tumors with Mismatch-Repair Deficiency. N Engl J Med 2015;372(26):2509–20.

[112] Marcus L, Lemery SJ, Keegan P, et al. FDA Approval Summary: Pembrolizumab for the Treatment of Microsatellite Instability-High Solid Tumors. Clin Cancer Res 2019;25(13):3753–8.

[113] FDA approves first cancer treatment for any solid tumor with a specific genetic feature. 2018. Available at: https://www.fda.gov/news-events/press-announcements/fda-approves-first-cancer-treatment-any-solid-tumor-specific-genetic-feature. Accessed March 18, 2020.

[114] FDA grants accelerated approval to pembrolizumab for first tissue/site agnostic indication. 2017. Available at: https://www.fda.gov/drugs/resources-information-approved-drugs/fda-grants-accelerated-approval-pembrolizumab-first-tissuesite-agnostic-indication. Accessed March 18, 2020.

[115] Ta RM, Hecht JL, Lin DI. Discordant loss of mismatch repair proteins in advanced endometrial endometrioid carcinoma compared to paired primary uterine tumors. Gynecol Oncol 2018;151(3):401–6.

[116] Shen X, Zhao B. Efficacy of PD-1 or PD-L1 inhibitors and PD-L1 expression status in cancer: meta-analysis. BMJ 2018;362:k3529.

[117] Planchard D, Popat S, Kerr K, et al. Metastatic non-small cell lung cancer: ESMO Clinical Practice Guidelines for diagnosis, treatment and follow-up. Ann Oncol 2018;29(Suppl 4):iv192–237.

[118] Herbst R, Lopes G, Kowalski M, et al. Association between tissue TMB (tTMB) and clinical outcomes with pembrolizumab monotherapy (pembro) in PD-L1-positive advanced NSCLC in the KEYNOTE-010 and -042 trials. Ann Oncol 2019;30(Suppl 5):v916–7.

[119] Paz-Ares L, Langer C, Novello S, et al. Pembrolizumab (pembro) plus platinum-based chemotherapy (chemo) for metastatic NSCLC: tissue TMB (tTMB) and outcomes in KEYNOTE-021, 189, and 407. Ann Oncol 2019;30(Suppl 5):v917–8.

Advances in Molecular Pathology 3 (2020) 189–198

ADVANCES IN MOLECULAR PATHOLOGY

PIK3CA and Breast Cancer

New Insights and Therapeutic Strategies

Andrea Ferreira-Gonzalez, PhD

Division Molecular Diagnostics, Department of Pathology, Virginia Commonwealth University, 403 North 13th Street, CSC Building 2nd Floor Room 247, Richmond, VA 23298-0248, USA

KEYWORDS

- Breast cancer • Hormone receptor • HER-2 • *PIK3CA* • PI3K tyrosine inhibitors • Real-time PCR
- Digital droplet PCR   • Next Generation Sequencing

KEY POINTS

- Due to the crucial role of PI3K, activating alterations in this signaling pathway is one of the most frequent genetic events in cancer and a major focus for drug development.
- Detection of *PIK3CA* mutations in refractory advanced breast cancer can help identify patients that could benefit from PI3K tyrosine kinase inhibitor treatment.
- Detection of *PIK3CA* mutations in cell-free tumor DNA is preferable for initial testing for eligibility for PI3K inhibitors.

INTRODUCTION

Breast cancer (BC) remains the most common cancer type among women in the world, affecting 12% of women. There were an estimated 268,600 new cases and 41,600 deaths in the United States in 2019. Despite significant advances in detection and treatment, BC remains the second leading cause of death for women in the United States, with most of the mortality attributed to the development of the metastatic disease. Breast malignancies are classified into 4 major clinical subtypes according to hormone (HR) and human epidermal growth factor receptor 2 (HER2) expression and triple-negative. Even though 5-year survival for localized BC is 98.7%, the 5-year survival rate for advanced BC (ABC) is a dismal 27%. More than 80% of BC is classified as hormone receptor-positive (HR+) BC [1]. These patients have benefited from significant scientific advances, and the fact that new targeted drug labels now include pharmacogenomics information constitutes evidence of it. Current therapeutic strategies for HR + BC comprise endocrine therapy (eg, tamoxifen, aromatase inhibitors), mammalian target of rapamycin (mTOR), or cyclin-dependent kinase 4/6 inhibition. These therapies have improved outcomes of patients, especially ABC, which compromises inoperable locally advanced and metastatic stage IV BC. Even though endocrine therapy is often initially successful in treating BC and ABC, disease progression, metastasis, and drug resistance develop eventually [2]. The mechanisms of endocrine resistance in HR + ABC are overexpression of HR, and diverse pathways (eg, *RAS/MAPK*, *NFKB*, or *PI3K/AKT/mTOR*) get involved in drug resistance to current therapy [3]. Phosphatidylinositol 3-kinase (PI3K)/AKT/mTOR is the most frequently altered pathway in HR + BC. With increasing treatment options for ABC, familiarity with the genomic landscape of BC and ABC, and how to incorporate tumor genomic findings onto patient care is critical.

E-mail address: andrea.ferreira-gonzalez@vcuhealth.org

https://doi.org/10.1016/j.yamp.2020.07.020

PHOSPHATIDYLINOSITOL 3-KINASES

PI3Ks are a highly conserved family of intracellular heterodimeric lipid kinases that regulate important cellular processes that respond to nutrition, growth factors, and other environmental cues. This plays a critical role in regulating many biological functions, including cell growth, proliferation, survival, differentiation, metabolism, motility, genomic stability, protein synthesis, and angiogenesis [1,3]. PIK3 is broadly divided into 3 classes (I–III) based on the structural and biochemical properties, such as substrate specificity. Class I PI3Ks is a heterodimer composed of a regulatory and a catalytic subunit that is known to drive oncogenesis. This class is further divided into subclasses IA and IB based on functional and structural biochemical differences. Class IA PI3Ks are heterodimers of a p100 catalytic subunit (α, β, γ, or δ) and a p85 regulatory subunit that receives upstream activation signals from the receptor tyrosine kinases and G protein-coupled receptors. The genes *PIK3CA*, *PIK3CB*, and *PIK3CD*, encode 3 highly homologous class IA catalytic isoforms: p100 α, p100 β, and p100 δ. Even though p100 α and β isoforms are very similar in their catalytic regulatory domains, they seem to play distinct roles in cellular signaling, growth, and tumorigenesis. Under normal physiologic conditions, activation of PI3K Class IA requires coupling to growth factors receptor tyrosine kinases (RTKs), including members of the human epidermal growth factor receptor (HER) family, and insulinlike growth factor 1 (IGF-1) receptor (Fig. 1). PI3K phosphorylates phosphatidylinositol 4,5-biphosphate (PIP_2) to phosphatidylinositol 3,4,5-triphosphate (PIP_3). The Src-homology 2 (SH2) domain serves to recruit the p85-p100 heterodimer to the plasma membrane, where its substrate PIP2 resides, as well as to relieve the basal inhibition of p110 by p85 and phosphorylates to PIP3. Accumulation of PIP_3 at the plasma membrane results in the recruitment of both AKT, a downstream serine/threonine kinase, and phosphoinositide-dependent kinase 1 (PDK1), an essential enzyme for the phosphorylation of AKT at Ser 308. Once phosphorylated, AKT interacts with many different effectors, including the TSC complex, constitutive inhibitor of mTORC1, thereby regulating RNA translation, cell growth, autophagy, and protein synthesis. A suppressor of this pathway is the tumor suppressor protein phosphatase and tensin homolog (PTEN), which catalyzes the de-phosphorylation of PIP3 to PIP2. Cellular PIP3 levels depend, therefore, on the competition between PI3K and PTEN [1,4].

Because of the crucial role of PI3K, activating alterations in the PI3K signaling is one of the most frequent genetic events in cancer and a major focus for drug development. In the wild-type PI3K holoenzyme, p85 inhibits p100α through an intermolecular interaction, and its inhibition is relieved by a conformational change induced by the engagement of the p85 aminoterminal SH2 domain with phosphotyrosines. Two classes of *PIK3CA* mutations promote PI3K signaling through distinct mechanisms. Somatic activating mutations were identified in the class A PI3K catalytic subunit, p100α in various solid malignancies. Most of the mutations cluster in the helical and kinase domain, including the 3 hot spot mutations, E545K, E542K in exon 9, DH1047R/L in exon 20, which activate the PI3K enzyme activity, leading to constitutive, unopposed phosphorylation of AKT and its downstream effectors. Both types of mutations were shown to be gain-of-function mutations and have transforming capacity. Exon 9 mutations are in the helical domain of the p100α, and mimic activation by RTK phosphopeptides and are dependent on RAS, which is considered to facilitate p100 alpha escape from the inhibitory effect of p85 via the SH2 domain. Exon 20 mutations are located near the activation loop in the kinase domain and increase lipid membrane binding promoting access to PIP_2 substrate and are Ras-independent [5,6].

The Relevance of *PIK3CA* Mutations in Breast Cancer

Alterations in the PI3K signaling pathway play essential roles in tumor initiation and survival, angiogenesis, and development of resistance to cancer therapies [7]. Mutations in the *PIK3CA* have been associated with resistance to endocrine therapy, HER2-directed therapy, and cytotoxic therapy. Many retrospective studies, including a large meta-analysis of more than 10,000 patients, found that *PIK3CA* mutations are commonly found in several types of BC. The clinical incidence of *PIK3CA* mutation differs according to BC subtype. The incidence has ranged from 28% to 47% in HR+ primary and ABC, 23% to 33% in HER2+ breast, and 8% to 25% in basal-like triple-negative BC. Although *PIK3CA* alterations appear to be associated with the presence of HR expression, the associations with prognostic outcomes have not been consistent and could also differ according to BC types. In a recent study of 590 patients with primary invasive BC (all subtypes, nearly all stage I-I disease) who had undergone surgery for primary BC, the presence of *PIK3CA* mutations conferred significant improvement in overall survival and BC-specific survival. The association between

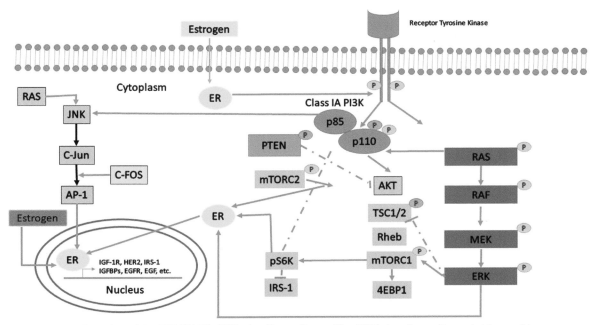

FIG. 1 Overview of the PI3K/AKT/mTOR signaling pathway. The PI3K signaling pathway is triggered by activation of receptor tyrosine kinase. Activating nodes (PI3K, AKT, PDK1, mTORC1, and mTORC2) and negative regulators (PTEN, TSC complex) are highlighted. Interaction with RAS and LKB1/AMPK pathways is also displayed.

PIK3CA mutation and a positive prognosis was further supported by a large pooled analysis of 19 cohorts with 10,319 patients with early-stage BC. However, the investigators found a weaker association on multivariate analysis compared with that found on univariate analysis, perhaps owing to the association of PIK3C mutations with favorable characteristics. In contrast, in a meta-analysis of 1929 patients with BC (all subtypes and various disease stages) who had received neoadjuvant chemotherapy, antiHER2 therapy, endocrine therapy, or a combination of these, the presence of *PIK3CA* mutations was associated with reduced progression-free survival, disease-free survival, and overall survival. The patient population in the meta-analysis was highly diverse, with different disease stages and multiple treatment lines and treatment types, in contrast to other studies that had included primary tissue from patients with earlier disease stage [8–15].

Several studies have evaluated the correlation of *PIK3CA* mutations with clinicopathological parameters, such as estrogen receptor (ER)/progesterone receptor (PR) positivity, the presence of lymph node metastases, and response to therapy in BC. Saal and colleagues [16]

were the first to report a definite clinical-pathological correlate of *PIK3CA* mutations in BC. They reported that *PIK3CA* mutations were frequently seen in tumors with typically expressed PTEN, ER, PR, and ERBB2 genes, as well as in tumors with nodal involvement. In a recent study, Wu and colleagues [17] showed that *PIK3CA* mutations were positively associated with ER + PR+ and low Ki67 labeling index and negatively correlated with the triple-negative BC subtype. *PIK3CA* mutations were not associated with the age of diagnosis, tumor stage, lymph node status, tumor size, or HER2 status. Various contradictory studies exist regarding the effect of *PIK3CA* mutation status on disease prognosis; *PIK3CA* mutations were reported to be correlated with poor survival rates. Barbareschi and colleagues [18] reported different effects based on mutation loci. They reported that those in exon 9 are associated with poor prognosis, whereas those occurring in exon 20 are associated with better prognosis. Deng and colleagues [19] demonstrated that *PIK3CA* mutation significantly reduced disease-free survival compared with wild-type *PIK3CA* in patients with ER+ tumors. Subsequent studies reported that *PIK3CA* mutations were highly associated with morphology, race, ER status, PR status, and HER2 status in BC. Furthermore, co-mutations of TP53 and PIK3CA were found to be associated with poor survival in residual disease after neoadjuvant chemotherapy in BC [15]. Also, studies have reported exon 9 mutations independently associated with early recurrence and death, whereas exon 20 PIK3CA mutations are associated with optimal prognosis. A contrary report highlighted that there is no association of PIK3CA mutation status with a prognosis of BC. Another important clinicopathological correlate of PIK3CA mutation is that they are more frequently found in lobular BCs as compared with ductal BCs. Barbareschi and colleagues [18] reported that this observation was specific for patients with exon 9 mutations. PIK3CA mutations have also been correlated with response to therapy in BC. An analysis of the outcomes and molecular landscape of patients with PIK3CA mutated metastatic BC from the SAFIR02 trials showed that patients with PIK3CA-mutated hormone receptor-positive/HER2 negative tumors have a poor outcome and resistance to chemotherapy [20].

HER2 is amplified/overexpressed in approximately 20% to 25% of BC cases and is associated with increased tumor aggressiveness. Although trastuzumab has provided significant clinical benefits to patients with HER2+ BC, de novo or acquired resistance to HER2 therapies remains a major obstacle. PI3K is the major pathway downstream of HER2, and PIK3CA mutations occur in nearly 25% of HER2+ BC cases. These PK3CA mutations can confer resistance to HR-2 targeted therapy and has been associated with poorer outcomes. Berns and colleagues reported that mutations in PIK3CA make BC resistant to antibody-based therapeutics trastuzumab. Overactivation of the PIK3CA due to oncogenic mutations rendered BC cells refractory to the anti-HER2 agent Lapatinib. PIK3CA mutations were shown to reduce sensitivity to neoadjuvant chemotherapy [12,14].

Patients with PIK3CA-mutated triple-negative BC present a better overall survival. This could be explained by the enrichment of PIK3CA mutations in luminal BC, which lost HR expression in the metastatic setting. A total of 649 patients with metastatic BC (MBC) from the SAFIR02 trial had PIK3CA mutational status available. The prognostic value of fPIK3CA mutations during chemotherapy was assessed in plasma samples from 44 patients by next-generation sequencing (NGS) and digital polymerase chain reaction (PCR). PIK3CA mutations were found in 28% of HR+/HER2− tumors and 10% of Triple Negative breast cancer (TNBC).

PIK3CA-mutated HR+/HER2− MBC was less sensitive to chemotherapy and presented worse overall survival compared with PIK3CA wild type. In metastatic TNBC, the median overall survival in patients with PIK3CA mutations was 24 versus 14 months for the PIK3CA wild type [17,19].

PI3K tyrosine kinase inhibitors

Given that hyperactivation of the PI3K pathway is one of the most common signaling abnormalities observed in BC, a substantial effort has been made to develop agents targeting this signaling cascade, particularly for HR+ BC. There are several general classes of agents that target the PI3K network: pan-PI3K inhibitors, isoform-specific PI3K inhibitors [21–24]. One of the major recent advances in treating HR+ metastatic BC has been the US Food and Drug Administration (FDA) approval of alpelisib (Piqray, Novartis). Alpelisib is an alfa-specific phosphoinositidide 3-kinase (PI3K) inhibitor that was approved for use in combination with fulvestrant (Faslodex, AstraZeneca) in patients with HR+, HER2− advanced or metastatic BC that tests positive for the PIK3CA mutation. The approval of alpelisib was based on the results of phase III SOLAR-1 trial. The study was enriched with tumors harboring a PIK3CA mutation but included a cohort of PIK3CA wild type as a proof of concept of activity in this group. Patients were stratified before randomization by PIK3CA mutation status. The addition of alpelisib to fulvestrant resulted in a significant improvement in progression-free survival (PFS) in this subgroup, increasing from 5.7 months in the placebo arm to 11.0 months in the alpelisib arm (hazard ratio 0.65; $P = .0065$). Furthermore, in patients with measurable disease and PIK3CA mutations, the overall response was markedly better in the alpelisib group than in the placebo group, at 35.7% versus 16.2%, respectively [25].

More recently, preliminary studies trying to elucidate the mechanism for PI3Ki resistance have been recently published. The study by Razavi and colleagues [26] attempted to interpret the spatial and temporal distribution of discrete genomic alterations that mediate resistance to PIK3CA PI3Ki therapy from samples acquired during a clinical trial of alpelisib in combination with letrozole or exemestane treatment in HR+ ABC. They performed analyses from tumors, and longitudinal circulating free tumor DNA (ctDNA) from patients enrolled in the study. They were able to determine that patients who progressed after only 2 months on therapy had pretreatment and posttreatment preexisting PTEN loss of function as well as ESR1 mutations that helped accelerate tumor progression. Furthermore, additional genomic alterations in *PTEN* and *ERS1* acquired during treatment might have led to the PI3Ki resistance. Resistance to PI3Ki could be mediated by activation of alternative pathways that drive cell proliferation (MAPK, ER, HER2, AXL, PIM-1, FOXO transcription factors); by signaling via other PI3K isoforms when specific subunits are blocked; by activation of downstream effectors in the PI3K pathway such as AKT and mTOR; by loss of regulation of PI3K signaling such as PTEN; or by epigenetics cross-talk between PI3K and ER pathways, resulting in upregulation of the ER-dependent transcription on PI3K inhibition (see Fig. 1). Considering these findings, *PIK3CA* mutations alone might not always predict sensitivity to PI3Ki, perhaps owing to the presence of simultaneous mutations mediating resistance. Ongoing research into the mechanism of primary and secondary resistance to PI3Ki should lead to novel clinical trial strategies and patient stratification [26].

Detection of PIK3CA mutations

Several technologies have been developed and evaluated in different settings as to their ability to detect mutations in the *PIK3CA* gene. These technologies include droplet digital PCR (BioRad, Hercules, CA), BEAMing (Beads, Emulsion, Amplification, Magnetics digital PCR) technology (Inostics Sysmex, Hamburg, Germany), real-time PCR such as therascreen *PIK3CA* RGQ mutation detection (Qiagen, Manchester, Ltd, Hilden, Germany), cobas *PIK3CA* (Roche, Moyaland, France), NGS such as Illumina (San Diego, CA) based assays and Oncomine pan-cancer (ThermoFisher, Waltham, MA); and laboratory-developed tests (LDT) such as the FDA cleared Foundation One CDx (Foundation Medicine, Cambridge, MA) and Guardant 360 (Guardant Health, Redwood City, CA) among others [27–32] (Table 1).

Currently, high-sensitivity PCR assays are suitable for the detection of genomic alterations at high sensitivity and specificity. These include real-time

---

TABLE 1
Comparison of Strengths and Limitations of Technologies for PIK3CA Mutation Detection

Categories of Genotyping Technologies	Type of Alterations	Advantages	Disadvantages
PCR-based			
Real-time PCR	SNV, small indels	Ease of use Lower cost	Lower sensitivity Only detects limited genomic alterations and loci
ARMS-Scorpions	SNV, small indels	Ease of use Lower cost	Lower sensitivity Only detects limited genomic alterations and loci
Digital PCR-based			
BEAMing	SNV	Moderate complexity High sensitivity	Only detects limited genomic alterations and loci
Droplet-based digital PCR	SNV	Moderate complexity High sensitivity	Only detects limited genomic alterations and loci
Microfluidic digital PCR	SNV	Moderate complexity High sensitivity	Only detects limited genomic alterations and loci
Targeted deep sequencing			
Panel PCR-NGS targeted	SNV, indels, CNV	High complexity When using molecular barcodes- High sensitivity	Expensive Low sensitivity Needs Bioinformatics support
Hybridization NGS targeted	SNV, indels, CNV	High complexity When using molecular barcodes- High sensitivity	Expensive Low sensitivity Needs bioinformatics support

Abbreviations: ARMS, amplification-refractory mutation system; BEAMing, beads, emulsion, amplification, magnetics; indel, insertion-deletion; CNV, copy number variation; NGS, next-generation sequencing; PCR, polymerase chain reaction; SNV, single-nucleotide variant.

quantitative PCR-based techniques such as the Intplex Q-PCR method and amplification-refractory mutations system (ARMS), among others. The ARMS assay is based on the use of sequence-specific PCR primers to identify single base changes or small deletions. Because the primers only work when they are complementary to a given DNA sequence, except for the 3-terminus, amplification is observed only if the target is contained within a sample. Digital PCR technology has been used with great success, and recent advances such as digital droplet PCR (ddPCR) have deeply enhanced the sensitivity for detection of point mutations at low allelic fractions (0.01% vs 5% in the previous techniques). ddPCR is characterized by the discretization and amplification of each DNA template in a single emulsion droplet. The separation of DNA molecules in many compartments through a microfluidic system enables high-throughput analysis by reducing the reaction volume for each compartment to nano/picoliter scale. By creating individual reaction chambers, the cross-contamination between neighboring compartments could be avoided to achieve precise quantification of targets in each sample. ddPCR is limited by its inability to detect unknown genotypes or rearrangements and difficulty multiplexing to determine the number of genetic variants. BEAMing is an alternative sensitive approach that provides molecular information about mutations with a frequency of more than 1/100. This technology allows for the detection of single-nucleotide variants, duplications, insertions, and deletions. It combines emulsion PCR with magnetic beads and flow cytometry for the detection and quantitation of target DNA copies. After the amplification step, each droplet contains a bead that is coated with thousands of copies of a single DNA molecule. Then, the beads are magnetically recovered and analyzed within minutes using flow cytometry or optimal scanning instruments. In this way, the DNA diversity present in the template population can be accurately characterized and used to determine the fraction of mutated DNA.

Amplicon-capture NGS allows for the detection of single-base substitutions, duplications, insertions, and deletions and consists of multiplexed PCR amplification of regions of interest, followed by NGS and a bioinformatic analysis. In hybridization-capture NGS, genomic DNA fragments are hybridized to specific probes and amplified. This technology allows for the detection of all the genomic alterations that amplicon-capture NGS detects and for exon duplications, deletions, and gene copy number changes. NGS allows for the detection of new or rare somatic variants with reasonable sensitivity. However, the potential

exists for false-negative results owing to low copies of mutated in patients with small tumors. However, it is expensive and requires sophisticated bioinformatic analyses of the data outputs. Description of NGS and modification have been covered in other articles.

Tissue-based detection of PIK3CA mutations

Detection of PIK3CA mutations in paraffin-embedded tissue has been performed by different methods from real-time PCR and ddPCR to more advanced and comprehensive NGS methods. Although studies on the diagnostic performance of these platforms have been published and even approved by the US FDA, there is yet no gold standard method available against which to evaluate these evolving tests. High sensitivity, specificity, and concordance using formalin-fixed paraffin-embedded (FFPE) tissue-based testing have been observed with the FDA-cleared CDx therascreen PIK3CA RGQ PCR compared with a hybrid capture NGS LDT assay used as part of the SOLAR I clinical trial. The FDA cleared a companion diagnostic test, the therascreen PIK3CA RGQ PCR (Qiagen) that detects 11 mutations in the PIK3CA gene in exon 7, 9, and 20. The accuracy of the assay for FFPE tissue was established by comparing the results of 379 cases tested with an LDT NGS assay with a positive percent agreement (PPA) of 99%, a negative percent agreement (NPA) of 90% for an overall percent agreement (OPA) of 94% [25]. These results have also been observed in other studies, which tend to indicate that NGS-based assays might be more sensitive compared with PCR-based assays, as they can detect common mutations and also a spectrum of alterations. Further studies with 3 different real-time PCR assays for detection of PIK3CA mutations (cobas PIK3CA mutation test) and 2 LDT assays (PCR amplification-refractory mutation system Scorpio ARMS and high-resolution melting curve PCR) found similar results [28].

It has been demonstrated that PIK3CA mutations can be acquired during disease progression. Analysis of mutational profiles of primary breast tissue and paired metastases in one study (n = 23) found high interpatient mutational concordance in most patients [27]. Another study assessed PIK3CA mutation status in exon 9 and/or exon 20 in tumor tissue samples from primary and paired asynchronous metastatic lesions from 104 patients. The frequency of PIK3CA mutations in the primary tumors was 45% compared with 53% in the paired metastatic tumors. One-third of these patients had different mutational status in their primary and asynchronous metastatic lesions, with a change to mutant from wild type predominantly. That analysis was subsequently supported by the conclusions of another study, which reported that the overall percentage of *PIK3CA* mutations (determined from tissue samples; n = 19) between the primary and metastatic lesions was similar (40.4% vs 42.0%, respectively). However, both gain (8%) and loss (10%) of *PIK3CA* mutations were detected in individual patients [33,34]. Although these conclusions are limited by the small sample sizes and potential differences in testing methodologies, discordance between primary and metastatic tumor testing could have important clinical implications to consider.

Caveats

Tumor biopsy is still considered the gold standard for the retrieval of crucial diagnostic, prognostic, and predictive information in diagnostic pathology. Notwithstanding that positive evidence supports traditional biopsy, several caveats often limit this procedure, hindering a precision-medicine approach. Tumor tissue is limited by sample availability and biopsy procedure risk. The static nature of this technique represents one of the primary limits because it is not able to capture both the inherent biological heterogeneity of the tumor and the dynamic adaptations caused by anticancer treatments. Moreover, because of intratumoral heterogeneity, the use of tumor tissue to obtain an accurate genomic landscape of BC could be challenging. Accurate determination of the genomic landscape of breast tumors is essential to identify driver mutations that may make them susceptible to targeted antitumor agents, but also to determine whether subclones within the metastasis subsequently acquire additional mutations that render the lesion drug-resistant, leading to disease progression. Metastatic lesions are unlike primary tumors, generally not surgically accessible, and must be treated with systematic therapies. The predictive value of alterations in *PIK3CA* might depend on the timing of the tissue collection and the technology used to determine molecular alteration status. It has been suggested that analyses of biomarkers should focus on both primary tumors and metastatic lesions to account for inherent disease heterogeneity, which only increases with disease progression. Moreover, longitudinal or simultaneous multisite testing is simply not feasible due to the clinical complications associated with seriate tissue sampling and its effects on a patient's quality of life.

Circulating free tumor DNA

ctDNA has recently emerged as a sensitive, minimally invasive tool to evaluate the *PIK3CA* mutation status of a tumor [31]. Compared with archival tumor tissue, ctDNA mutational analysis can provide a more dynamic assessment of tumor heterogeneity, because it putatively integrates DNA shed from multiple tumor sites. As body fluids can easily be obtained, liquid biopsy is considered a noninvasive and repeatable test that allows a dynamic assessment of specific molecular markers capable of intercepting the onset of disease recurrence or treatment and potentially predict treatment response and prognosis. Cell-free DNA (cfDNA) is released from both normal and cancer cells into the circulation. A rapid turnover of tumor cells is thought to result in a consistently increased release of ctDNA. Tumor cells actively release several types of nucleic acids, including DNA, that is, cfDNA and ctDNA, microRNAs, noncoding RNA, and microvesicles such as exosomes as a result of their spread both as single cells or clusters. The ctDNA amount is influenced by the extent of the distribution, including tumor burden. Generally, very little tumor DNA is present in the circulation in early-stage BC compared with other advanced stages [32]. The development of novel high-throughput technologies has already brought liquid approaches to the standard treatment of solid tumors, demonstrating their utility for a tissue-free cancer characterization.

Liquid biopsy has the potential to overcome several practical issues, such as hardly accessible primary and metastatic lesions, patients' refusal to invasive procedures, not feasible serial sampling, or inadequate material for molecular analysis. The analysis of ctDNA has the potential to capture both biological heterogeneity of the advanced disease and the dynamic adaptations caused by anticancer treatments. However, the detection frequency of actionable mutations and the consistency between different analytical approaches and platforms are still much debated.

Kodahl and colleagues [35] analyzed the presence of *PIK3CA* mutations in FFPE metastatic tissue, and corresponding ctDNA in the serum of patients with advanced BC using a highly sensitive, optimized ddPCR assay. Interestingly, they found that 83% of patients with *PIK3CA* mutation in metastatic tumor tissue had detectable *PIK3CA* mutations in corresponding serum ctDNA [35]. Similar studies were carried out in the SOLAR-1 clinical trial. The plasma results were compared with the tissue results for a total of 328 patients. Agreement between the plasma and tissue results were calculated using the tissue results as a reference. The point estimates were 55% for PPA, 97% for NPA, and 72% for OPA. Further clinical utility analysis for the positive plasma patients showed an estimated 46% risk reduction in disease progression or death (hazard ratio 0.54, 95% confidence interval [CI] 0.33–0.88) PFS for the alpelisib in combination with fulvestrant arm compared with the placebo plus fulvestrant arm. In comparison, the PFS HR in the therascreen PIK3CA RGQ tissue positive population was 0.65 (95% CI 0.50–0.85) in the SOLAR-1 PIK3CA mutant cohort [25]. The PFS for the patients who had tissue and plasma positive results was 0.53 (95% CI 0.33–0.84). Concordance of the plasma therascreen PIK3CA RGQ with the tissue results for NPA was 97% and demonstrated a low risk of false positives. This might be because of the amount of ctDNA that could be influenced by the extent of the disease, including tumor burden. Generally, very little tumor DNA is present in the circulation in early-stage BCs compared with advanced stages [25]. However, ctDNA containing PIK3CA mutations has been suggested to be a promising biomarker of patients with cancer with advanced disease both for the early detection of recurrence and to monitor treatment response.

Studies with ctDNA compared with tissue-based mutational analysis using an NGS-based assay showed a 75% concordance among 13 of 17 cases studied. Additional studies carried out in the BELLE-2 and BELLE-3 clinical trials using the BEAMining PCR assay, showed similar concordance of PIK3CA mutation status using this method in ctDNA and tumor tissue analysis (77% and 83%, respectively) [36]. More recently, in the SOLAR I phase III clinical trial, the therascreen PIK3CA RGQ PCR assay was able to detect ctDNA mutations in 75% of the patients whose tissue carried a PIK3CA mutation (PPA 55%, NPA 97%, and OPA 72%) [25]. Furthermore, a subgroup analysis from the SOLAR I phase III clinical trial evaluated PFS by PIK3CA mutation in ctDNA that resulted in an even more significant clinical benefit compared with Tissue based testing (median PFS from 3.7 months to 10.9 months). Negative results in plasma specimens with positive tissue results were associated with a low allelic fraction in tissue specimens. On the other hand, negative results in tissue samples with positive plasma results were associated with tumor heterogeneity or tumor evolution. Based on these results, the easy accessibility of ctDNA and the good correlation of PIK3CA mutation status determined by ctDNA and tumor tissue makes it plausible to use ctDNA initially and to carry out mutation testing for PIK3CA in the tumor tissue in the case of ctDNA negativity.

To demonstrate the accuracy of the therascreen PIK3CA RGQ assay in ctDNA, a study was conducted with plasma specimens from the SOLAR-1 clinical trial relative to a validated NGS assay. The therascreen PIK3CA RGQ and the NGS assay were analyzed for 542 samples, which showed a 97.39% PPA, a 91.26% NPA for an overall 92.99% overall agreement. Considering these findings, the FDA recommended to carry out the test in ctDNA initially, and if the test is negative for PIK3CA mutations in plasma, patients should undergo testing for PIK3CA mutations in tumor tissue. A subgroup analysis for the SOLAR-1 phase III trial evaluating PFS by PIK3CA mutational analysis status measured in ctDNA observed that assessing mutational status via liquid biopsy resulted in an even more significant clinical benefit compared with a tissue biopsy, with improvements of median PFS from 3.7 months to 10.9 months. Indeed, although patients with PIK3CA mutations evaluated in tissue sample had a 35% reduction in risk for disease progression, the risk reduction was 45% for the patients with PIK3CA mutations identified in ctDNA [25].

Moreover, in the combined analysis from the BELLE-2 and BELLE-3 clinical trials, PIK3CA-mutant tumors derived more benefit from buparlisib treatment as compared with PIK3CA wild type. However, this benefit seemed to be numerically higher when the PIK3CA mutation was identified by BEAMing in ctDNA as compared with those identified by PCR in tumor tissue. Based on these results, the easy accessibility of ctDNA and the excellent correlation of PIK3CA mutation status determined by ctDNA and tissue tumor makes it plausible to use ctDNA initially and to carry out testing from tissue in case of ctDNA negativity [35]. Subsequent studies by Gerratana and colleagues [37] compared tests with similar analytical capabilities with an established clinically validated ctDNA testing platform to investigate concordance in the detection of genomic abnormalities of samples from patients with metastatic BC. The investigators evaluated plasma form 15 patients with MBC using NGS high-throughput technologies to compare the performance of the Guardant 360 NGS-based assay (Guardant Health Inc, Redwood City, CA) with the PredicinePlus (Predicine Inc, Hayward, CA). The comparison of both technologies was investigated across the most frequently mutated genes, and a high agreement was observed for all genes ($k = 1$–0.81 with P values ranging from $P = 0.001$ to $P = 0.0001$) [37].

Furthermore, some cases and limited studies have supported the potential use of ctDNA mutation assessment as a minimally invasive method to identify the current molecular status of tumor burden and to detect changes that might be occurring over time [38,39].

Caveats

The sensitivity of the cfDNA sequencing can depend on the amount of tumor DNA shedding, which can be influenced by disease type, tumor burden, and therapy. It has been suggested that cfDNA may account for tumor heterogeneity by potentially capturing genomic alterations present at multiple sites compared with tissue sampling, which is limited from a single biopsy site. Another issue relates to the timing of the assessment: most clinical trials tested biomarkers on archived tissue, usually the primary breast tumor.

As already mentioned, given that *PIK3CA* mutations can be acquired with disease progression, it is generally recommended that testing of ctDNA be performed as the first step in the evaluation. One of the advantages of ctDNA is that it is present in peripheral blood and can be obtained by normal venipuncture. Although this is considered a minimally invasive procedure, it still has preanalytical requirements that are needed to ensure the quality of the ctDNA. ctDNA is smaller fragments of DNA, usually166 base pairs in length, that are released from tumor cells due to necrosis, apoptosis, or active release from viable tumor cells in the circulation. When blood is collected in EDTA tubes and stored, the white blood cells begin to lyse and release genomic wild-type DNA into the sample in quantities typically folds higher than the ctDNA is present. This makes the detection of mutations or other ctDNA biomarkers more difficult. The use of commercially available cell stabilization tubes can prevent or delay the lysis of white cells, thereby reducing the dilution effect of the ctDNA [40].

SUMMARY

The PI3K pathway is the most frequently mutated in BC. These mutations lead to hyperactivation of kinase activity of the PI3K pathway, resulting in deregulated cell proliferation. Also, these mutations have implications in the effectiveness of treatment and prognosis of early and metastatic BC. However, the prognostic and predictive value of these mutations remains unclear at present. Different clinical trials and, in particular, for alpelisib have successfully reported usefulness for PI3K inhibitors in ABC, showing a significant positive association with prognostic parameters, such as PFS and OS. More extensive prospective studies should be conducted further to elucidate the role of PIK3CA mutations in BC. Further studies and standardized testing practices are required to better characterize alterations in *PIK3CA* during BC progression. ctDNA has recently emerged as a sensitive, minimally invasive tool to evaluate the *PIK3CA* mutation status of a tumor. Failure to reassess *PIK3CA* status and to reevaluate treatment suitability in the metastatic setting could result in the exclusion of individual therapeutic options (ie, a patient with newly acquired *PIK3CA* mutations might benefit from PI3K-targeted therapy), which could substantially alter the clinical outcomes.

DISCLOSURE

The author has nothing to disclose.

REFERENCES

[1] Li A, Schleicher SM, Andre F, et al. Genomic alteration in metastatic breast cancer and its treatment. Am Soc Clin Oncol Educ Book 2020;40:1–14.

[2] Tarantino P, Morganti S, Curigliano G. Biologic therapy for advanced breast cancer: recent advances and future directions. Expert Opin Biol Ther 2020;21:1–15.

[3] Giridhar KV, Liu MC. Available and emerging molecular markers in the clinical management of breast cancer. Expert Rev Mol Diagn 2019;19:919–28.

[4] Verret B, Cortes J, Bachelot T, et al. Efficacy of PI3K inhibitors in advanced breast cancer. Ann Oncol 2019; 30(Suppl 10):x12–20.

[5] Brandão M, Caparica R, Eiger D, et al. Biomarkers of response and resistance to PI3K inhibitors in estrogen receptor-positive breast cancer patients and combination therapies involving PI3K inhibitors. Ann Oncol 2019; 30(Suppl 10):x27–42.

[6] Schwartzberg LS, Vidal GA. Targeting PIK3CA alterations in hormone receptor-positive, human epidermal growth factor receptor-2-negative advanced breast cancer: new therapeutic approaches and practical considerations. Clin Breast Cancer 2020 S1526-8209(20)30032-X.

[7] Vasan N, Toska E, Scaltriti M. Overview of the relevance of PI3K pathway in HR-positive breast cancer. Ann Oncol 2019;30(Suppl 10):x3–11.

[8] Condorelli R, Mosele F, Verret B, et al. Turner NC genomic alterations in breast cancer: level of evidence for actionability according to ESMO Scale for Clinical Actionability of molecular Targets (ESCAT). Ann Oncol 2019;30:365–73.

[9] Wang M, Li J, Huang J, et al. The predictive role of *PIK3CA* mutation status on *PI3K* inhibitors in *HR+* breast cancer therapy: a systematic review and meta-analysis. Biomed Res Int 2020;2020:1598037.

[10] Zardavas D, Te Marvelde L, Milne RL, et al. Tumor PIK3CA genotype and prognosis in early-stage breast cancer: a pooled analysis of individual patient data. J Clin Oncol 2018;36:981–90.

[11] Sobhani N, Roviello G, Corona SP, et al. The prognostic value of PI3K mutational status in breast cancer: a meta-analysis. J Cell Biochem 2018;1:4287–92.

[12] Alqahtani A, Ayesh HSK, Halawani H. PIK3CA gene mutations in solid malignancies: association with clinico-pathological parameters and prognosis. Cancers (Basel) 2019;12:93.

[13] Dirican E, Akkiprik M, Özer A. Mutation distributions and clinical correlations of PIK3CA gene mutations in breast cancer. Tumour Biol 2016;37:7033–45.

[14] Dey N, De P, Leyland-Jones B. PI3K-AKT-mTOR inhibitors in breast cancers: from tumor cell signaling to clinical trials. Pharmacol Ther 2017;175:91–106.

[15] Shatsky R, Parker BA, Bui NQ, et al. Next-generation sequencing of tissue and circulating tumor DNA: the UC San Diego Moores Center for Personalized Cancer Therapy Experience with Breast Malignancies. Mol Cancer Ther 2019;18:1001–11.

[16] Saal LH, Holm K, Maurer M, et al. PIK3CA mutations correlate with hormone receptors, node metastasis, and ERBB2, and are mutually exclusive with PTEN loss in human breast carcinoma. Cancer Res 2005;65(7):2554–9.

[17] Wu H, Wang W, Du J, et al. The distinct clinicopathological and prognostic implications of PIK3CA mutations in breast cancer patients from Central China. Cancer Manag Res 2019;11:1473–92.

[18] Barbareschi M, Buttitta F, Felicioni L, et al. Different prognostic roles of mutations in the helical and kinase domains of the PIK3CA gene in breast carcinomas. Clin Cancer Res 2007;13(20):6064–9.

[19] Deng L, Chen J, Zhong XR, et al. Correlation between activation of PI3K/AKT/mTOR pathway and prognosis of breast cancer in Chinese women. PLoS One 2015; 10(3):e0120511.

[20] Mosele F, Stefanovska B, Lusque A, et al. Outcome and molecular landscape of patients with PIK3CA-mutated metastatic breast cancer. Ann Oncol 2020;31:377–86.

[21] Ellis H, Ma CX. PI3K inhibitors in breast cancer therapy. Curr Oncol Rep 2019;2:110.

[22] Juric D, Janku F, Rodón J, et al. Alpelisib plus fulvestrant in PIK3CA-altered and PIK3CA-wild-type estrogen receptor-positive advanced breast cancer: a phase 1b clinical trial. JAMA Oncol 2019;5:e184475.

[23] Mayer IA, Abramson VG, Formisano L, et al. A phase Ib study of alpelisib (BYL719), a PI3Kα-specific inhibitor, with letrozole in ER+/HER2- metastatic breast cancer. Clin Cancer Res 2017;23:26–34.

[24] Mayer IA, Prat A, Egle D, et al. A phase II randomized study of neoadjuvant letrozole plus alpelisib for hormone receptor-positive, human epidermal growth factor receptor 2-negative breast cancer (NEO-ORB). Clin Cancer Res 2019;25:2975–87.

[25] André F, Ciruelos E, Rubovszky G, et al, SOLAR-1 Study Group. Alpelisib for PIK3CA-mutated, hormone receptor-positive advanced breast cancer. N Engl J Med 2019;380:1929–40.

[26] Razavi P, Dickler MN, Shah PD, et al. Alterations in *PTEN* and *ESR1* promote clinical resistance to alpelisib plus aromatase inhibitors. Nature Cancer 2020;1: 382–93.

[27] Shimoi T, Hamada A, Yamagishi M, et al. PIK3CA mutation profiling in patients with breast cancer, using a highly sensitive detection system. Cancer Sci 2018;109(8): 2558–66.

[28] Lambert A, Salleron J, Lion M, et al. Comparison of three real-time PCR assays for the detection of PIK3CA somatic mutations in formalin-fixed paraffin embedded tissues of patients with breast carcinomas. Pathol Oncol Res 2019;25(3):1117–23.

[29] O'Leary B, Hrebien S, Beaney M, et al. Comparison of BEAMing and droplet digital PCR for circulating tumor DNA analysis. Clin Chem 2019;65:1405–13.

[30] Buono G, Gerratana L, Bulfoni M, et al. Circulating tumor DNA analysis in breast cancer: is it ready for prime time? Cancer Treat Rev 2019;73:73–83.

[31] Tay TKY, Tan PH. Liquid biopsy in breast cancer: a focused review. Arch Pathol Lab Med 2020;10:5858.

[32] Rossi G, Mu Z, Rademaker AW, et al. Cell-free DNA and circulating tumor cells: comprehensive liquid biopsy analysis in advanced breast cancer. Clin Cancer Res 2018;24:560–8.

[33] Bertucci F, Finetti P, Guille A, et al. Comparative genomic analysis of primary tumors and metastases in breast cancer. Oncotarget 2016;7(19):27208–19.

[34] Chae YK, Davis AA, Jain S, et al. Concordance of genomic alterations by next-generation sequencing in tumor tissue versus circulating tumor DNA in breast cancer. Mol Cancer Ther 2017;16:1412–20.

[35] Kodahl AR, Ehmsen S, Pallisgaard N, et al. Correlation between circulating cell-free PIK3CA tumor DNA levels and treatment response in patients with PIK3CA-mutated metastatic breast cancer. Mol Oncol 2018;12: 925–35.

[36] Nathan MR, Schmid P. A review of fulvestrant in breast cancer. Oncol Ther 2017;5(1):17–29.

[37] Gerratana L, Zhang Q, Shah AN, et al. Performance of a novel next generation sequencing circulating tumor DNA (ctDNA) platform for the evaluation of samples from patients with metastatic breast cancer (MBC). Crit Rev Oncol Hematol 2020;145:102856.

[38] Chung JH, Pavlick D, Hartmaier R, et al. Hybrid capture-based genomic profiling of circulating tumor DNA from patients with estrogen receptor-positive metastatic breast cancer. Ann Oncol 2017;28:2866–73.

[39] Tzanikou E, Markou A, Politaki E, et al. PIK3CA hotspot mutations in circulating tumor cells and paired circulating tumor DNA in breast cancer: a direct comparison study. Mol Oncol 2019;13:2515–30.

[40] Moynahan ME, Chen D, He W, et al. Correlation between PIK3CA mutations in cell-free DNA and everolimus efficacy in HR+, HER2- advanced breast cancer: results from BOLERO-2. Br J Cancer 2017;116: 726–30.

Identity/HLA

Advances in Molecular Pathology 3 (2020) 199–205

ADVANCES IN MOLECULAR PATHOLOGY

HLA Typing by Next-Generation Sequencing

Lessons Learned and Future Applications

Caleb Cornaby, PhD[a], Eric T. Weimer, PhD[a,b,*]

[a]McLendon Clinical Laboratories, UNC Hospitals, 101 Manning Drive, Chapel Hill, NC 27514, USA; [b]Department of Pathology and Laboratory Medicine, University of North Carolina at Chapel Hill School of Medicine, Chapel Hill, NC 27514, USA

KEYWORDS

- HLA • Next-generation sequencing • Nanopore • HLA regulation • Transplant diagnostics

KEY POINTS

- HLA typing by molecular methods have evolved from sequence-specific oligonucleotide probes to next-generation sequencing (NGS).
- Introduction of NGS-based HLA typing significantly reduced the number of ambiguities observed through full HLA gene sequencing.
- HLA enrichment methods will continue to improve the speed of HLA typing and enable additional content to be evaluated for hematopoietic cell transplant patients as well as solid organ transplant patients.
- Application of NGS to the HLA region will further the study of HLA regulation and expression as it has an impact on transplant outcomes.
- Long-read HLA sequencing will enhance understanding of HLA haplotypes and alter how laboratories perform high-resolution HLA typing.

INTRODUCTION

The HLA region on chromosome 6p21 covers more than 224 annotated genes, covering a span of more than 3.6 megabases. Although that may seem large, it comprises less than 0.15% of the whole human genome [1]. This region has been one of the most studied regions of the human genome since its discovery [2] and contains a plethora of genes that are crucial for immune cell function and regulation [3,4]. The major histocompatibility complex (MHC) class I molecules, encoded by *HLA-A*, *HLA-B*, and *HLA-C*, are used by nearly all cells in the human body to express endogenous proteins on their surface for immune cell surveillance [5]. Through this mechanism the

immune system can identify defective and pathogen infected cells [6]. MHC class II molecules, encoded by HLA loci *DPB1*, *DM*, *DO*, *DQB1*, *DQA1*, *DRB1*, and *DRA* among others, are used by antigen-presenting leukocytes to exhibit pathogenic peptides for T-lymphocyte examination and recruitment [7]. Additionally, the HLA region encodes the complement system proteins vital for the innate immune response, which is responsible for opsonization and neutralization of pathogens [8].

HLA typing is essential for assessment and treatment of a variety of medical conditions, including hematologic, rheumatologic, autoimmune, and cardiologic, among other diseases. The prevalence of hematologic

---

*Corresponding author. 101 Manning Drive, Room 1032 East Wing, Chapel Hill, NC 27514. *E-mail addresses:* eric.weimer@med.unc.edu; Twitter: @ericweimer (E.T.W.)

https://doi.org/10.1016/j.yamp.2020.07.015
2589-4080/20/

malignancy in the general population has been observed to be greater than 63 per 100,000 people [9]. Although there are a variety of treatment regimens for these malignancies, hematopoietic cell transplant (HCT) often is the treatment. Some patients can benefit from an autologous transplant; however, a large portion of patients need an HCT allotransplant. HLA typing is required to find an appropriate HLA match even if the HCT allotransplant donor is a sibling or other blood relative [10]. In patients receiving a solid organ transplant, HLA typing has been observed to be most beneficial, particularly in cases where sensitized transplant patients have developed allele specific antibodies [11]. Lack of appropriate typing, particularly at the *HLA-A*, *HLA-B*, and *HLA-DRB1* loci, puts these patients at risk of transplant rejection and possible chronic systemic disease.

Typing of HLA allele variants is associated with a diverse array of human diseases. There are a host of autoimmune diseases associated with HLA variants, including systemic lupus erythematosus, psoriasis, multiple sclerosis, and sarcoidosis, among others. For some of these autoimmune diseases, HLA-associated risk alleles have been identified as strong genetic predictors of disease development. Other diseases associated with HLA alleles include type II diabetes, schizophrenia, Parkinson disease, and coronary artery disease [12]. Furthermore, there are HLA alleles correlated with adverse drug reactions. Some examples include abacavir in patients with the HLA-B*57:01 allele and carbamazepine and oxcarbazepine in patients with the HLA-B*15:02, HLA-B15:11, or HLA-A*31:01 allele [13]. From the numerous examples available in the literature to date, typing of the HLA region has become a crucial part for diagnosing disease as well as a vital component of transplant medicine and treatment regimen implementation [14,15].

HLA TYPING IN THE BEGINNING

One of the first, and for decades considered the gold standard of, HLA typing is serologic typing [16]. This approach uses serologic and deductive methods to identify the patient HLA type. To perform this type of HLA typing, isolated recipient lymphocytes are placed in wells with dye, complement, and different sera with affinity for characterized HLA alleles. If the recipient lymphocytes display the HLA type that the sera are characterized for, then complement is able to bind to the cells and compromise the cell membrane. This permeabilization allows the cells to take up the dye. Cells in each well with the different sera are inspected under a microscope for dye. By identifying which combination of sera caused cell lysis, the HLA type for the recipient can be determined.

The advantage of this method in the past was the speed at which typing could be achieved. In several hours, a basic HLA typing could be assigned. The disadvantage to this method was that serologic typing has poor sensitivity for the detection of small amino acid differences in HLA proteins, which can elicit a significant immune response. Also, a laboratory could use only previously characterized sera for known HLA alleles. This becomes increasingly difficult as novel alleles are continuing to be identified and largely has been abandoned with the adoption of molecular typing techniques.

MOLECULAR-BASED HLA TYPING ERA

As molecular methods for HLA typing became available, they soon began to be employed in HLA typing laboratories. One of the earliest molecular typing techniques utilized was restriction fragment length polymorphism [17,18]. This technique uses DNA restriction endonucleases to cleave isolated genomic DNA, which then is run on an agarose gel and transferred to a membrane for probing with HLA locus unique primers. Although having continual problems with cross-hybridization issues, another disadvantage was that not all alleles could be differentiated using this technique alone [18]. Later, when polymerase chain reaction (PCR) technology became available, the 2 techniques were utilized together. PCR-amplified HLA alleles could be digested with restriction enzymes to ascertain appropriate HLA typing. This was used for many years to help resolve ambiguous HLA typing results [19].

A variety of other typing methodologies became available with the advent of PCR. With the ability to amplify DNA, probes for specific HLA alleles could be developed. This technique was referred to as sequence-specific oligonucleotide probe (SSOP) typing. Key to SSOP is immobilization of amplified DNA, typically to a paper or membrane; then the probes can be applied. Visualization of the bound primers can be done by chemiluminescence or fluorescence. By observing the developed blots, an HLA typing then could be established [18,20,21].

Another PCR-based method using HLA allele–specific primers during amplification of genomic DNA commonly was used for typing, referred to as sequence-specific primer typing [22,23]. This method was useful because 1 of the primers could be used universally for many different alleles of a single HLA loci, whereas the second primer of the set could be variable, sometimes by just 1 nucleotide, to allow the specific amplification of only certain alleles. These reactions could be validated in house or purchased in kits of varying complexities, depending on the resolution of results that needed to be achieved [24]. Depending on the locus of interest for typing, a laboratory could have results after only a couple hours [25].

Direct sequencing of the alleles of interest, or sequence-based typing (SBT), involves identifying the nucleotide sequence at specific HLA loci and comparing it to a database of allele sequences confirmed by SBT to identify the patient HLA type. For several years, SBT was performed exclusively using Sanger dideoxynucleotide sequencing [26]. Although there are different platforms that perform Sanger sequencing, the principle of identifying the nucleotide sequence of interest is similar. Depending on the protocol, the isolated genomic DNA is PCR amplified using HLA loci–specific primers. Postamplification, the DNA is amplified again, using only 1 primer and dideoxynucleotides. Dideoxynucleotides act to terminate the PCR process for that strand. The resultant solution contains partially amplified fragments of all lengths that then can be length separated using a gel system or capillary electrophoresis. The termination labeled nucleotides then are read for each separated band and the nucleotides are identified and placed in sequence [27].

As can be imagined, SBT has many advantages over previous molecular methods. Although PCR methods can be faster, be less labor intensive, and work as a closed system, confirmatory testing often is required, and results often can still be ambiguous. In many cases, typing never is resolved fully. Sanger sequencing, on the other hand, can query every base pair. This ability allowed for more rapid discovery of novel HLA alleles than at any time previous. Typing also could be done with a new level of confidence because bases could be matched to show the differences between alleles. The ability to judge how well a transplant candidate was for a match could be weighed against the mismatch of the donor HLA loci. Setting the scene for this terminology and field of HLA research that still is of great import today. Sanger sequencing also has its disadvantages. Compared with some of the previous methods, it was both time consuming and labor intensive to obtain typing by SBT.

SBT has become virtually synonymous with Sanger sequencing, which has been the standard for providing high-resolution typing. There are many laboratories that continue to use Sanger sequencing as the method of choice for high-resolution typing due to

instrumentation costs, implementation costs, and low volumes. Although those are valid reasons for continuing with Sanger sequencing, the declining costs of next-generation sequencing (NGS) coupled with the higher resolution, phasing, and elimination of ambiguities will result in continued expansion of these new sequence-based methods within clinical laboratories.

NEXT-GENERATION SEQUENCING–BASED HLA TYPING

With the advent of NGS technologies for sequencing, it did not take long for these methodologies to be applied to HLA typing. Almost as soon as NGS technology became more economically feasible for research, some of the earlier studies of the HLA locus were done using NGS methods, such as pyrosequencing [1,28]. Soon thereafter, several clinical HLA laboratories received American Society of Histocompatibility and Immunogenetics approval to utilize NGS-based HLA typing methods [29]. Since that time, the number of clinical HLA laboratories that use NGS for HLA typing has only increased. With the rising use of NGS in HLA typing, there has been a proportional expansion of NGS HLA typing assays, novel allele discoveries, and disease associations with HLA alleles [30,31].

Although the technique used for massive parallel sequencing might be slightly different, depending on the platform and assay used for HLA typing, the fundamentals of NGS are very similar and can be divided into several major steps. The first step requires the amplification or targeted concentration of isolated genomic DNA from the patient. This is followed by DNA clean up, fragmentation, adapter and index ligation, normalization, and sample pooling. The order and operation of these steps depends on the NGS protocol and technique used for library preparation [32]. Once the samples are loaded onto the NGS platform of choice and sequencing is performed, the final step in the process is the bioinformatic analysis to compile and parse reads to obtain the actual base pair sequence [33].

Of the methodologies utilized in target enrichment, HLA laboratories currently using NGS-based HLA typing typically employ either short-range PCR [34,35], long-range PCR [36–38], or hybrid capture-based methods [39,40]. These approaches enable HLA enrichment so that a depth of coverage adequate for high-resolution HLA typing can be achieved. Short-range PCR generally has the advantage of speed and higher depth of coverage compared with long-range PCR. A disadvantage of short-range PCR is the potential loss of phasing over longer stretches of DNA/RNA.

Long-range PCR uses HLA loci primers to specifically amplify the HLA regions of interest, most commonly whole-gene amplification. Sometimes primer sets used can amplify sequences that include the introns, and-many untranslated regions. The major advantage of long-range PCR is amplification of the entire HLA gene at the expense of time. There now are commercial long-range PCR products, however, that amplify the HLA genes within 3 hours [41,42]. For practicality in the clinical HLA laboratory, assays often use multiplexed primers that amplify only regions of interest. These HLA loci of interest often include *HLA-A*, *HLA-B*, *HLA-C*, *HLA-DPA1*, *HLA-DPB1*, *HLA-DQA1*, and *HLA-DRB1* [43,44].

Short-range and long-range PCR-based HLA enrichment methods have been used for years in the clinical HLA setting with reliable performance. There is greater opportunity and reliability in identifying novel alleles during HLA typing, with substantially fewer ambiguities. With NGS-based typing methods, laboratories also can perform better quality control. Minor allele fractions can be calculated to ensure that there is no allele bias and provide a haplotype estimate. There are potential drawbacks, however, with PCR-based enrichment. As with all PCR-based strategies, there is potential for allele bias amplification and, importantly for HLA typing, PCR can contribute to allele dropout or allele imbalance [1,32,45]. Typically, allele dropout is due to sequence variation at primer binding sites or preferential allele amplification. Allele dropout (approximately 1%) is a rare observation within clinical HLA laboratories due to quality assurance practices and the high-quality assays available for HLA typing [46,47].

An alternative HLA enrichment method to PCR-based approaches is hybridization of a probe to specific HLA loci during library preparation. In short, complementary nucleic acid sequences, RNA or DNA, for HLA loci bound to magnetic beads are used to specifically select for these regions during DNA purification. Using this method, hybridization probes can target capture class I and class II HLA loci with lower-risk allele dropout or allele imbalance compared with PCR amplification methods [48,49]. Also, removing the majority of nonspecific reads that otherwise would be discarded during bioinformatic analysis ensures a larger portion of the DNA used for sequencing will be from HLA loci of interest for typing. A beneficial byproduct of this method is that it also allows for sequencing coverage of other HLA loci besides the traditional loci targeted using PCR. Furthermore, hybrid capture NGS assays can be done in significantly less time than some long-range PCR-based NGS

because there is no need for PCR amplification prior to library preparation.

FUTURE FOR CLINICAL NEXT-GENERATION SEQUENCING HLA TYPING

Adoption of NGS for HLA typing in the clinical setting has continued to rise, typically in laboratories evaluating solid organ transplant patients and donors, and these laboratories have realized several benefits of HLA typing by NGS. Transplanted recipients benefit from NGS HLA typing by having high-resolution HLA typing available on donors to improve donor-specific antibody assessments [41,50]. In addition, NGS HLA typing can enhance virtual crossmatch assessment and aid in interpretation of physical crossmatch results by providing the level HLA expression [41,51]. For example, rs9277534, a single-nucleotide polymorphism within HLA-DPB1 that has regulatory function and impact on HCT outcomes, has been suggested to have an impact on B-cell flow cytometric crossmatches [52]. Additionally, rs9267649 has been associated with DNA methylation of *HLA-DRB*1 and reduced expression of *HLA-DRB1* [53]. Taken together, the application of NGS to HLA typing has demonstrated the importance of HLA regulation and expression and the subsequent impact on clinical outcomes. The continued expansion of HLA typing by NGS will serve to increase this growing field of study.

The future of clinical HLA (or immunogenetics in general) relies on connection of the vast amount of data captured by NGS to clinical outcomes. The current standard of care for HCT patients requires only a particular group of HLA loci to be typed. Additionally, the standard of care requires only the antigen-binding domain (ABD) to be sequenced. Although there are some reports that indicate that sequencing the ABD is sufficient [54] there also are reports that the information beyond the ABD influence clinical outcomes [55–57]. There is increasing evidence that other regions, beyond the antigen recognition domain, may influence patient outcomes. For example, Petersdorf and colleagues [58], found that exon 1 (leader peptide) of HLA-B informed graft-versus-host disease risk and permits risk stratification–based HLA matching for HCT patients. Additionally, Petersdorf and colleagues [59] found that HLA-DRB1 amino acid repertoire influenced transplant survivorship. These studies and others demonstrate there is still much to learn out of traditional HLA typing for improved transplant outcomes.

An area of continued exploration is extending the IMGT/HLA reference sequences. The lack of full-length reference sequences is a substantial roadblock in establishing unambiguous HLA genotypes. Recently, the Anthony Nolan Research Institute has addressed this issue by extending reference sequences for 95 HLA class I alleles [60]. In addition, the HLA Informatics Group at Anthony Nolan Research Institute, who maintain the IMGT/HLA database, now are receiving more full-length HLA class I submission than partial gene sequences with the continued adoption of HLA typing by NGS [61].

With the advent of the third-generation sequencing methods, including Pacific Biosciences' Single-Molecule Real-Time (SMRT) DNA sequencing [Menlo Park, CA, USA] and Oxford Nanopore Technologies (ONT) [Oxford, UK], sequencing laboratories have begun long-read sequencing. Long-read sequencing enables laboratories to sequence DNA/RNA sequences beyond the capability of traditional Illumina or Ion Torrent platforms. There is a growing list of clinical laboratories employing third-generation sequencing technologies to provide single-molecule HLA typing. The main advantage is single-molecular sequencing generates long reads, often greater than 20 kilobases, which enables the entire HLA class I and II genes to be sequenced [62]. At the moment, there are several clinical laboratories using SMRT methodologies for HLA genotyping, there are fewer laboratories using ONT sequencing, particularly for HLA class II genotyping. A recent publication by De Santis and colleagues [42], however, demonstrated the feasibility of rapid, high-resolution HLA genotyping using ONT sequencing within 4 hours.

The potential application of ONT sequencing for HLA genotyping may enable true epitope-based matching algorithms. The current approach has been inferenced HLA genotypes based on ethnicity and haplotype information. Although inference-based HLA genotype has an accuracy ranging from 80% to 100%, depending on ethnicity and bioinformatics approach [63–66], optimal epitope determination is based on high-resolution HLA genotyping data. Advancements, such as rapid, high-resolution HLA genotyping for deceased donors, will have a significant impact on patient outcomes [50].

By combining rapid, high-resolution HLA genotyping, HLA expression, and virtual crossmatch, HLA laboratories may improve recipient and donor matching along with patient outcomes for solid organ recipients. The HLA community continues to make significant strides in expanding knowledge of the HLA region beyond ABD and the implications for patients.

DISCLOSURE

Dr E.T. Weimer reports a grant from Omixon and personal fees from CareDx during the conduct of this review. Dr C. Cornaby has nothing to disclose.

REFERENCES

[1] Hosomichi K, Shiina T, Tajima A, et al. The impact of next-generation sequencing technologies on HLA research. J Hum Genet 2015;60:665–73.

[2] Horton R, Wilming L, Rand V, et al. Gene map of the extended human MHC. Nat Rev Genet 2004;5:889–99.

[3] Crux NB, Elahi S. Human Leukocyte Antigen (HLA) and immune regulation: How do classical and non-classical HLA alleles modulate immune response to human immunodeficiency virus and hepatitis C virus infections? Front Immunol 2017;8:832.

[4] Reeves E, James E. Antigen processing and immune regulation in the response to tumours. Immunology 2017;150:16–24.

[5] Dendrou CA, Petersen J, Rossjohn J, et al. HLA variation and disease. Nat Rev Immunol 2018;18. https://doi.org/10.1038/nri.2017.143.

[6] Montgomery RA, Tatapudi VS, Leffell MS, et al. HLA in transplantation. Nat Rev Nephrol 2018;14. https://doi.org/10.1038/s41581-018-0039-x.

[7] Miles JJ, Mccluskey J, Rossjohn J, et al. Understanding the complexity and malleability of T-cell recognition. Immunol Cell Biol 2015;93:433–41.

[8] Kulski JK, Shiina T, Inoko H, et al. An update of the HLA genomic region, locus information and disease associations: 2004. Tissue Antigens 2019;64:631–49.

[9] Li J, Smith A, Crouch S, et al. Estimating the prevalence of hematological malignancies and precursor conditions using data from Haematological Malignancy Research Network (HMRN). Cancer Causes Control 2016;27:1019–26.

[10] Edgerly CH, Weimer ET. The past, present, and future of HLA typing in transplantation. Methods Mol Biol 1802;(2018):1–10.

[11] Duquesnoy RJ, Kamoun M, Baxter-Lowe LA, et al. Should HLA mismatch acceptability for sensitized transplant candidates be determined at the high-resolution rather than the antigen level? Am J Transplant 2015;15:923–30.

[12] Trowsdale J, Knight JC. Major histocompatibility complex genomics and human disease. Annu Rev Genomics Hum Genet 2013;14:301–23.

[13] Fan W-L, Shiao M-S, Hui RC-Y, et al. Review Article HLA association with drug-induced adverse reactions. J Immunol Res 2017. https://doi.org/10.1155/2017/3186328.

[14] Kawai T, Cosimi AB, Spitzer TR, et al. HLA-mismatched renal transplantation without maintenance immunosuppression from the transplantation unit. N Engl J Med 2008;358(4):353–61.

[15] Kamburova EG, Wisse BW, Joosten I, et al. Differential effects of donor-specific HLA antibodies in living versus deceased donor transplant. Am J Transplant 2018;18: 2274–84.

[16] Althaf MM, El Kossi M, Jin JK, et al. Human leukocyte antigen typing and crossmatch: A comprehensive review. World J Transplant 2017;7:339–48.

[17] Bidwell JL, Bidwell EA, Savage DA, et al. A DNA-RFLP typing system that positively identifies serologically well-defined and ill-defined HLA-DR and DQ alleles, including DRw10. Transplantation 1988;45:640–6.

[18] Gerlach JA. Human lymphocyte antigen molecular typing how to identify the 1250 alleles out there. Arch Pathol Lab Med 2002;126(3):281–4.

[19] Hui KM, Bidwell JL. Handbook of HLA Typing Techniques. Boca Raton, FL: Google Books, CRC Press; 1993. (n.d.).

[20] Wordsworth P. Techniques used to define human MHC antigens: polymerase chain reaction and oligonucleotide probes. Immunolog Letters 1991;29(1-2):37–9.

[21] Suberbielle-Boissel C, Chapuis E, D.C.-T. Comparative study of two methods of HLA-DR typing: serology and PCR/dot blot reverse. Transplant Proceedings 1997; 29(5):2335–6.

[22] Metcalfe P, Waters AH. HPA-1 typing by PCR amplification with sequence-specific primers (PCR-SSP): a rapid and simple technique. Br J Haematol 1993;85: 227–9.

[23] Bunce M, Taylor CJ, Welsh KI. Rapid HLA-DQB typing by eight polymerase chain reaction amplifications with sequence-specific primers (PCR-SSP). Hum Immunol 1993;37:201–6.

[24] Bunce M, O'Neill CM, Barnardo MCNM, et al. Phototyping: comprehensive DNA typing for HLA-A, B, C, DRB1, DRB3, DRB4, DRB5 & DQB1 by PCR with 144 primer mixes utilizing sequence-specific primers (PCR-SSP). Tissue Antigens 1995;46:355–67.

[25] Olerup O, Zetterquist H. HLA-DR typing by PCR amplification with sequence-specific primers (PCR-SSP) in 2 hours: an alternative to serological DR typing in clinical practice including donor-recipient matching in cadaveric transplantation. Tissue Antigens 1992;39. https://doi.org/10.1111/j.1399-0039.1992.tb01940.x.

[26] Sanger F, Nicklen S, Coulson AR. DNA sequencing with chain-terminating inhibitors. Proc Natl Acad Sci U S A. 1977;74(12):5463-7.

[27] Dunn PPJ. Human leucocyte antigen typing: techniques and technology, a critical appraisal. Int J Immunogenet 2011;38:463–73.

[28] Bentley G, Higuchi R, Hoglund B, et al. High-resolution, high-throughput HLA genotyping by next-generation sequencing. Tissue Antigens 2009;74:393–403.

[29] Montgomery MC, Petraroia R, Weimer ET. Buccal swab genomic DNA fragmentation predicts likelihood of successful HLA genotyping by next-generation sequencing. Hum Immunol 2017;78:634–41.

[30] Ingram KJ, O'Shields EF, Kiger DF, et al. NGS and HLA: The long road ahead. Hum Immunol 2020. https://doi.org/10.1016/j.humimm.2020.03.001.

[31] Shieh M, Chitnis N, Monos D. Human Leukocyte Antigen and Disease Associations: A Broader Perspective. Clin Lab Med 2018;38(4):679-93.

[32] Profaizer T, Kumánovics A. Human Leukocyte Antigen Typing by Next-Generation Sequencing. Clin Lab Med 2018;38(4):565-78.

[33] Klasberg S, Surendranath V, Lange V, et al. Bioinformatics strategies, challenges, and opportunities for next generation sequencing-based HLA genotyping. Transfus Med Hemother 2019;46:312–25.

[34] Nelson WC, Pyo CW, Vogan D, et al. An integrated genotyping approach for HLA and other complex genetic systems. Hum Immunol 2015;76:928–38.

[35] Smith AG, Pyo CW, Nelson W, et al. Next generation sequencing to determine HLA class II genotypes in a cohort of hematopoietic cell transplant patients and donors. Hum Immunol 2014;75:1040–6.

[36] Holcomb CL, Hoglund B, Anderson MW, et al. A multisite study using high-resolution HLA genotyping by next generation sequencing. Tissue Antigens 2011;77: 206–17.

[37] Ehrenberg PK, Geretz A, Sindhu RK, et al. High-throughput next-generation sequencing to genotype six classical HLA loci from 96 donors in a single MiSeq run. HLA 2017;90:284–91.

[38] Weimer ET, Montgomery M, Petraroia R, et al. Performance characteristics and validation of next-generation sequencing for human leucocyte antigen typing. J Mol Diagn 2016;18:668–75.

[39] Wittig M, Anmarkrud JA, Kassens JC, et al. Development of a high-resolution NGS-based HLA-typing and analysis pipeline. Nucleic Acids Res 2015;43:e70.

[40] Lank SM, Golbach BA, Creager HM, et al. Ultra-high resolution HLA genotyping and allele discovery by highly multiplexed cDNA amplicon pyrosequencing. BMC Genomics 2012;13:378.

[41] Liu C, Duffy BF, Weimer ET, et al. Performance of a multiplexed amplicon-based next-generation sequencing assay for HLA typing. PLoS One 2020;15:e0232050.

[42] De Santis D, Truong L, Martinez P, et al. Rapid high-resolution HLA genotyping by MinION Oxford nanopore sequencing for deceased donor organ allocation. HLA 2020. https://doi.org/10.1111/tan.13901.

[43] Montgomery M, Berka J, immunology EW-H, et al. Suitability of dried DNA for long-range PCR amplification and HLA typing by next-generation sequencing. Hum Immunol 2019;80(2):135–9.

[44] Ehrenberg PK, Geretz A, Baldwin KM, et al. High-throughput multiplex HLA genotyping by next-generation sequencing using multi-locus individual tagging. BMC Genomics 2014;15:864.

[45] Walsh PS, Erlich HA, Higuchi R. Preferential PCR amplification of alleles: mechanisms and solutions. PCR Methods Appl 1992;1(4):241-50.

[46] Osoegawa K, Vayntrub TA, Wenda S, et al. Quality Control Project of NGS HLA Genotyping for the 17th International HLA and Immunogenetics Workshop. Hum Immunol 2019. https://doi.org/10.1016/j.humimm.2019.01.009.

[47] Montgomery MC, Weimer ET. Clinical validation of next generation sequencing for HLA typing using trusight HLA. Hum Immunol 2015;76:139.

[48] Gandhi MJ, Ferriola D, Huang Y, et al. Targeted next-generation sequencing for human leukocyte antigen typing in a clinical laboratory: metrics of relevance and considerations for its successful implementation. Arch Pathol Lab Med 2017;141:806–12.

[49] Wittig M, Juzenas S, Vollstedt M, et al. High-resolution HLA-typing by next-generation sequencing of randomly fragmented target DNA. Methods Mol Biol 2018;63–88.

[50] Senev A, Emonds M, Van Sandt V, et al. The clinical importance of extended 2nd field high-resolution HLA genotyping for kidney transplantation. Am J Transplant 2020. https://doi.org/10.1111/ajt.15938.

[51] Badders JL, Jones JA, Jeresano ME, et al. Variable HLA expression on deceased donor lymphocytes: Not all crossmatches are created equal. Hum Immunol 2015;76:795–800.

[52] Soe NN, Yin Y, Valenzuela NM, et al. OR3 HLA-DPB1 single nucleotide polymorphism determines DP molecule expression and B lymphocyte crossmatch results. Hum Immunol 2017;78:3.

[53] Kular L, Liu Y, Ruhrmann S, et al. DNA methylation as a mediator of HLA-DRB1 15:01 and a protective variant in multiple sclerosis. Nat Commun 2018;9:1–15.

[54] Hurley CK, Ng J. Continue to focus clinical decision-making on the antigen recognition domain for the present. Hum Immunol 2019;80:79–84.

[55] Mayor NP, Hayhurst JD, Turner TR, et al. Recipients receiving better hla-matched hematopoietic cell transplantation grafts, uncovered by a novel hla typing method, have superior survival: a retrospective study. Biol Blood Marrow Transplant 2019;25:443–50.

[56] Shieh M, Chitnis N, Clark P, et al. Computational assessment of miRNA binding to low and high expression HLA-DPB1 allelic sequences. Hum Immunol 2019;80:53–61.

[57] Thibodeau J, Moulefera MA, Balthazard R. On the structure–function of MHC class II molecules and how single amino acid polymorphisms could alter intracellular trafficking. Hum Immunol 2019;80:15–31.

[58] Petersdorf EW, Carrington M, O'hUigin C, et al. Role of HLA-B exon 1 in graft-versus-host disease after unrelated haemopoietic cell transplantation: a retrospective cohort study. Lancet Haematol 2020;7:e50–60.

[59] Petersdorf EW, Stevenson P, Malkki M, et al. Patient HLA germline variation and transplant survivorship. J Clin Oncol 2018;36:2524–31.

[60] Hassall KB, Latham K, Robinson J, et al. Extending the sequences of HLA class I alleles without full-length genomic coverage using single molecule real-time DNA sequencing. HLA 2020;95:196–9.

[61] Robinson J, Barker DJ, Georgiou X, et al. IPD-IMGT/HLA Database. Nucleic Acids Res 2019;48:D948–55.

[62] Mayor NP, Robinson J, McWhinnie AJ, et al. HLA Typing for the Next Generation. PLoS One 2015;10:e0127153.

[63] Dilthey AT, Gourraud PA, Mentzer AJ, et al. High-accuracy hla type inference from whole-genome sequencing data using population reference graphs. PLoS Comput Biol 2016;12:e1005151.

[64] Xie C, Yeo ZX, Wong M, et al. Fast and accurate HLA typing from short-read next-generation sequence data with xHLA. Proc Natl Acad Sci U S A 2017;114:8059–64.

[65] Xie M, Li J, Jiang T. Accurate HLA type inference using a weighted similarity graph. BMC Bioinformatics 2010;11:S10.

[66] Huang Y, Dinh A, Heron S, et al. Assessing the utilization of high-resolution 2-field HLA typing in solid organ transplantation. Am J Transplant 2019;19:1955–63.

Advances in Molecular Pathology 3 (2020) 207–219

ADVANCES IN MOLECULAR PATHOLOGY

HLA and Autoimmune Disease

Samuel E. Weinberg, MD, PhD, Lawrence J. Jennings, MD, PhD*

Department of Pathology and Laboratory Medicine, Northwestern University Feinberg School of Medicine, 303 E Chicago Avenue, Chicago, IL 60611, USA

KEYWORDS
- HLA - MHC - Autoimmunity - Genetic association

KEY POINTS
- The known number of HLA variants has significantly expanded in recent years with increased availability of high-throughput DNA sequencing modalities.
- New statistical approaches used in combination with the increasing numbers of unique HLA alleles have continued to expand the known associations between specific HLA variants and autoimmune conditions.
- Despite the ever-expanding list of reported correlations between HLA variants and autoimmune diseases, the molecular mechanisms underlying these associations remain poorly understood.
- A combination of genetic and environmental factors influence an individuals susceptibility to autoimmune disease.
- Recent advances in our understanding of the immune system, suggest that HLA plays a significant role in the generation of immune tolerance.

INTRODUCTION

The HLA family of proteins was first described in the 1930s as a cellular antigen responsible for the rejection of tumors explanted into mice. Originally termed, *major histocompatibility complex* (MHC), in mice, the human homolog later was identified in the 1950s [1]. Not long after that discovery, the specific HLA serologic variants, HLA-B27 and HLA-DR2, were found to correlate with the development of ankylosing spondylitis and multiple sclerosis, respectively [2–4]. Initially, HLA variants were predominantly identified using limited-resolution serologic-typing techniques. With the increased availability of high-throughput DNA sequencing modalities, however, the number of known unique HLA variants has risen exponentially in recent years [5]. The increase in known alleles in combination with new statistical approaches has greatly expanded the number of associations between specific HLA variants and autoimmune conditions [6,7]. Yet, despite the ever-expanding list of reported correlations between

HLA variants and autoimmune diseases, the molecular mechanisms underlying these associations remain poorly understood.

THE GENETIC COMPONENT

It has long been recognized that autoimmune diseases often occur within families and seemingly have a genetic predisposition. This genetic association is exemplified through twin studies comparing disease concordance between monozygotic and dizygotic twins. Because monozygotic twins share virtually 100% of their DNA sequence whereas dizygotic twins share on average 50%, twin studies help define the genetic contribution of disease association. An analysis of available twin studies for autoimmune diseases shows the genetic contribution to be very high for some diseases and less for others (Table 1). There is a broad range of concordance for some diseases. This could be due to the limitations of these twin studies

---

*Corresponding author, *E-mail address:* L-Jennings@northwestern.edu

https://doi.org/10.1016/j.yamp.2020.07.016
2589-4080/20/

TABLE 1
Concordance Rates in Monozygotic and Dizygotic Twins in Various Autoimmune Diseases

Disease	Monozygotic Pairwise Concordance	Dizygotic Pairwise Concordance
Systemic lupus erythematosus	11–40	0–4
Rheumatoid arthritis	0–21	0–8.8
Type 1 diabetes mellitus	13–47.4	3.8–11.6
Multiple sclerosis	0–50	0–16.7
Autoimmune thyroid disease	17–22.2	0–1.9
Celiac disease	60–75	9.1–11
Psoriasis	35–64	10–14
Inflammatory bowel disease	20–50	0–6.5

Adapted from Bogdanos DP, Smyk DS, Rigopoulou EI, et al. Twin studies in autoimmune disease: genetics, gender and environment. J Autoimmun. 2012;38:J158–9; with permission.

(eg, self-reporting, small cohorts, and lack of follow-up) but also due to variable expressivity and penetrance. For all autoimmune diseases, an environmental contribution is evident. This environmental contribution could be due to pathogen exposure, diet, microbiome, epigenetics, or other environmental factors and greatly adds to the difficulty of understanding the molecular mechanisms of these diseases. Of all the genomic loci that have been associated with autoimmune disease, a vast majority of heritability can be attributed to the HLA genes, which have been associated with these diseases with remarkable statistical significance (Table 2). Moving from allele or haplotype association to the mechanisms of pathogenesis, however, has proved challenging.

THE BASIC BIOLOGY OF HUMAN LEUKOCYTE ANTIGEN

To begin to understand the challenges of linking specific HLA variants to autoimmune disease, the basic biology of HLA molecules must be discussed. HLAs comprise a large family of proteins, which are all encoded for by genes located in the MHC locus located on the short arm of chromosome 6. These proteins usually are subdivided into 2 main groups: classical and nonclassical HLAs (Fig. 1). Classical HLAs display significant polymorphisms across the population and function as antigen-presenting molecules to T cells and are the central focus of this review. Nonclassical HLAs are discussed briefly, however, because studies also link polymorphism in these molecules to various

autoimmune, inflammatory, infectious, and malignant diseases [8–10]. Nonclassical HLA proteins exhibit limited genetic variation compared with classical HLAs and do not directly participate in antigen presentation to T cells. Nonclassical HLAs can be subdivided further into those that participate in peptide loading onto classical HLA molecules versus those with other unique biological roles, such as activation of natural killer cells and immune modulation.

Classical HLAs are separated into 2 distinct subtypes (class I and II) based on the T-cell subsets they present antigens to. Class I HLAs display antigens to cytotoxic $CD8^+$ T cells, whereas class II molecules interact with the TCRs on helper $CD4^+$ T cells. Both class I and class II HLA molecules display extreme amounts of genetic polymorphism. This polymorphism is thought to benefit the host by increasing possible pathogen recognition by the immune system [11–13]. Variation in HLA molecules allows for the presentation of a different set of unique peptides, typically referred to as the antigen repertoire.

In their simplest form, classical HLA molecules function as the education and surveillance system for the adaptive immune systems. Information in the form of short peptide sequences, termed *epitopes*, acquired from the intracellular or extracellular environment, is loaded onto the peptide-binding groove of maturing HLA molecules. Once present on the cell surface, the HLA-peptide complex can be recognized by a T cell via its T-cell receptor (TCR), resulting in T-cell activation and downstream effector function. Importantly, each individual T cell expresses only a single TCR with a

TABLE 2
Representative HLA and Disease Associations

Disease	HLA Association	Genome-Wide Association Study *P* Value
Psoriasis	HLA-C*06:02	4.5E-723
Myasthenia gravis	HLA-C*07:01	1.7E-114
Ankylosing spondylitis	HLA-B*27	5.0E-304
Idiopathic membranous nephropathy	HLA-DRB1*03	8.0E-93
Type 1 diabetes mellitus	DRB1*04-DQA1*03:01-DQB1*03:02; DRB1*03-DQA1*05:01-DQB1*02:01	1.0E-307
Rheumatoid arthritis (cyclic citrullinated peptide positive)	HLA-DRB1*04:01, HLA-DQA1*03:01	1.0E-300
Systemic lupus erythematosus	HLA-DRB1*03:01	2.0E-165
Multiple sclerosis	HLA-DRB1*05:01	3.8E-225
Systemic sclerosis (anti–topoisomerase-I antibody positive)	DRB1*11:04-DQA1*05:01-DQB1*03:01	9.2E-187
Systemic sclerosis (anticentromere antibody positive)	DRB1*11:04	1.1E-130
Pemphigus vulgaris	HLA-DQB1*03:01	7.7E-21
Narcolepsy	HLA-DQB1*06:02	6.0E-14
Ulcerative colitis	HLA-DRB1*11:01	4.7E-133
Graves disease	HLA-DRB1*03:01, HLA-DQA1*05:01	2.0E-65
Celiac disease	HLA-DQA1*05:01, HLA-DQB1*02:01	5.8E-209
Selective IgA deficiency	HLA-DQB1*02:01	3.0E-92

Adapted from Kennedy AE, Ozbek U, Dorak MT. What has GWAS done for HLA and disease associations? Int. J. Immunogenet. 2017;44:195–211; with permission.

unique peptide sequence out of billions of possibilities. Thus, in principle, each HLA-peptide combination should show a unique specificity for a corresponding TCR. A common misconception is that a TCR binds to a specific peptide sequence; however, TCRs recognize the 3-dimensional peptide-HLA complex. Thus, single amino acid polymorphisms in HLA molecules can alter peptide binding profoundly, having a drastic impact on which antigens are recognized by an individual's T cells. Although the basics of this process appear simple, the actual cellular and molecular events leading to successful antigen presentation comprise an exceedingly intricate system that is complicated further by the significant polymorphism observed among HLAs.

CHALLENGES WITH HLA–AUTOIMMUNE DISEASE ASSOCIATION

Although specific HLA variants are linked to several different diseases, identifying the particular HLA alleles driving an autoimmune condition is challenging. As discussed previously, the HLA complex is encoded by a 3–million base pairs cluster of genes on chromosome 6. Because of their close proximity to one another and

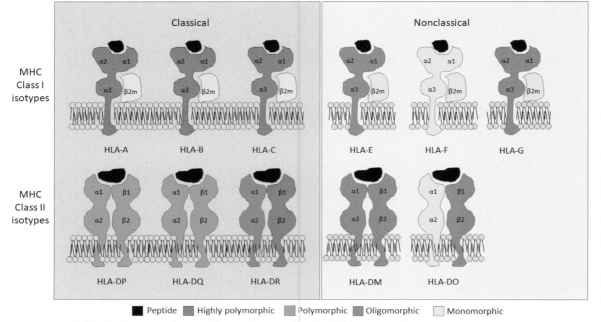

FIG. 1 Classical and nonclassical HLA molecules. Classical HLA proteins display significant polymorphism across the population and function as antigen-presenting molecules to T cells. Nonclassical HLA proteins exhibit less genetic variation and function to load peptide onto classical HLA molecules (class II) or other unique biological roles, such as activation of natural killer cells and immune modulation (class I).

resulting linkage disequilibrium, individuals tend to inherit common groups of HLA genes, termed *HLA haplotypes*. Thus, multiple HLA genes present in a single individual tend to all associate with the same autoimmune disease. Moreover, most autoimmune conditions display pathogenic CD4[+] and CD8[+] T-cell responses even though the 2 cell types respond to different HLA genes [14,15]. Thus, a majority of autoimmune disorders likely require the simultaneous expression of multiple HLA genes for disease development. Further complicating matters, because the quantity of organ transplants performed has increased drastically over the past 40 years, much of the focus on HLA biology shifted away from understanding the physiologic functions of HLA toward understanding the critical yet biologically artificial mechanisms of HLA-linked rejection. This gap severely limited knowledge of how HLA polymorphism shapes immune responses in homeostatic and diseased states. Luckily, in recent years there has been a re-emergence of the study of HLA variation and disease with the widespread adoption of unbiased, high-throughput proteomic and genetic approaches combined with innovative immune

models [16–19]. These tools just now are beginning to reshape understanding of the cellular mechanisms that may underlie HLA polymorphism and autoimmune disease correlation.

In simplified terms, the development of autoimmune disease requires a T-cell–driven response to a self-antigen, typically expressed in a tissue. In healthy individuals, peripheral T cells either never encounter these antigens or recognize them without promoting an effector response, a process termed, *tolerance*. In autoimmune conditions, however, T cells encounter these antigens and drive downstream inflammatory responses, ultimately resulting in tissue damage. Why tolerogenic mechanisms fail is, however, poorly understood. This is true even for celiac disease, which is the only autoimmune disease for which the molecular trigger has been identified.

PATHOGENESIS OF CELIAC DISEASE
Current understanding of the pathogenesis of celiac disease recently has been reviewed [20]. Although the protein and its peptide fragment that cause celiac disease

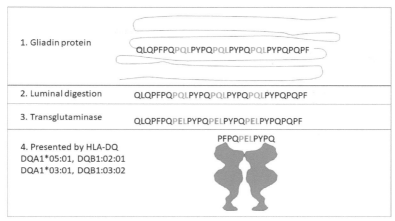

1. Gliadin protein	QLQPFPQPQLPYPQPQLPYPQPQLPYPQPQPF
2. Luminal digestion	QLQPFPQPQLPYPQPQLPYPQPQLPYPQPQPF
3. Transglutaminase	QLQPFPQPELPYPQPELPYPQPELPYPQPQPF
4. Presented by HLA-DQ DQA1*05:01, DQB1:02:01 DQA1*03:01, DQB1:03:02	PFPQPELPYPQ

FIG. 2 Mechanism of celiac disease activation. (1,2) Proline-rich regions of gliadin protein resists intestinal degradation. (3) Transglutaminase enzyme removes the amide functional group converting glutamine to glutamic acid. (4) The resultant peptide binds specific HLA molecules and is presented to its corresponding TCR. (*Adapted from* Stamnaes J, Sollid LM. Celiac disease: autoimmunity in response to food antigen. Semin Immunol. 2015;27(5):346; with permission.)

have been characterized, much of the pathogenesis remains poorly understood. As shown in Fig. 2, the gluten protein present in dietary wheat is broken down to shorter peptide fragments in the intestinal lumen before crossing the epithelium. It is modified by tissue transglutaminases to create the short antigenic peptides recognized by specific HLA-DQ heterodimers. More than 90% of celiac disease patients exhibit the DQA1*05:01, DQB1*02:01 heterodimer with the remainder exhibiting DQA1*03:01, DQB1*03:02 or at least 1 molecule of the DQA1*05:01, DQB1*02:01 heterodimer. After these initiating steps, however, the pathogenesis is less clear. The key steps are shown in Fig. 3. The antigen-presenting cells release activating cytokines (interleukin [IL]-12 and IL-15) and present the antigen to activate gluten-specific CD4$^+$ T cells. These activated T cells release proinflammatory cytokines (interferon [IFN]-γ, tumor necrosis factor α, and IL-21) and activate B cells that have internalized tissue transglutaminase in complex with the gluten peptide. Antibodies against the peptide and tissue transglutaminase are generated but damage to the epithelium seems to result from activation of the intraepithelial lymphocytes that up-regulate natural killer receptors and lyse epithelial cells expressing stress signals (HLA-E and MIC-A). The cytokines seem to inhibit or perhaps overwhelm the local regulatory T (Treg) cells, which should dampen the autoimmune response, but why this happens in some individuals but not others is not clear. Evidence indicates that the described peptide–HLA

molecule interaction is necessary but not sufficient to elicit the intestinal atrophy and malabsorption characteristic of celiac sprue, given that more than a third of the white population possesses these HLA-DQ molecules that predispose to celiac disease; yet only an estimated 1% develops the disease.

PROPOSED MECHANISMS OF PATHOGENESIS

For celiac disease, the antigen trigger is known and yet the other factors that lead to loss of tolerance remains obscure. For other autoimmune diseases, even the antigenic trigger remains unknown, which may seem surprising given the strong HLA associations and the number of studies attempting to elucidate the pathogenesis. It may be that celiac disease is more the exception than the rule and a single antigenic trigger will not be found because the pathogenesis of other autoimmune diseases is even more complex. The remainder of this review first focuses on how HLA polymorphism affects the cellular processes that generate mature HLA-peptide complexes. Through a discussion of specific molecular mechanisms, how different HLA variants can influence the expression of immunogenic self-antigens that alter the likelihood of generating a self-targeted T cell response is detailed. In contrast, the second part of the review highlights possible mechanisms by which HLA variants, in combination with environmental factors, can alter

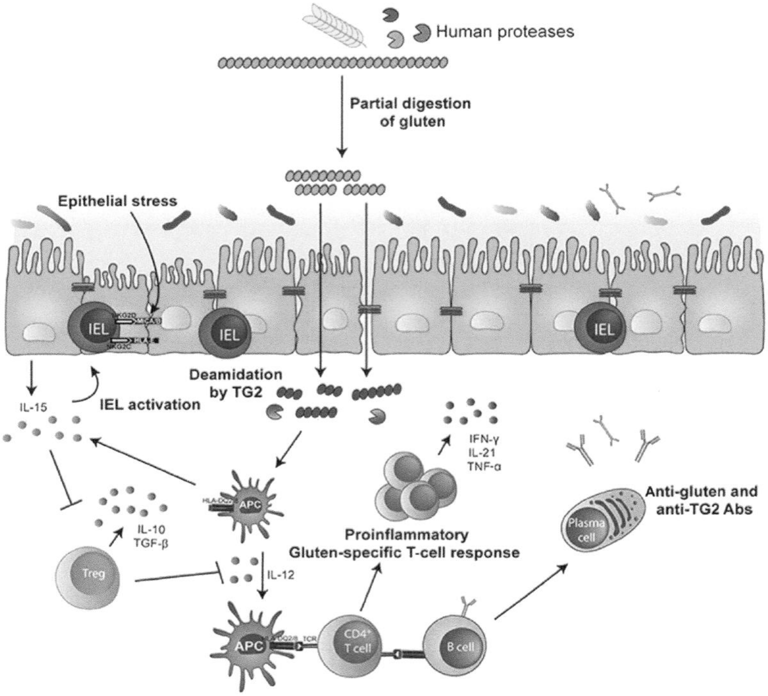

FIG. 3 Key steps in CeD pathogenesis. Gluten peptides containing T-cell epitopes resist gastrointestinal degradation. tTG catalyses the deamidation of gluten peptides, which then can bind more efficiently to the disease-relevant HLA-DQ molecules on APCs. Activated gluten-specific CD4+ T cells secrete a variety of proinflammatory cytokines, such as IFN-g and IL-21, that contribute to the intestinal lesion and promote activation of IELs and stimulate B-cell responses. Activated IELs transform into cytolytic NK-like cells that mediate destruction of enterocytes expressing stress signals. IL-15 renders effector T cells resistant to the suppressive effects of Tregs and, in the lamina propria, endows mucosal DCs with inflammatory properties promoting proinflammatory responses and preventing Treg differentiation. (*From* Tye-Din JA, Galipeau HJ, Agardh D. Celiac disease: a review of current concepts in pathogenesis, prevention, and novel therapies. Front. Pediatr. 2018;6:350.). APC, antigen presenting cell; CeD, Celiac Disease; IELs, intra-epithelial lymphocytes; NK, natural killer; TG, tissue transglutaminase 2; tTG, tissue transglutaminase.

immunologic tolerance, leading to the development of autoimmune pathology.

Changes in the HLA protein sequence, resulting from inherited HLA polymorphisms, likely result in changes in the quantity of self-antigen presented to the immune system, which provides perhaps the simplest hypothesis for the association of autoimmunity with unique HLA variants. This model is supported by data showing that a majority of HLA polymorphisms occur in the region of the genes that encode for the peptide-binding groove [21,22]. Furthermore, HLA molecules with only a single amino acid change in the peptide-binding groove show contrasting associations with the development of inflammatory arthritis, which suggests that

alterations in the peptide-binding groove structure may be permissive for the development of particular autoimmune diseases [23]. Despite the strong appeal of this model, numerous conflicting observations suggest a more complicated mechanism underlying the development of autoimmunity. For instance, many of the most polymorphic residues on HLA proteins exist outside of the peptide-binding groove, and these still result in an altered peptide-binding repertoire [24–26]. The next section discusses the molecular steps in the generation of classical HLAs to highlight how different HLA genetic polymorphisms potentially influence antigen presentation through multiple processes. This section is not intended to function as a comprehensive discourse on HLA formation and structure. Instead, a straightforward overview of mature HLA-antigen generation is provided, while emphasizing potential mechanisms of HLA-driven autoimmunity.

GENERATION AND FUNCTION OF CLASS I HLA

Class I HLA molecules present antigens from the intracellular environment to CD8$^+$ T cells and thus are expressed ubiquitously on almost all cells of the body, excluding red blood cells. This allows for continuous immune-mediated surveillance of tissues where presentation of cellular peptides (self) is tolerated while peptides corresponding to viruses or other intracellular pathogens (nonself) elicit an immune reaction. Viral infection is a classic example of this process; viral proteins contain unique peptide sequences that, when presented by class I HLA molecules, subsequently are recognized by CD8$^+$ T cells, leading to the destruction of the infected cell. Although class I HLAs are associated most commonly with protection from intracellular infections, the same fundamental mechanism occurs during other noninfectious processes, such as recognition of oncogenic proteins in immune-mediated tumor destruction and self-antigen presentation in cases of autoimmune diseases [27].

HLA class I molecules are encoded by 3 genes, HLA-A, HLA-B, and HLA-C. There are more than 3000 known variants of each of these 3 genes, which display codominant expression, meaning that an individual may express 6 distinct core HLA class I proteins [28]. On the cell surface, a mature HLA class I molecule is a heterodimer consisting of an HLA-A, HLA-B, or HLA-C protein in complex with a β_2-microglobulin. Importantly, β_2-microglobulin does not contribute to the peptide-binding groove of class I HLA molecules. Thus, the amino acid sequence of HLA-A, HLA-B, or HLA-C controls the antigen repertoire displayed to CD8$^+$ T cells. Evidence suggests that the molecular process of loading peptides onto class I HLA molecules plays an underlying role in the development of autoimmune diseases associated with multiple class I HLA variants.

The process begins in the cytoplasm, where proteasomal degradation of cellular proteins results in the formation of short peptides, 8 to 10 amino acids length. Different class I HLA variants show a binding bias toward distinct lengths of peptide sequences, thus resulting in unique antigen repertoires [29]. These peptides are transferred into the endoplasmic reticulum (ER) by the transporter associated with antigen processing (TAP) protein complex. The TAP protein complex binds

peptides in the cytoplasm and, using an adenosine triphosphate–dependent process, translocates the peptides into the ER lumen. Once the peptides reach the ER lumen, they are loaded onto a class I HLA molecule by the peptide loading complex. This complex consists of multiple proteins, including TAP, tapasin, calreticulin, calnexin, and Erp57, which stabilize maturing class I HLAs. Importantly, the process of loading a peptide onto a class I HLA molecule is optimized for the selection of a high-affinity peptide–HLA binding. Thus, the first peptide encounter by a type I HLA molecule in the ER lumen is not necessarily the peptide displayed to T cells on the cell surface. The iterative process of peptide selection onto an HLA molecule is controlled primarily by tapasin, which has potentially important biological ramifications. For example, different class I HLA variants display differential binding to tapasin, which results in altered antigen repertoires [30–32]. Furthermore, recent studies have demonstrated that other proteins, such as tapasin-related protein (TAPBPR), can influence peptide–class I HLA affinity selection outside of the classic peptide loading complex [33,34]. Similarly to tapasin, TAPBPR is known to show unique binding with different type I HLA variants [35]. These observations suggest that differential HLA affinities to the peptide loading machinery may be 1 potential mechanism underlying associations of type I HLA variants with autoimmune disease.

Before the class I HLA-peptide conjugate can be transported to the cell surface, the peptide loading complex must fully dissociate, and the HLA molecule must undergo post-translational modifications to produce a fully mature HLA complex. Post-translational modifications, such as glycosylation, begin in the ER lumen, but are carried out most extensively in the Golgi apparatus. Studies investigating these alterations are limited; yet, emerging data suggest that glycosylation of HLA molecules has functional consequences for the HLA antigen repertoires and downstream activation of T cells (reviewed by Ryan and colleagues [36]). New tools now exist, which allow for the high-throughput identification of modified residues on HLA molecules and may help identify new mechanisms leading to the development of autoimmunity [37]. After successful anterograde trafficking to the cell surface, type I HLA-peptide conjugates are available for binding to the TCR of CD8$^+$ T cells. During TCR binding, the CD8 molecule functions as a stabilizer of TCR-HLA binding, allowing for the stable formation of a specialized junction used for cell-cell communication, called an immune synapse. Multiple lines of evidence suggest that the duration and strength of immune synapse formation alter the downstream immunologic response, including the likelihood of cytotoxic T-cell–mediated target cell death [38]. CD8 molecules display different binding affinities for specific HLA variants. Thus, specific HLA polymorphisms may have an impact on the strength of immune synapse formation, potentially altering the efficiency of CD8+ cytotoxic T-cell–mediated killing. Thus, alterations in HLA-CD8 binding affinity provides another possible mechanism for the association of HLA with autoimmune diseases [39,40].

Class I HLA function is complicated further due to the unique nature of CD8+ T-cell activation, which requires not only TCR binding to a mature class I HLA but also a costimulatory signal that is provided by an antigen-presenting cell (APC). Prior to experiencing this second signal, HLA binding to a TCR on a CD8+ T cell does not result in the destruction of infected or damaged cells. This dual requirement, however, necessitates that APCs present an antigen that they currently are not expressing. For example, in the setting of a viral infection, an APC would have to be actively infected with a virus for HLA to display viral peptides to drive CD8+ T-cell activation. To overcome this paradox, APCs are able to obtain antigens from the environment, which then are displayed on class I HLAs, a process termed, *cross-presentation*. Cross-presentation is considerably understudied compared with classic HLA antigen presentation, but research suggests that 2 distinct pathways are involved. In 1 pathway, class I HLA molecules complex with antigen within the endosome/lysosome rather than in the ER (analogous to how class II HLA antigen loading occurs). In the second pathway, endosomal proteins are transported into the cytosol for proteasomal degradation and subsequently are loaded onto class I HLAs (the limited information known about these pathways is reviewed by Embgenbroich and Burgdorf [41]). Although there currently are no known links between different HLA variants and methods of cross-presentation, many of the processes having an impact on class I HLA-peptide loading, discussed previously could have an impact on this process, which ultimately may dictate the initial selection of a self-antigen in autoimmune conditions.

GENERATION AND FUNCTION OF CLASS II HLA

Unlike class I HLAs, class II molecules consist of alpha and beta subunits, which both contribute to the peptide-binding groove of mature class II HLAs. The 3 alpha subunits (DRA, DQA, and DPA) show relatively limited genetic variation and form dimers with their specific beta chains (DRB, DQB, and DPB, respectively). In contrast to the alpha subunits, the 3 beta chains show high amounts of genetic diversity; the allele with the smallest number of reported variants, DPB, still has greater than 800 unique polymorphs [28]. As with class I HLAs, there is a large body of literature linking specific HLA class II polymorphisms to disease [42,43].

Outside of the thymus, class II HLAs are expressed predominantly on APCs, including macrophages, dendritic cells, and B cells. In contrast to class I HLA, class II molecules only present antigens obtained from the external environment. The first step in the production of a mature class II HLA is the translation of the alpha and beta protein subunits in the rough ER. This process is complicated, however, by the fact that class II HLAs present exogenous antigens to CD4+ T cells but are produced in an environment full of endogenous peptides. To overcome this issue, the HLA class II histocompatibility antigen gamma chain, a nonclassical HLA molecule better known as the invariant chain, functions to bind and sequester the nascent class II HLA alpha and beta subunits, thus resulting in proper formation of the peptide-binding groove while simultaneously preventing HLA binding to self-peptide binding in the ER. The invariant chain also enables the transport of class II HLA from the ER to the endosome. HLA-containing endosomes fuse with lysosomes, where a cysteine protease, cathepsin S, cleaves 2 sites on the invariant chain. At this point, only a small portion of the invariant chain, termed, *class II invariant peptide* (*CLIP*), remains bound to the HLA molecule. Next, the additional nonclassical HLA proteins, HLA-DM and HLA-DO, catalyze the degradation of CLIP and subsequent antigen loading onto the class II HLA molecule. HLA-DM functions analogously to tapasin and TAPBPR in class I HLA molecules and facilitates the loading of high-affinity peptides onto class II HLA molecules. Similarly to tapasin and TAPBPR, HLA-DM and HLA-DO have been associated with numerous autoimmune conditions, although the molecular mechanisms underlying these correlations remain somewhat mysterious [44].

Alterations with invariant chain function and proper peptide loading are associated with numerous autoimmune diseases, suggesting that impairment of the invariant chain function may result in the presentation of self-antigen to CD4+ T cells (reviewed by Fortin and colleagues [45]). Single nucleotide polymorphisms in class II HLA beta subunits can influence the affinity of the invariant chain and CLIP binding affinity [46–48]. These studies suggest that unique class II molecules with impaired CLIP binding may be prone to the display of self-antigens. Additionally, class II HLA variants show altered interactions with HLA-DM that correlate with the presentation of distinct peptide sequences [49]. These data highlight how polymorphism in class I and II HLAs can result in the presentation of unique antigen repertoires that likely display different frequencies of self-antigen.

HLA POLYMORPHISM AND IMMUNE TOLERANCE

Despite the significant number of studies linking variants within class I and II HLA genes with alterations in the presentation of self-antigens, multiple lines of evidence demonstrate that presentation of self-antigen alone is not sufficient to explain most HLA–autoimmune disease correlations. A large portion of the population without underlying autoimmune conditions have T cells that recognize tissue-specific self-antigens [50–52]. Additionally, different HLA alleles associated with the same autoimmune condition can display entirely different antigen repertoires, making it unlikely that the presentation of a common epitope underlies disease development [53]. Instead, these data suggest that a potential failure in immunologic tolerance, in combination with varied expression of self-antigens, results in the development of autoimmune pathologies.

T-cell–mediated immune tolerance occurs via 2 mechanisms: central and peripheral. Central tolerance involves the removal of CD4+ and CD8+ T cells that display high-affinity binding to HLA–self-antigen complexes, termed, *negative selection*. In this process, thymic epithelial cells display enormous numbers of antigens on class I and class II HLA molecules to maturing T cells. This exposure results in a Goldilocks-style selection process, whereby T cells that fail to bind and those displaying high-affinity interactions, thus posing a high risk for self-antigen recognition, are removed from the developing T-cell pool [54,55]. Importantly, the amount of peripheral T cells that display high-affinity binding to self-antigen correlates with expression of specific class I and II HLA variants [56–58]. The precise molecular mechanisms of how T cells avoid negative selection, termed *thymic escape*, are unknown. The best evidence, however, implicates HLA polymorphism in this process [59,60].

The past few decades have seen the discovery of a previously unknown mechanism of tolerance, Treg cells. Treg cells are a distinct population of CD4+ T cells that are defined by the expression of the transcription factor Foxp3 and are responsible for suppression of T-cell–mediated immune responses. Individuals with mutations in Foxp3 lack Treg cells and consequentially develop a profound autoimmune disease, termed *immunodysregulation polyendocrinopathy enteropathy X-linked syndrome*, within the first year of life [61,62]. The precise mechanisms of Treg cell development and suppressive function are beyond the scope of this review; however, it is essential to highlight the emerging role that HLA polymorphism plays in these processes. For instance, a specific HLA variant, HLA-DR1, is known to induce the formation of anti–basement membrane–specific Treg cells, which protect against the development of Goodpasture syndrome [63]. Similar studies also have found correlations between unique HLA variants and increased Treg cell function that protect from the development of autoimmune diabetes and inflammatory arthritis [64,65].

Along with Treg cells, which function predominantly outside of the thymus, circulating effector T cells have cell autonomous mechanisms to limit autoimmunity. The most well studied of these processes is characterized by T cells entering an extended period of hyporesponsiveness after TCR recognition of an HLA-peptide conjugate, termed *T-cell anergy*. Defects in T-cell anergy have long been associated with the development of autoimmune disease in animal models. Recent studies have identified significant numbers of anergic autoreactive T cells in healthy individuals, suggesting that T-cell anergy also may have an impact on human disease [66–68]. In addition, specific HLA variants have been linked to intrinsic differences in T-cell anergy. This finding came from the observation that there are different rates of genetic polymorphism among class I HLA molecules. HLA-B shows the highest amount of polymorphism and thus generally is considered the immunodominant class I HLA molecule [69,70]. Despite their increased amount of variation, however, HLA-B molecules show less diverse antigen repertoires with lower antigen binding affinities compared with HLA-A complexes [71,72]. In combination, these data suggest that HLA-B molecules function primarily in driving inflammatory CD8+ T-cell responses. In contrast, higher-affinity HLA-A–peptide conjugates may work to promote anergic and tolerogenic responses. Moreover, specific HLA variants show differential cell surface stability and expression levels, which correlate with an individual's risk of autoimmune disease development [73,74]. These observations suggest that the balance between multiple unique HLA polymorphisms may influence an individual's susceptibility to autoimmune pathology.

Taken together, emerging data highlight the huge variety of HLA polymorphisms and the extreme complexity these introduce into the immune system. The processes, discussed previously, are just a few of the possible mechanisms by which unique class I and II variants can influence the development of autoimmune disease. Data from the literature suggest that in most autoimmune conditions, a single HLA allele is unlikely to dictate a binary outcome of a healthy or diseased state. Instead, increased understanding of the interplay of tolerogenic immune mechanisms and unique HLA variants highlights that the development of autoimmune disease likely depends on the full complement of HLA proteins. An individual may possess multiple HLA variants that promote immune tolerance while simultaneously expressing other HLA molecules with a heightened propensity for the expression of self-antigens. Future studies to further characterize the relationship between individual HLA polymorphisms and specific immune system functions are greatly needed, thus allowing better quantification of the relative balance between these distinct immune processes within patients.

ENVIRONMENTAL FACTORS IMPACTING HLA POLYMORPHISM

One of the earliest proposed models for the development of autoimmunity was a mechanism by which infection with specific pathogens generated a misplaced or hyperactive immune response. One process underlying an overactive immune response is molecular mimicry, in which the activation of T cells against bacterial or viral antigen results in an autoreactive T-cell response. Thus, after the clearance of an infection, a pool of self-reactive T cells remains, which are defective in the tolerogenic mechanisms, described previously. Not every individual exposed to the same pathogen, however, develops an autoimmune disease, hinting that unique HLA variants could be uniquely capable of generating self-reactivity. Studies dating back decades have implicated HLA-B27–associated spondyloarthropathy and autoimmune diabetes with an initiating infectious event [75–78]. Recent data indicate that specific TCRs can tolerate considerable variability in the HLA-peptide binding complex, provided that a core binding motif of 2 to 3 peptides remains conserved [79,80]. In this process, termed *hot spot molecular mimicry*, specific HLA variants induce weak binding to a short peptide sequence present in microbial proteins, but high-affinity binding to this same peptide sequence displayed in the setting of a self-antigen [79]. Different pathogens can cause T-cell activation through the same hot spots [81,82]. These data imply a potentially new model in which the specific HLA variant and not a particular infectious agent might promote a similar autoimmunological response.

In addition to hot spot molecular mimicry, other lines of evidence have further supported the role of microbes in the development of autoimmune pathologies. Multiple recent studies have demonstrated that microbiome alterations can promote the thymic escape of self-reactive T cells and the development of autoimmunity in animal models of disease [83,84]. Additionally, individuals with particular HLA variants show unique gut microbiome compositions that correlate with the development of autoimmune disease [85] (https://www.biorxiv.org/content/10.1101/2020.01.14.907196v1). These observations raise the possibility that HLA variation may dictate the formation of a microbiome that is permissive for the development of autoimmunity potentially through the maintenance of a pool of self-reactive T cells early in life. The same tolerogenic mechanisms that prevent autoimmunity, described previously, also are proposed to function in selection of an individual's microbiome. Further studies are required to formally test these models in order to determine how HLA polymorphism truly has an impact on microbial composition and its causal role in development of autoimmunity.

SUMMARY

The strong associations of HLA alleles with autoimmune diseases have clearly been established. For celiac disease, specific HLA alleles are shown to be directly involved in the pathogenesis. For other autoimmune diseases, however, this connection is not as apparent. It is perhaps more probable that a single HLA allele–antigen pathway does not exist but rather that a combination of HLA alleles or haplotypes drives pathogenesis. Variants in other genes of the MHGC as well as other genomic loci also have been associated with autoimmune disease and likely work in concert in these multifactorial diseases. But, as evidenced by twin studies, environmental factors must play a role in the pathogenesis. These environmental factors include pathogens, the microbiome, diet, and epigenetic modifications and may introduce an antigenic trigger but likely also contribute to the pathogenesis of autoimmune disease through the loss of tolerance. A deeper understanding of these environmental factors and how they affect the immune response will provide opportunities for avoiding and managing these devastating diseases.

DISCLOSURE
The authors have nothing to disclose.

REFERENCES

[1] Thorsby E. A short history of HLA. Tissue Antigens 2009; 74:101–16.

[2] Jersild C, Fog T, Hansen GS, et al. Histocompatibility determinants in multiple sclerosis, with special reference to clinical course. Lancet 1973;2:1221–5.

[3] Schlosstein L, Terasaki PI, Bluestone R, et al. High association of an HL-A antigen, W27, with ankylosing spondylitis. N Engl J Med 1973;288:704–6.

[4] Brewerton DA, Hart FD, Nicholls A, et al. Ankylosing spondylitis and HL-A 27. Lancet 1973;1:904–7.

[5] Robertson J, Guethlein LA, Cereb N, et al. Distinguishing functional polymorphism from random variation in the sequences of >10,000 HLA-A, -B and -C Alleles. PLoS Genet 2017;13. https://doi.org/10.1371/JOURNAL.PGEN.1006862.

[6] Kennedy AE, Ozbek U, Dorak MT. What has GWAS done for HLA and disease associations? Int J Immunogenet 2017;44:195–211.

[7] Thorsby E. Invited anniversary review: HLA associated diseases. Hum Immunol 1997;53:1–11.

[8] Moscoso J, Serrano-Vela JI, Pacheco R, et al. HLA-G, -E and -F: allelism, function and evolution. Transpl Immunol 2006;17:61–4.

[9] Kochan G, Escors D, Breckpot K, et al. Role of non-classical MHC class I molecules in cancer immunosuppression. Oncoimmunology 2013;2:e26491.

[10] Rizzo R, Bortolotti D, Bolzani S, et al. HLA-G molecules in autoimmune diseases and infections. Front Immunol 2014;5:592.

[11] Prugnolle F, Manica A, Charpentier M, et al. Pathogen-driven selection and worldwide HLA class I diversity. Curr Biol 2005;15:1022–7.

[12] Vogel TU, Evans DT, Urvater JA, et al. Major histocompatibility complex class I genes in primates: co-evolution with pathogens. Immunol Rev 1999;167:327–37.

[13] Hughes AL, Nei M. Pattern of nucleotide substitution at major histocompatibility complex class I loci reveals overdominant selection. Nature 1988;335:167–70.

[14] Bluestone JA, Bour-Jordan H, Cheng M, et al. T cells in the control of organ-specific autoimmunity. J Clin Invest 2015;125:2250–60.

[15] Pilli D, Zou A, Tea F, et al. Expanding Role of T Cells in Human Autoimmune Diseases of the Central Nervous System. Front Immunol 2017;8:652.

[16] Huang M, Zhang W, Guo J, et al. Improved Transgenic Mouse Model for Studying HLA Class I Antigen Presentation. Sci Rep 2016;6:33612.

[17] Vieira-Sousa E, van Duivenvoorde LM, Fonseca JE, et al. Review: animal models as a tool to dissect pivotal pathways driving spondyloarthritis. Arthritis Rheumatol 2015;67:2813–27.

[18] Salimi N, Fleri W, Peters B, et al. The immune epitope database: a historical retrospective of the first decade. Immunology 2012;137:117–23.

[19] Hosomichi K, Shiina T, Tajima A, et al. The impact of next-generation sequencing technologies on HLA research. J Hum Genet 2015;60:665–73.

[20] Tye-Din JA, Galipeau HJ, Agardh D. Celiac disease: A review of current concepts in pathogenesis, prevention, and novel therapies. Front Pediatr 2018;6. https://doi.org/10.3389/fped.2018.00350.

[21] van Deutekom HWM, Keşmir C. Zooming Into the Binding Groove of HLA molecules: which positions and which substitutions change peptide binding most? Immunogenetics 2015;67. https://doi.org/10.1007/S00251-015-0849-Y.

[22] Wieczorek M, Abualrous ET, Sticht J, et al. Major Histocompatibility Complex (MHC) Class I and MHC Class II proteins: conformational plasticity in antigen presentation. Front Immunol 2017;8. https://doi.org/10.3389/FIMMU.2017.00292.

[23] Fiorillo MT, Greco G, Maragno M, et al. The naturally occurring polymorphism Asp116–>His116, differentiating the ankylosing spondylitis-associated HLA-B*2705 from the non-associated HLA-B*2709 subtype, influences peptide-specific CD8 T cell recognition. Eur J Immunol 1998;28:2508–16.

[24] Macdonald WA, Purcell AW, Mifsud NA, et al. A naturally selected dimorphism within the HLA-B44 supertype alters class I structure, peptide repertoire, and T cell recognition. J Exp Med 2003;198:679–91.

[25] Herman J, Jongeneel V, Kuznetsov D, et al. Differences in the recognition by CTL of peptides presented by the HLA-B*4402 and the HLA-B*4403 molecules which differ by a single amino acid. Tissue Antigens 1999;53:111–21.

[26] Williams AP, Peh CA, Purcell AW, et al. Optimization of the MHC class I peptide cargo is dependent on tapasin. Immunity 2002;16:509–20.

[27] Malekzadeh P, Pasetto A, Robbins PF, et al. Neoantigen screening identifies broad TP53 mutant immunogenicity in patients with epithelial cancers. J Clin Invest 2019;129:1109–14.

[28] Robinson J, Barker DJ, Georgiou X, et al. The IPD and IMGT/HLA database: allele variant databases. Nucleic Acids Res 2015;43:D423–31.

[29] Rist MJ, Theodossis A, Croft NP, et al. HLA peptide length preferences control CD8+ T cell responses. J Immunol 2013;191:561–71.

[30] Park B, Lee S, Kim E, et al. A single polymorphic residue within the peptide-binding cleft of MHC class I molecules determines spectrum of tapasin dependence. J Immunol 2003;170:961–8.

[31] Peh CA, Burrows SR, Barnden M, et al. HLA-B27-restricted antigen presentation in the absence of tapasin

reveals polymorphism in mechanisms of HLA class I peptide loading. Immunity 1998;8:531–42.

[32] Wiiliams AP, CA P, AW P, et al. Optimization of the MHC class i peptide cargo is dependent on tapasin. Immunity 2002;16. https://doi.org/10.1016/S1074-7613(02)00304-7.

[33] Hermann C, van Hateren A, Trautwein N, et al. TAPBPR alters MHC class I peptide presentation by functioning as a peptide exchange catalyst. Elife 2015;4. https://doi.org/10.7554/eLife.09617.

[34] Boyle LH, Hermann C, Boname JM, et al. Tapasin-related protein TAPBPR is an additional component of the MHC class I presentation pathway. Proc Natl Acad Sci U S A 2013;110:3465–70.

[35] Ilca FT, Drexhage LZ, Brewin G, et al. Distinct Polymorphisms in HLA Class I molecules govern their susceptibility to peptide editing by TAPBPR. Cell Rep 2019;29:1621–32.e3.

[36] Ryan SO, Cobb BA. Roles for major histocompatibility complex glycosylation in immune function. Semin Immunopathol 2012;34:425–41.

[37] Hart GW, Copeland RJ. Glycomics hits the big time. Cell 2010;143:672–6.

[38] Dustin ML. The immunological synapse. Cancer Immunol Res 2014;2:1023–33.

[39] Wooldridge L, Lissina A, Vernazza J, et al. Enhanced immunogenicity of CTL antigens through mutation of the CD8 binding MHC class I invariant region. Eur J Immunol 2007;37:1323–33.

[40] Salter RD, Norment AM, Chen BP, et al. Polymorphism in the alpha 3 domain of HLA-A molecules affects binding to CD8. Nature 1989;338:345–7.

[41] Embgenbroich M, Burgdorf S. Current Concepts of Antigen Cross-Presentation. Front Immunol 2018;9:1643.

[42] Matzaraki V, Kumar V, Wijmenga C, et al. The MHC locus and genetic susceptibility to autoimmune and infectious diseases. Genome Biol 2017;18:76.

[43] Tsai S, Santamaria P. MHC class II polymorphisms, autoreactive T-cells, and autoimmunity. Front Immunol 2013;4:321.

[44] Mellins ED, Stern LJ. HLA-DM and HLA-DO, key regulators of MHC-II processing and presentation. Curr Opin Immunol 2014;26:115–22.

[45] Fortin J-S, Cloutier M, Thibodeau J. Exposing the Specific Roles of the Invariant Chain Isoforms in Shaping the MHC Class II Peptidome. Front Immunol 2013;4:443.

[46] Doebele RC, Pashine A, Liu W, et al. Point mutations in or near the antigen-binding groove of HLA-DR3 implicate class II-associated invariant chain peptide affinity as a constraint on MHC class II polymorphism. J Immunol 2003;170:4683–92.

[47] Freund C, Höfer T. A Missing Switch in Peptide Exchange for MHC Class II Molecules. Front Immunol 2019;10:2513.

[48] Anczurowski M, Yamashita Y, Nakatsugawa M, et al. Mechanisms underlying the lack of endogenous processing and CLIP-mediated binding of the invariant chain by HLA-DP84Gly. Sci Rep 2018;8:4804.

[49] Álvaro-Benito M, Wieczorek M, Sticht J, et al. HLA-DMA polymorphisms differentially affect MHC class II peptide loading. J Immunol 2015;194. https://doi.org/10.4049/JIMMUNOL.1401389.

[50] Legoux FP, Lim J, Cauley AW, et al. CD4+ T Cell Tolerance to Tissue-Restricted Self Antigens Is Mediated by Antigen-Specific Regulatory T Cells Rather Than Deletion. Immunity 2015;43:896–908.

[51] Hogquist KA, Jameson SC. The self-obsession of T cells: how TCR signaling thresholds affect fate "decisions" and effector function. Nat Immunol 2014;15:815–23.

[52] Danke NA, Yang J, Greenbaum C, William W Kwok. Comparative Study of GAD65-specific CD4+ T Cells in Healthy and Type 1 Diabetic Subjects. J Autoimmun 2005;25. https://doi.org/10.1016/J.JAUT.2005.08.007.

[53] Merino E, Montserrat V, Paradela A, et al. Two HLA-B14 subtypes (B*1402 and B*1403) differentially associated with ankylosing spondylitis differ substantially in peptide specificity but have limited peptide and T-cell epitope sharing with HLA-B27. J Biol Chem 2005;280:35868–80.

[54] Luo X, Miller SD, Shea LD. Immune Tolerance for Autoimmune Disease and Cell Transplantation. Annu Rev Biomed Eng 2016;18:181–205.

[55] Schwartz RH. Historical overview of immunological tolerance. Cold Spring Harb Perspect Biol 2012;4:a006908.

[56] Gascoigne NRJ, Palmer E. Signaling in thymic selection. Curr Opin Immunol 2011;23:207–12.

[57] Dendrou CA, Petersen J, Rossjohn J, et al. HLA variation and disease. Nat Rev Immunol 2018;18:325–39.

[58] Dyall R, Messaoudi I, Janetzki S, et al. MHC polymorphism can enrich the T cell repertoire of the species by shifts in intrathymic selection. J Immunol 2000;164:1695–8.

[59] Böhme J, Schuhbaur B, Kanagawa O, et al. MHC-linked protection from diabetes dissociated from clonal deletion of T cells. Science 1990;249:293–5.

[60] Schloss J, Ali R, Racine JJ, et al. HLA-B*39:06 efficiently mediates type 1 diabetes in a mouse model incorporating reduced thymic insulin expression. J Immunol 2018;200:3353–63.

[61] Sakaguchi S. Regulatory T cells: history and perspective. Methods Mol Biol 2011;707:3–17.

[62] Romano M, Fanelli G, Albany CJ, et al. Past, present, and future of regulatory T cell therapy in transplantation and autoimmunity. Front Immunol 2019;10:43.

[63] Ooi JD, Petersen J, Tan YH, et al. Dominant protection from HLA-linked autoimmunity by antigen-specific regulatory T cells. Nature 2017;545:243–7.

[64] Tsai S, Serra P, Clemente-Casares X, et al. Antidiabetogenic MHC class II promotes the differentiation of MHC-promiscuous autoreactive T cells into FOXP3+ regulatory T cells. Proc Natl Acad Sci U S A 2013;110:3471–6.

[65] Wen X, Yang J, James E, et al. Increased islet antigen-specific regulatory and effector CD4+ T cells in healthy individuals with the type 1 diabetes-protective haplotype. Sci Immunol 2020;5. https://doi.org/10.1126/sciimmunol.aax8767.

[66] Maeda Y, Nishikawa H, Sugiyama D, et al. Detection of self-reactive CD8+ T cells with an anergic phenotype in healthy individuals. Science 2014;346:1536–40.

[67] Kalekar LA, Schmiel SE, Nandiwada SL, et al. CD4(+) T cell anergy prevents autoimmunity and generates regulatory T cell precursors. Nat Immunol 2016;17:304–14.

[68] Saibil SD, Deenick EK, Ohashi PS. The sound of silence: modulating anergy in T lymphocytes. Curr Opin Immunol 2007;19:658–64.

[69] Bihl F, Frahm N, Di Giammarino L, et al. Impact of HLA-B alleles, epitope binding affinity, functional avidity, and viral coinfection on the immunodominance of virus-specific CTL responses. J Immunol 2006;176:4094–101.

[70] Kiepiela P, Leslie AJ, Honeyborne I, et al. Dominant influence of HLA-B in mediating the potential co-evolution of HIV and HLA. Nature 2004;432:769–75.

[71] Harari A, Cellerai C, Enders FB, et al. Skewed association of polyfunctional antigen-specific CD8 T cell populations with HLA-B genotype. Proc Natl Acad Sci U S A 2007;104:16233–8.

[72] Rao X, Costa AICAF, van Baarle D, et al. A comparative study of HLA binding affinity and ligand diversity: implications for generating immunodominant CD8+ T cell responses. J Immunol 2009;182:1526–32.

[73] Miyadera H, Ohashi J, Lernmark Å, et al. Cell-surface MHC density profiling reveals instability of autoimmunity-associated HLA. J Clin Invest 2015;125:275–91.

[74] Kaur G, Gras S, Mobbs JI, et al. Structural and regulatory diversity shape HLA-C protein expression levels. Nat Commun 2017;8:15924.

[75] Pugliese A. Autoreactive T cells in type 1 diabetes. J Clin Invest 2017;127:2881–91.

[76] Morse ZJ, Horwitz MS. Innate Viral Receptor Signaling Determines Type 1 Diabetes Onset. Front Endocrinol (Lausanne) 2017;8:249.

[77] Martin R, Gran B, Zhao Y, et al. Molecular mimicry and antigen-specific T cell responses in multiple sclerosis and chronic CNS Lyme disease. J Autoimmun 2001;16:187–92.

[78] López-Larrea C, González S, Martinez-Borra J. The role of HLA-B27 polymorphism and molecular mimicry in spondylarthropathy. Mol Med Today 1998;4:540–9.

[79] Harkiolaki M, Holmes SL, Svendsen P, et al. T cell-mediated autoimmune disease due to low-affinity crossreactivity to common microbial peptides. Immunity 2009;30:348–57.

[80] Cole DK, Bulek AM, Dolton G, et al. Hotspot autoimmune T cell receptor binding underlies pathogen and insulin peptide cross-reactivity. J Clin Invest 2016;126:2191–204.

[81] Nielsen TR, Rostgaard K, Askling J, et al. Effects of infectious mononucleosis and HLA-DRB1*15 in multiple sclerosis. Mult Scler 2009;15:431–6.

[82] Wucherpfennig KW, Strominger JL. Molecular mimicry in T cell-mediated autoimmunity: viral peptides activate human T cell clones specific for myelin basic protein. Cell 1995;80:695–705.

[83] Sprouse ML, Bates NA, Felix KM, et al. Impact of gut microbiota on gut-distal autoimmunity: a focus on T cells. Immunology 2019;156:305–18.

[84] Yadav SK, Boppana S, Ito N, et al. Gut dysbiosis breaks immunological tolerance toward the central nervous system during young adulthood. Proc Natl Acad Sci U S A 2017;114:E9318–27.

[85] Russel JT, Roesch LWF, Ördberg M, et al. Genetic risk for autoimmunity is associated with distinct changes in the human gut microbiome. Nat Commun 2019;10. https://doi.org/10.1038/S41467-019-11460-X.

Moving?

Make sure your subscription moves with you!

To notify us of your new address, find your **Clinics Account Number** (located on your mailing label above your name), and contact customer service at:

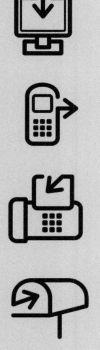

Email: journalscustomerservice-usa@elsevier.com

800-654-2452 (subscribers in the U.S. & Canada)
314-447-8871 (subscribers outside of the U.S. & Canada)

Fax number: 314-447-8029

Elsevier Health Sciences Division
Subscription Customer Service
3251 Riverport Lane
Maryland Heights, MO 63043

*To ensure uninterrupted delivery of your subscription, please notify us at least 4 weeks in advance of move.